Urinary Tract Infections

Detection, Prevention, and Management

Fifth Edition

Urinary

Tract

Infections

Detection, Prevention, and Management

Fifth Edition

Calvin M. Kunin, M.D., F.A.C.P.

Pomerene Professor of Medicine

Department of Internal Medicine

The Ohio State University School of Medicine

Columbus, Ohio

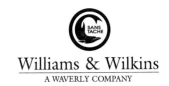

Williams & Wilkins
A WAVERLY COMPANY

BALTIMORE • PHILADELPHIA • LONDON • PARIS • BANGKOK
BUENOS AIRES • HONG KONG • MUNICH • SYDNEY • TOKYO • WROCLAW

Editor: Jonathan W. Pine, Jr.
Managing Editor: Leah Ann Kiehne Hayes
Production Coordinator: Linda Carlson and Carol Eckhart
Copy Editor: Kathy Gilbert
Cover Designer: Silverchair Science & Communications, Inc.
Typesetter: Peirce Graphic Services, Inc.
Printer & Binder: R.R. Donnelly & Sons

351 West Camden Street
Baltimore, Maryland 21201-2436 USA

Rose Tree Corporate Center
1400 North Providence Road
Building II, Suite 5025
Media, Pennsylvania 19063-2043 USA

Accurate indications, adverse reactions and dosage schedules for drugs are provided in this book, but it is possible that they may change. The reader is urged to review the package information data of the manufacturers of the medications mentioned.

Printed in the United States of America

First Edition, 1972
Second Edition, 1974
Third Edition, 1979
Fourth Edition, 1987

Library of Congress Cataloging-in-Publication Data

Kunin, Calvin M., 1929–
    Urinary tract infections : detection, prevention, and management / Calvin M. Kunin. — 5th ed.
        p.   cm.
    Rev. ed. of: Detection, prevention, and management of urinary tract infections / Calvin M. Kunin. 4th ed. 1987.
    Includes bibliographical references and index.
    ISBN 0-683-18102-5
    1. Urinary tract infections.   I. Kunin, Calvin M., 1929– Detection, prevention, and management of urinary tract infections.   II. Title.
    [DNLM: 1. Urinary Tract Infections. WJ 151 K96d 1997]
RC901.8.K86 1997
616.6—dc20
DNLM/DLC
for Library of Congress   96-26585
                                                                                                    CIP

The publishers have made every effort to trace the copyright holders for borrowed material. If they have inadvertently overlooked any, they will be pleased to make the necessary arrangements at the first opportunity.

To purchase additional copies of this book, call our customer service department at **(800) 638-0672** or fax orders to **(800) 447-8438**. For other book services, including chapter reprints and large quantity sales, ask for the Special Sales department.

Canadian customers should call **(800) 268-4178,** or fax **(905) 470-6780**. For all other calls originating outside of the United States, please call **(410) 528-4223** or fax us at **(410) 528-8550**.

Visit *Williams & Wilkins* on the Internet: http://www.wwilkins.com or contact our customer service department at **custserv@wwilkins.com**. Williams & WIlkins customer service representatives are available from 8:30 am to 6:00 pm, EST, Monday through Friday, for telephone access.

97 98 99
1 2 3 4 5 6 7 8 9 10

This book is dedicated to the memory of my mentors, Maxwell Finland, M.D., and Edward Kass, M.D., Ph.D., who introduced me to this field and provided invaluable counsel for many years.

Preface

This book has grown during the past 25 years from a short manual to a wide-ranging synthesis of the literature on urinary tract infections. The current edition has been entirely rewritten, but the core concepts remain unchanged. The title has been changed slightly to emphasize the focus on urinary tract infections. Each chapter is designed to be read as an independent account of a particular issue with its own set of references. Some of the important concepts are reiterated in each chapter to provide a brief review or for special emphasis. Several new features have been added. These include an Overview at the beginning of each chapter, Key Points About . . . clinical topics, and summary tables of important concepts. The goal is to provide the reader with a synthesis of the current concepts in this field regardless of his or her clinical or basic science discipline.

Although this book was prepared by a single author it is based on the work of many contributors to the field whose work is interpreted here. The seminal investigators include Beeson on pathogenesis; Kass and Sanford on significant bacteriuria; Stamey, Fowler, and Schaeffer on acquisition of infection; McCabe, Jackson, and Vosti on host factors; Hodson, Rolleston, Ransley, Smellie, Jodal, Koff, and Rushton on vesicoureteral reflux; O'Grady and Cattell on urokinetics; Brumfitt, Hamilton-Smith and Washington, on laboratory management; Asscher and Kaye, on growth of bacteria in urine; Andriole, Braude, Sanford, Freedman, Roberts and O'Hanley, on experimental infection and vaccines; Kimmelstiel, Cotran and Heptinstall, on pathology; Bailey, Rubin and Ronald, on single dose therapy; Turck, Ronald, Thomas, Kincaid-Smith and Fairley, on localization of infection; Freeman, Gleckman, Nicolle and Kaye, on treatment of males and the elderly; Ofek, Beachey, Hanson, Winberg, Svanborg, Mäkelä and numerous Scandinavian investigators, on uropathic *Escherichia coli;* Mobley, on Proteus; Soriano, on *Corynebacterium urealyticum;* Dukes, Gillespie, Guttmann, Lapides, Burke, and Warren, on catheter care; Stamm, Johnson (and their numerous colleagues in Seattle), Pfau, Sobel, Stansfeld, Little and Norrby, on rationalization of therapy; Maki, Wenzel, and Schaberg, on nosocomial infection; Hinman, Bruce, Reid, Parsons, Mulholland and Uehling, on novel concepts of vaginal interference and the bladder defense mechanism; Musher and Aronson, on urease inhibitors; and Marrie, Foxman and

Schlager, on recurrent infection. Many other outstanding investigators are recognized in the citations to their work and in the text. Missing from the list, but acknowledged here, are the innovative scientists in the pharmaceutical industry who developed the drugs that are essential for management. I owe a special debt to Jay Gillenwater and Albert Paquin for educating me about urology.

Finally, I wish to acknowledge the lessons I have learned from my patients who have helped me to better appreciate the natural history and management of urinary tract infections.

Calvin M. Kunin, M.D., F.A.C.P.

Contents

An Overview of Urinary Tract Infections

Definitions and General Concepts

Urinary tract infection is a broad term used to describe microbial colonization of the urine and infection of the structures of the urinary tract. The epithelial surfaces of the urinary tract are contiguous, extending from the site
at which urine is formed in the renal glomerulus to its exit at the urethral
meatus. In the absence of infection, these structures are bathed in a common stream of sterile urine. The infectious process may involve the kidney,
renal pelvis, ureters, bladder, and urethra, as well as adjacent structures
such as the perinephric fascia, prostate, and epididymis. All of these structures are at risk of acquiring infection from the common urinary stream.

Urinary tract infections encompass a wide variety of clinical entities.
These entities include urethritis, prostatitis, epididymitis, cystitis, acute and
chronic pyelonephritis, and perinephric abscess. Often the condition is clinically silent (asymptomatic bacteriuria or asymptomatic funguria) and can
be detected only by the finding of large numbers of microorganisms in the
urine. Microorganisms may colonize the urine without an apparent inflammatory response. When pus cells are present (*pyuria*), the condition is considered to be an *asymptomatic infection.* Asymptomatic individuals are at increased risk of developing symptomatic infections.

The clinical diagnosis can be established readily from the history and microscopic examination of the urine. Highly effective drugs are available for
treatment or prophylaxis for all but the most intractable infections. Asymptomatic infections are common but are detected readily by quantitative urine
culture. The ability to arrive at a specific diagnosis, detect correctable lesions,
council the patient, and provide effective therapy makes care of urinary tract
infections one of the most gratifying experiences in medical practice.

The laboratory hallmark of infection is the presence of the invading mi-
crobe(s) and inflammatory cells in the urine. This makes it possible to identify the causative microorganism, perform antimicrobial susceptibility tests,
and prescribe specific therapy. Microscopic examination of the urine and
quantitative cultures also provide clear endpoints to assess cure or failure
and to detect recurrent infection. Under certain circumstances, the site of infection may not be in contact with the urinary stream, and the voided urine
may be sterile (Table 1.1). These situations can be suspected from the history and clinical presentation.

The most common causative microorganisms are bacteria and yeasts
that grow well in urine. The urinary tract can also be invaded by mycobacteria, fungi, parasites, and viruses. Infections produced by each of these microorganisms will be dealt with separately. Urinary tract infections are not
restricted to humans, but can occur in domestic and farm animals and fish.
Experimental models in animals have provided important information
about the pathogenesis of the disease.

The urinary tract is remarkably resistant to infection. Susceptibility is in-

Table 1.1. Examination of the Urine of Patients with Urinary Tract Infections

Hallmarks of Infection
  Microorganisms (usually >100,000 colony forming units, cfu/ml)*
  Polymorphonuclear leukocytes (usually >20 per cubic millimeter)
Voided Urine May be Sterile Despite Active Urinary Tract Infection
  During the early phase of metastatic infection to the kidney
  When the kidney is infected, but the ureter is blocked by a stricture or stone
  With perinephric abscesses
  With chronic prostatitis or prostatic abscesses
  During treatment with effective antimicrobial drugs
Routine Culture May be Negative in the Presence of Infection
  With fastidious microorganisms (*Hemophilus influenzae*)
  With renal tuberculosis (*Mycobacterium tuberculosis*)

*Lower counts may be present during the initial phase of the "pyuria-dysuria" syndrome.

creased when any one of the structures is damaged or when the free flow of urine is obstructed. Microorganisms may enter the urinary tract from the distal portions of the urethra, from instruments inserted into the urethra and bladder (*ascending infection*), or from the blood stream (*descending or hematogenous infection*). Host factors are the major determinants of infection and response to therapy. This point will be emphasized throughout this book. Some microbes are inherently more virulent than others and can produce invasive infection in otherwise healthy hosts. These microbes are considered to be *uropathogens*. The clinical distinction between *uncomplicated* and *complicated* urinary tract infections is of paramount importance in determining the severity of infection, clinical outcome, and therapeutic strategies. Noninvasive procedures are now available to detect the presence of structural abnormalities or obstruction to the flow of urine. Many of these abnormalities can be corrected by modern urologic surgery.

The pathogenesis, microbiology, epidemiology, and natural history of urinary tract infections in humans have been the subject of intense investigation over the past 40 years. Strategies have been developed to aid diagnosis, assess the underlying problems, and determine the potential risks for renal damage. A great deal of folklore and misunderstanding still exists about how urinary tract infections are acquired and how they are best treated. The role of sexual intercourse, feminine hygiene, and fluid intake remains controversial. The relation of urinary tract infections to vesicoureteral reflux, hypertension, prematurity, end-stage renal disease, and to issues such as whether to treat asymptomatic bacteriuria are still debated.

The goal of this book is to provide clinicians, microbiologists, and other health care workers with a practical approach to the diagnosis, prevention, and management of urinary tract infections based on an understanding of the nature of the invading microbes, the host response, and the pathogenesis of infection.

Distinction from Sexually Transmitted and Vaginal Infections

Sexually transmitted diseases and vaginal infections are considered separately from urinary tract infections because they are usually limited to the male and female genital structures, are produced by a different set of microbes, have distinctly different epidemiologic characteristics, and require different forms of therapy. It may be difficult at times to distinguish gonococcal or chlamydial urethritis from urinary tract infections because they also produce urethral irritation. Some patients with vaginitis have pyuria and dysuria. It also may be difficult at times to differentiate vaginitis from sexually transmitted diseases and urinary tract infections without appropriate cultures.

Epidemiology

Urinary tract infections are among the most common conditions encountered in office practice, hospitals, and extended care facilities. They occur in both sexes and at all ages (Fig. 1.1). Urinary tract infections in males tend to occur more frequently in the very young and very old and among homosexuals. They are an important cause of prostatitis and epididymitis. Urinary tract infections in females occur throughout life and increase with age. They produce considerable morbidity among those who are prone to recurrent infections. About half of adult women report that they have had a urinary tract infection at some time during their life. Approximately 2,500,000 women in the United Kingdom experience an attack of dysuria and frequency each year, and 100,000 suffer recurrent infections (1). In the United States, there were 5,740,000 office visits to physicians in 1990 for one of the following primary complaints: painful urination, frequency and urgency, or urinary tract infection (2). Most of the visits (75.8%) were made by females to general physicians. There were about 280,000 visits to urologists for urinary tract infections in the United States during 1989–1990 (3).

An overview of urinary tract infections as seen in relation to age, sex and predisposing factors is shown in Figure 1.1. Note that the frequency of asymptomatic and symptomatic infections parallel each other with age, and that the pattern of infection differs in males and females. Infections in males are most common at the extremes of life. In contrast, infections in females increase with age. Asymptomatic bacteriuria (to be discussed in the next chapter) appears as the hidden portion of the iceberg in the lower portion of the figure and may become symptomatic. Infection from urinary catheters can occur at any age. Catheters are used most commonly in hospitalized patients, in males with prostatic hypertrophy, and in elderly incontinent females.

The quantitative count of bacteria in urine has proven to be a useful tool

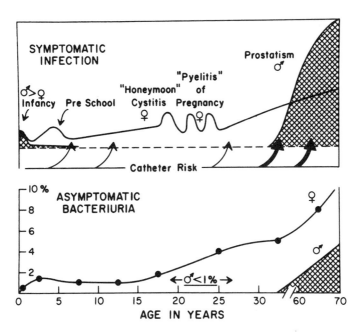

Figure 1.1. Overview of the frequency of urinary tract infections and prevalence of significant bacteriuria according to age and sex. (Modified from the original concept of Jawetz.)

to define the reservoir of subclinical urinary tract infections in large populations (4,5). The prevalence of asymptomatic bacteriuria according to age and sex is shown in the bottom portion of Figure 1.1. The rate is about 1% to 2% in newborns. Newborn males are infected more often than females, and uncircumcised males are at higher risk (6). After the first year of life, infections are more common in females. During the ages 5 to 18 years, the prevalence is 1.2% in girls and 0.03% in boys (7). The incidence in girls is 0.4% per year, is linear with time throughout the school years, and is unaffected by menarche. The cumulative frequency of asymptomatic infection in girls during the school years is about 5%. Bacteriuria in girls is independent of socioeconomic status and race and is not increased in diabetics. The prevalence of bacteriuria in females rises about 1% per decade and may be as high as 10% or more in elderly women (8). Females with asymptomatic bacteriuria are at increased risk of developing symptomatic infections when they become sexually active or pregnant. The frequency of bacteriuria during pregnancy varies from 2% to 6%, depending upon age, parity, and socioeconomic group. Detection and treatment of bacteriuria early in pregnancy has been shown to prevent acute pyelonephritis during the third trimester (9).

Major Clinical Problems

Urinary tract infections are important complications of pregnancy, diabetes, polycystic renal disease, renal transplantation, sickle cell anemia, and in patients with structural and neurological conditions that impede the free flow of urine. They are the leading cause of gram negative sepsis in hospitalized patients. About half of all hospital-acquired infections originate in the urinary tract in association with the urinary catheter and urologic procedures. Urinary catheters are used in about 10% of patients admitted to hospitals and long-term care facilities in the United States. Catheter-associated urinary tract infections have been shown to increase mortality threefold in a general hospital (10) and to be an independent risk factor for death among patients in long-term care facilities (11). Some of the major clinical problems are listed in Table 1.2.

Common Microorganisms

Microorganisms that produce urinary infections generally grow well in urine. The most common are gram negative bacteria that belong to the family *Enterobacteriacea*. Members of the family include *Escherichia coli*, Klebsiella, Enterobacter, Proteus, Salmonella, and Shigella. Other important gram negative bacteria include *Pseudomonas aeruginosa*, Acinetobacter, and

Table 1.2. Major Clinical Problems in Urinary Tract Infection

Disseminated gram-negative bacterial infection and pyelonephritis in the newborn
Circumcision as a means of preventing urinary tract infections in boys
Urinary tract infection superimposed on genitourinary malformations, vesico-ureteral reflux and neurologic disorders of bladder function in children
Morbidity of recurrent urinary tract infection among females with uncomplicated infection
Acute, uncomplicated pyelonephritis in females
Chronic pyelonephritis
Urinary tract infections during pregnancy; implications for the fetus
Urinary tract infection complicating diabetes, renal transplantation, polycystic renal disease, urinary stones, obstructive uropathy, neurologic and neoplastic disease in adults
Urinary tract infections in older males with prostatic hypertrophy
Prostatitis and epididymitis
Infections produced by instrumentation of the urinary tract with catheters and other devices
The urosepsis syndrome and endotoxemia
Metastatic infections to the kidney by virulent microorganisms

related species. The most common gram positive bacteria are *Staphylococcus aureus* and coagulase-negative staphylococci, including *Staphylococcus saprophyticus* (which has a special role in young women) and group B streptococci and enterococci. The most common yeast is *Candida albicans,* but other species of yeasts and invasive fungi may produce urinary tract infections. Commensal organisms that colonize the urethra, such as Lactobacilli, most Corynebacteria species, Gardnerella, alpha streptococci, and strict (obligate) anaerobes, grow poorly in urine and are considered as urethral or vaginal contaminants. They cannot be dismissed entirely because at times they may be recovered from the blood and renal abscesses in patients with long-standing infection, but this is distinctly unusual. Gonococci readily infect the urethra and genital tract but do not multiply and often are killed rapidly in urine.

"Uropathogens"

The term "uropathogens" is commonly used to describe the microorganisms, listed previously, that are found most frequently in patients with urinary tract infections. Some authors prefer to reserve the term "uropathogens" for individual strains or clones that possess special virulence properties. These clones will be referred to in this book as "uropathogenic" or "invasive" *E. coli.* Urease-producing microbes, such as Proteus, Providencia, Morganella, and *Corynebacterium urealyticum,* are particularly pathogenic because of their ability to produce urease and predispose to urinary calculi.

Pathogenesis

Ascending Infection

The most common route of infection is by the *ascending route.* Uropathic microbes colonize the urethra and enter the bladder via the urinary stream or along the mucosal sheath. Invasive infection occurs when the microorganisms grow in urine, attach to urothelial cells, and penetrate the urothelial lining. Gram negative bacteria may release endotoxin locally and induce the production of interleukins. The microorganism may ascend to the ureters and kidneys. Ascent is generally thought to occur by Brownian motion but may be augmented by motile flagella and, in some cases, by the spread of a extracellular glycocalyx. Ascending infection is by far the most common route in females and the one most commonly associated with instrumentation in both sexes. Infection of the kidney begins in the renal pelvis and caliceal fornices. It then progresses to involve one or more renal segments. This progression accounts for the pie or wedge-shaped distribution of infection. A residual scar may form when the process is healed.

Hematogenous Infection

Infections may also occur by the hematogenous or blood-borne route. The kidney is well-supplied by blood vessels and, at any one time, receives one quarter of the cardiac output. Any systemic infection can lead to seeding of the kidney, but certain microorganisms are particularly invasive. *Staphylococcus aureus* bacteremia is associated commonly with spread to the kidney and may produce cortical abscesses. The process may extend to the perirenal fat and produce perinephric abscesses. Systemic candidiasis arising from an intravascular device or from the gastrointestinal tract in a neutropenic patient may produce extensive metastatic infection in the kidney. Occasionally, a hematogenous focus may arise from the kidney itself. In this case, microorganisms are disseminated from the kidney to the bloodstream and reinfect the kidney, producing multiple small abscesses throughout the organ.

Other Pathways of Infection

Some workers have postulated that a pathway may exist from the intestines to the kidney by way of lymphatic channels. Franke in 1910 (12) demonstrated channels between the appendix and rectum and right kidney, but direct lymphatic channels have not been convincingly demonstrated between the lower urinary tract and the kidneys. Some investigators report passage of india ink particles from the lower to upper tract in animals, but this remains to be confirmed. Beeson pointed out that lymphatic drainage of a region generally follows its blood supply and venous drainage (13). The arteries and veins of the urinary tract are segmentally distributed even at different levels of the ureter. Drainage from the bladder wall and ureter is not toward the kidney, but into the common iliac glands. Therefore, Beeson doubts that the postulated pathway from lower to upper tract via the lymphatics exists at all.

Unanswered Questions Concerning the Routes of Infection

Although the ascending route of infection appears to be the most satisfactory explanation of infection in females, some troubling features of urinary infection remain to be explained. For example, how do males who have not been instrumented develop prostatic infection and pyelonephritis? How do anaerobic bacteria that are occasionally isolated from renal abscesses get there? Although the evidence remains incomplete, a study by Schwarz in dogs (14) provides suggestive evidence of translocation of *E. coli* from the traumatized bowel to the kidney. He inoculated *E. coli* 0119 by submucosal injection and subsequently recovered the organisms from the kidney of dogs whose ureters had been ligated. The route by which the bacteria reached the kidney is not clear from these experiments.

Major Risk Factors for Infection

The clinical distinction between uncomplicated and complicated urinary tract infections is of paramount importance (see the following definitions). Host factors are the key determinants of the role of invasive properties of the microorganisms, localization of infection, extent of renal damage, bacteremia, dissemination, therapeutic, prophylactic and immune strategies, development of resistance, and the ultimate prognosis. The major predisposing factors are linked with their most important effect in Figure 1.2.

Uncomplicated (Medical) Infection

Uncomplicated urinary infections are defined as those in which no underlying structural or neurological lesions can be detected. They occur most commonly in otherwise healthy females, but also in uncircumcised infants and homosexual males. Most uncomplicated infections, even acute, uncomplicated pyelonephritis, respond readily to treatment with antimicrobial

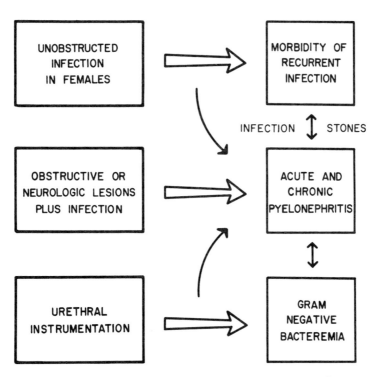

Figure 1.2. Current concept of the relation between predisposing factors and the outcome of urinary tract infection.

drugs to which the invading microbes are susceptible. The long-term prognosis for preservation of renal function is excellent. The major problem is the considerable morbidity suffered by some women who have recurrent, symptomatic infections. A small number of well-documented cases exist in which patients with acute, uncomplicated pyelonephritis develop permanent renal damage, but this situation is rare (15–18).

The reasons why some otherwise healthy females are particularly prone to acquire urinary tract infections continues to be investigated (see Chapter 10). The key factors appear to be the short, but complex, structure of the female urethra, the ability of uropathogenic bacteria (especially adhesive, fimbriated, strains of E. coli) to colonize the periurethral zone, and the presence of specific receptors to the adhesive strains on urothelial cells. The roles of sexual activity, feminine hygiene, and fluid intake continue to be debated. The microorganisms that are commonly found in uncomplicated infections are shown in Table 1.3. Uncomplicated infections may become complicated in patients who are infected with urease-producing bacteria, such as Proteus mirabilis. Urease splits urea into ammonia and carbon dioxide, producing an alkaline urine. This favors the precipitation of struvite stones that may obstruct the urinary tract.

Complicated (Surgical) Infection

Complicated (or surgical) infections occur in individuals of both sexes who have structural or functional abnormalities of the voiding mechanism, prostatic calculi, or underlying diseases which predispose the kidney to infection. These diseases include diabetes mellitus, sickle cell anemia, polycystic renal disease, and renal transplantation. Infections caused by an indwelling

---

Table 1.3. Microorganisms Found in Uncomplicated Infections*

Most Common
  Escherichia coli—accounts for about 80%–90% of cases
  Staphylococcus saprophyticus—accounts for about 10%–20% of cases in young women,
    with the highest frequency during the late summer and early fall
Less Common
  Other *Enterobacteriaceae*—Klebsiella, Enterobacter, Proteus, Salmonella and Shigella
  Other gram positive bacteria—*Staphylococcus aureus,* group B streptococci and
    enterococci
Common Contaminants
  Lactobacilli
  Anaerobic streptococci
  Diphtheroids
  Coagulase negative staphylococci

---

*These microbes tend to be susceptible to antimicrobial drugs. The frequency of resistant strains depends on the extent of use of antimicrobial drugs in the population.

Table 1.4. Microorganisms in Complicated Infections*

Enterobacteriaceae
Escherichia coli accounts for about 20% of cases; other species include Klebsiella, Enterobacter, Proteus, Providencia, Morganella
Other gram negative bacilli
Pseudomonas, Acinetobacter
Gram positive bacteria
Staphylococcus aureus, coagulase-negative staphylococci (other than *Staphylococcus saprophyticus*), group B streptococci, enterococci, *Corynebacterium urealyticum*
Yeasts and fungi
Candida, Torulopsis
Parasites
Schistosoma haematobium (Bilharzia)

*These microorganisms tend to be resistant to antimicrobial drugs. The frequency of resistance depends on the selective pressure of antimicrobial drugs and transmission of resistant strains.

urinary catheter or other drainage devices are considered to be complicated. Complicated infections may be exceedingly difficult to eradicate with antimicrobial drugs without correction of the underlying defect. The microorganisms that are commonly found in complicated infections are shown in Table 1.4. These microorganisms consist of less pathogenic or virulent stains of *E. coli* and other gram negative and gram positive bacteria. The microorganisms are often resistant to multiple antimicrobial drugs because of the selective pressure of antibiotic use. Complicated infections are exceedingly difficult to treat unless the underlying structural or functional problems are corrected. Patients with complicated infections are more likely to develop severe renal damage, bacteremia, sepsis, and an increased mortality.

Metastatic Infection

The urinary tract may be invaded from a distant site by way of the blood stream. The kidney is most often involved, but infection may occur in any part of the tract, including the prostate. Metastatic infections may be an expression of a generalized infection produced by 1) virulent microorganisms in an otherwise healthy host, 2) opportunistic microorganisms in hosts compromised by immune deficiency, neutropenia, or an infected foreign body located at a distant site, 3) mycobacterial and endemic mycoses, and 4) viral infections. At times, microorganisms can enter the bloodstream from an infected kidney and reinvade the organ. The source of anaerobic bacteria found in long-standing renal abscesses is unknown, but is most likely by means of the bloodstream. The microorganisms that are commonly found in metastatic infections in relation to host factors are shown in Table 1.5.

Table 1.5. Microorganisms That Produce Metastatic Infections of the Urinary Tract, According to Host Factors and Epidemiologic Settings

Virulent microorganisms in an otherwise healthy host
   Staphylococcus aureus
   Eschericia coli—Invasive clones among newborn children
Opportunistic microorganisms in compromised hosts
   Candida albicans
   Aspergillus fumigatus
   Zygomycetes (*mucor* spp., *Rhizopus* spp.)
Mycobacteria and endemic mycoses
   Mycobacterium tuberculosis
   Histoplasma capsulatum, Blastomyces dermatitidis, Coccidioides immitis
Viruses
   Herpes-type: *Herpes simplex, Herpes zoster,* Cytomegalovirus
   Adenoviruses: type 4 and 11
   Papova, Polyoma, JC and JK virus in immunocompromised hosts
   Coxsackie and ECHO viruses

Clinical Classification

The clinical significance of a urinary tract infection is determined best by the history and the clinical, laboratory, and radiologic findings. Terms such as asymptomatic bacteriuria, urethritis, cystitis, prostatitis, and pyelonephritis are incomplete and may be misleading unless they are placed within the appropriate epidemiologic setting and clinical context. For example:

- Asymptomatic bacteriuria caused by *Pseudomonas aeruginosa* in a young girl with recurrent infections, complicated by a neurogenic bladder, **has an entirely different meaning than:**
- Asymptomatic (persistent) bacteriuria caused by *Pseudomonas aeruginosa* in an elderly man, complicated by prostatic obstruction and an indwelling urinary catheter.
- Acute (first episode, uncomplicated) pyelonephritis caused by *E. coli* in an otherwise healthy young woman **has an entirely different meaning than:**
- Acute (recurrent, complicated) pyelonephritis caused by *E. coli* in an elderly diabetic woman; course complicated by sepsis.

To provide more meaningful descriptions of patients with urinary tract infections, a simple classification scheme is presented in Table 1.6. This scheme can be adopted, like a Chinese menu, to describe individual cases. The causative microorganism and complications are added when known. Additional descriptive characteristics are placed in brackets. This framework provides clinical meaning to expressions such as asymptomatic bacteriuria

Table 1.6. Framework for Clinical Classification of Urinary Tract Infections

Category	Findings
Clinical presentation	Asymptomatic
	Urethritis, Prostatitis, Cystitis, Pyelonephritis
History	First or recurrent episodes
	Persistent infection
Disease activity	Acute or chronic
	Active or inactive
Etiologic microorganism(s)	Bacteria, yeasts, fungi, viruses
Route of infection	Ascending or metastatic
Host structure	
Uncomplicated	Healthy female or homosexual male
Complicated	Neurogenic bladder, reflux, urinary catheter
Host factors	
Demographic	Age, sex, hospital, nursing home
Underlying disease(s)	Pregnant, diabetic, renal transplant
Complications	Bacteremia, Sepsis syndrome

or pyelonephritis and can be used to design therapeutic or prophylactic strategies and predict prognosis.

Examples of Diagnoses Based on the Clinical Classification Framework

1. A 20-year-old, previously healthy, pregnant woman is admitted because of chills, fever (103.4° F), and left flank pain. The white blood count is 20,000mm³, with 80% neutrophils and 5% bands. Microscopic examination of the uncentrifuged urine reveals 10–15 white blood cells and 20–40 gram negative bacteria per high powered field (HPF). She appears acutely ill but is normotensive, and the serum creatinine is 0.9 mg/dL. A renal ultrasound reveals a diffusely enlarged left kidney and a normal right kidney. No evidence of stone or obstruction exists, and the bladder empties completely. Urine culture reveals $> 10^5$ colony forming units (cfu) of *E. coli*. The blood culture taken on admission is positive for the same organism.

Diagnosis: Acute (first episode, symptomatic, ascending, uncomplicated) pyelonephritis during pregnancy caused by *E. coli;* course complicated by bacteremia.

2. A 40-year-old woman with severe multiple sclerosis is admitted to a hospital for the third time within a year because of progressive obtundation, poor intake of fluids, and low-grade fever (100° F). She is difficult to arouse. The neurologic findings of multiple sclerosis have not changed since her last admission. A urinary catheter is in place. It is removed and is found to be heavily encrusted at the tip, and the lumen is blocked by impacted mu-

cous. Her blood pressure on arrival to the hospital is 80/40 mm Hg and she appears dehydrated. The BUN is 60 mg/dL and the creatinine is 2.8 mg/dL. The white blood count is 9,000 mm Hg with 78% neutrophils and 8% bands. Microscopic examination of the uncentrifuged urine reveals 10–15 white blood cells and 20–40 gram negative bacteria/HPF. The pH of the urine is 8.0. CT scan of the head is normal. An abdominal CT reveals a normal left kidney. The right kidney is diffusely enlarged with a staghorn calculus in the pelvis. Urine culture reveals $> 10^5$ cfu/ml of *Proteus mirabilis*. The blood culture is positive for the same organism.

Diagnosis: Acute and chronic (recurrent, symptomatic, ascending) pyelonephritis caused by *Proteus mirabilis* in a woman with multiple sclerosis, complicated by a right staghorn calculus and an indwelling urinary catheter; course complicated by bacteremia and the sepsis syndrome.

3. An 80-year-old woman is well except for senile dementia. She is incontinent of urine but does not have an indwelling urinary catheter. She resides in a long-term care facility. A urine culture performed 1 year previously contained large numbers of bacteria. An ultrasound of the kidney and bladder obtained at that time was reported to be normal. On a routine monthly visit, her physician notes that she is afebrile and her condition has not changed. He obtains a routine urinalysis, urine culture, hemogram, electrolytes, and renal function studies. The hemoglobin is 12.5 mg/dL, white blood cell count 5,600 mm^3, and the creatinine is 0.7 mg/dL. The urine is positive by the leukocyte esterase and nitrite tests, and culture reveals $> 10^5$ cfu/ml of *Klebsiella pneumoniae*.

Diagnosis: Chronic, uncomplicated bladder infection (persistent, asymptomatic bacteriuria with pyuria) caused by *Klebsiella pneumoniae*, in an incontinent, elderly woman with senile dementia residing in a nursing home.

Common Questions and Answers Based on the Clinical Classification Framework

Questions about urinary tract infections can be addressed only within the appropriate clinical context. The answers usually require additional information about the patient. For example:

Question: Should asymptomatic bacteriuria be treated?

Answer: Yes, during pregnancy; No, in the elderly; No, in a patient with a long-term urinary catheter; Probably, in a woman with highly recurrent symptomatic infections.

Question: What is the drug of choice and appropriate duration of therapy for cystitis?

Answer: To answer this question, one needs to know that the "cystitis" is bacterial and not caused by something else. Other causes of cystitis include radiation therapy to the bladder or prostate, interstitial cystitis, and use of beta lactam antibiotics. One also needs to know whether this is the first or one of several recurrent infections, what antimicrobial drugs were used before this episode, and whether the patient has an important underlying disease such as diabetes. Let us assume that this is one of several intermittent infections in an otherwise healthy, nonpregnant, young woman. The drugs that should be considered include trimethoprim alone or trimethoprim/sulfamethoxazole or nitrofurantoin, or the least expensive fluoroquinolone, to be taken for 3 days.

Question: How long should a patient with pyelonephritis be treated with intravenous antibiotics?

Answer: To answer this question, one needs to know whether the patient has acute, uncomplicated or complicated pyelonephritis, whether this is the first or one of many infections, and whether the patient is able to tolerate oral drugs. A gram stain of the urine is needed to make a presumptive diagnosis of the most likely causative microorganism. Let us assume that this is an elderly woman who was brought in from a nursing home with hypotension, fever, and leukocytosis, has a urinary catheter in place, and whose gram stain shows innumerable pus cells and gram negative rods. She is known to be allergic to penicillin and cephalosporins. The catheter should be removed and she should be treated intravenously with an aminoglycoside antibiotic. Therapy should be changed to a less toxic intravenous drug as soon as susceptibility data are available. The drug should be given orally as soon as she can take food without difficulty.

Question: How extensive should the work-up be for an outpatient with urinary tract infection?

Answer: To answer this question, more details of the clinical history need to be provided. One needs to know whether the patient is a child or adult or elderly, male or female, and whether this is the first or one of several recurrent infections. Let us assume that the patient is an otherwise healthy teenaged female with recurrent infections who has undergone extensive radiologic investigations in the past, all of which have been normal. No further tests are needed.

Question: How should a study be designed to evaluate a new drug for the treatment of urinary tract infections?

Answer: It depends on the claims to be made for the product. The most favorable results will be obtained by limiting the patient population to adult females with uncomplicated infections. Worse results will be obtained with elderly patients in nursing homes. Even worse results will be obtained in patients managed with indwelling urinary catheters.

Question: Doctor, if my little girl continues to have repeated attacks of urinary tract infections, will she end up on the artificial kidney?

Answer: No, because an ultrasound of her kidney and bladder were entirely normal and she only has had a few scattered episodes of urinary tract infection. These infections are very common and rarely, if ever, damage the kidney.

The key point of these examples is that helpful answers can be provided only when the details of the case are known. This approach to case management will be presented in greater detail in the chapter on Management.

Mortality and End-Stage Renal Disease Associated with Urinary Tract Infections

Urinary tract infections occur more frequently in females than in males throughout most of life. It would be expected that if urinary tract infections produced significant renal damage, women would have higher death rates from renal disease than would men. Actually, however, the life expectancy of women exceeds that of men, and the rates of end-state renal disease are higher in males (54.3%) (19). These facts imply that either urinary tract infections in females do not have a significant impact on renal disease and mortality, or the data are obscured by other factors.

Mortality Statistics

The number of deaths attributed to infections of the kidney in the United States in 1993 was 0.4 per 100,000 (20). The rate was higher in females (0.6 per 100,000) than in males (0.2 per 100,000) and about the same in whites and blacks. The highest rate was in the very old (29.3 per 100,000 in people > 85 years) (21). Complications of prostatic obstruction is the most likely contributory cause of death in males. Urinary catheters are the most likely contributory cause of death in elderly women. Women account for over 80% of the elderly in nursing homes. Similar age-related data have been reported in the United Kingdom and Israel (22,23) (Figs. 1.3 and 1.4).

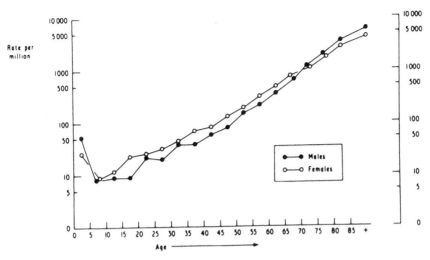

Figure 1.3. Death rates for infections of the kidney in males and females in England and Wales. Reproduced with permission from Waters WE (22).

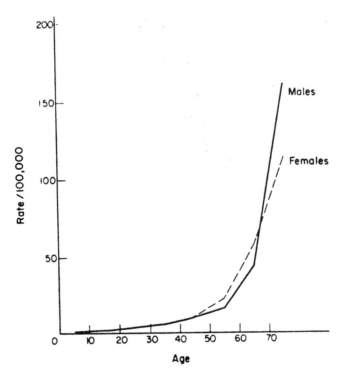

Figure 1.4. Mean annual renal mortality rate from primary renal disease (excluding malignancies and polycystic kidney disease) in Israel by age and sex, per 100,000. Reproduced with permission from Modan B, Moore BP, Paz B (23).

Factors That Might Obscure the Association Between Urinary Tract Infections, Renal Failure, and Mortality

Urinary tract infections are common in diabetics and the elderly. These patients frequently have several life-threatening diseases, including hypertension, renal failure, and strokes and may be managed with indwelling urinary catheters during their final days. It is difficult to distinguish between the role of infection and the underlying diseases as the ultimate cause of death. Death certificates identify major underlying diseases, such as congenital abnormalities, diabetes, paraplegia, surgical procedures, dementia, cancer, stroke, and cardiovascular disease. They may not provide adequate information concerning concomitant urinary tract infections.

Examples In Which the Role of Urinary Tract Infections Might be Missed or Disregarded on Death Certificates

1. An elderly man with severe prostatic obstruction is managed with an indwelling urinary catheter. He then undergoes a prostatectomy. His course is complicated by septic shock and multi-system failure. The septic episode responds to antimicrobial drugs; he is intubated, develops pneumonia, gastritis, a myocardial infarction, and dies. The death certificate states the cause of death as myocardial infarction. The underlying cause is coronary artery disease. Associated causes of death might include pneumonia, bleeding ulcers, and sepsis. Actually, all of these events were precipitated by "urosepsis" several weeks earlier.
2. An elderly female diabetic has renal disease secondary to diabetic nephrosclerosis. She also suffers from recurrent episodes of urinary tract infection, which are treated with multiple courses of antimicrobial drugs, including β lactam antibiotics and amphotericin B for candiduria. She eventually dies of renal failure. An autopsy is not done. The death certificate lists the cause of death as renal failure secondary to diabetes mellitus. It may not state that the patient had superimposed urinary tract infections and that nephrotoxic drugs were used to treat the infections.

Data from Dialysis and Transplant Programs

There were 150,650 patients on chronic renal dialysis and 55,261 with a functioning renal transplant in the United States in 1992. In the same year, 55,377 new cases of end-stage renal disease (ESRD) were reported to the USRDS registry (19). There were 4352 children under the age of 20 years with ESRD during the same general period. The annual incidence of new cases is about 9.1% per year. The most common causes of ESRD in adults and children are shown in Table 1.7. Pyelonephritis is not mentioned in this analysis, but it is undoubtedly a major complication of diabetes, obstructive

Table 1.7. The Ten Most Common Causes of End-Stage Renal Failure Managed by Dialysis or Transplantation, 1989–1992

Primary Disease	All Ages %	<20 years %
Diabetes	36.2	1.4
Hypertension	30.1	5.5
Glomerulonephritis	12.9	36.0
Cystic kidney diseases	3.1	4.4
Interstitial nephritis	3.1	4.4
Obstructive nephropathy	2.1	7.9
Collagen vascular diseases	2.2	9.4
Malignancies	1.3	0.3
Metabolic diseases	0.5	1.3
Congenital diseases*	0.7	18.5

From USRDS 1995 Annual Data Report (19).
*Includes congenital obstructive uropathy, renal agenesis and dysplasia, and Alport's syndrome.

nephropathy, and congenital diseases. Many of the cases ascribed to interstitial nephritis are probably caused by reflux nephropathy.

Pyelonephritis as a Cause of End-Stage Renal Failure

Complicated pyelonephritis accounted for 26.1% of cases of renal failure among patients awaiting transplantation (24). The underlying lesions included vesicoureteral reflux (66.7%), analgesic abuse (14.3%), nephrolithiasis (11.9%), and obstruction (7.2%). Similarly, interstitial nephritis was found to be the major lesion in 27% of patients with end-stage renal failure (25). Over half of these patients had urinary obstruction, vesicoureteral reflux, or other structural abnormalities of the urinary tract.

Mortality in the Elderly

Several studies in the early literature suggested that a relationship might exist between bacteriuria and mortality in the aged (26,27). These observations have not been substantiated even by some of the original investigators (28). In a controlled trial of long-term prophylaxis of urinary tract infection in ambulatory men, treatment had no effect on mortality (29). Similar results were obtained among elderly men in nursing homes (30). More recently, a prospective cohort study, combined with a controlled clinical trial of treatment of elderly women without urinary catheters, demonstrated that urinary tract infection was not an independent risk factor for mortality and that treatment did not lower the mortality rate (31). These observations have led to a more relaxed attitude towards treatment of uncomplicated, asymptomatic bacteriuria in the elderly.

> **Key Points About Mortality and End-Stage Renal Diseases Associated With Urinary Tract Infections and Pyelonephritis**
>
> • The major causes of end-stage renal disease are diabetes, hypertension, glomerulonephritis and polycystic renal disease.
> • Uncomplicated urinary tract infections rarely cause end-stage renal disease.
> • Treatment or prophylaxis of uncomplicated urinary tract infections at all ages may decrease morbidity, but has no effect on mortality.
> • Complicated urinary tract infections are major causes of morbidity and contribute to mortality in patients with diabetes, polycystic renal disease, congenital abnormalities of the urinary tract, neurologic disorders, and those with urinary catheters.

References

1. Brumfitt W, Hamilton-Miller JMT. Prophylactic antibiotics for recurrent urinary tract infections. J Antimicrob Chemother 1990;25:505–512.
2. Schappert SM. National ambulatory medical survey: 1990 summary. Advance data from vital and health statistics: no. 213. Hyattsville, Maryland: National Center for Health Statistics, 1992:1–12.
3. Woodwell DA. Office visits to urologists: United States, 1989–90. Advance data from vital and health statistics: no. 234. Hyattsville, Maryland: National Center for Health Statistics, 1992:1–12.
4. Kass EH. Asymptomatic infections of the urinary tract. Trans Assoc Am Physicians 1956;69:56–63.
5. Boshell BR, Sanford JP. A screening method for the evaluation of urinary tract infection in female patients without catheterization. Ann Intern Med 1958;48:1040–1045.
6. Wiswell TE, Smith FR, Bass JW. Decreased incidence of urinary tract infections in circumcised male infants. J Pediatr 1985;75:901–903.
7. Kunin CM, Deutscher R, Paquin AJ. Urinary tract infection in school children: epidemiologic, clinical and laboratory study. Medicine 1964;43:91–130.
8. Evans DA, Williams DN, Laughlin LW, et al. Bacteriuria in a population-based cohort of women. J Infect Dis 1978;138:768–773.
9. Gratacos E, Torres PJ, Vila J, et al. Screening and treatment of asymptomatic bacteriuria in pregnancy prevent pyelonephritis. J Infect Dis 1994;169:1390–1392.
10. Platt R, Polk BF, Murdock B, et al. Mortality associated with nosocomial urinary-tract infection. N Engl J Med 1982;307:637–642.
11. Kunin CM, Douthitt S, Dancing J, et al. The association between the use of urinary catheters and morbidity and mortality among elderly patients in nursing homes. Am J Epidemiol 1992;135:291–301.
12. Franke K. Uber die lymphgefasse des dickdarmes. Arch Anat Physiol (Lpz.) Anatom Abt. 1910;191.
13. Beeson PB. Factors in the pathogenesis of pyelonephritis. Yale J Biol Med 1955;28:81–104.
14. Schwarz H. Renal invasion by E. coli via a mucosal lesion of the sigmoid colon: a demonstration utilizing methods of autoradiography and group-specific serologic typing. Invest Urol 1968;6:98–113.
15. Bailey RR, Little PJ, Rolleston GL. Renal damage after acute pyelonephritis. Br Med J 1969;1:550–551.
16. Baker LRI, Cattell WR, Fry IKF, et al. Acute renal failure due to pyelonephritis. Q J Med 1979;68:603–612.
17. Jones SR. Acute renal failure in adults with uncomplicated acute pyelonephritis: case reports and review. Clin Infect Dis 1992;14:243–246.
18. Johansson B, Troll S, Berg U. Renal parenchymal volume during and after acute pyelonephritis measured by ultrasonography. Arch Dis Child 1988;63:1309–1314.
19. USRDS 1995 Annual data report. Am J Kidney Dis 1995;26:S1-S186.

20. National Center for Health Statistics, Advance Report of Final Mortality Statistics 1993; 44:No. 7, 1996.
21. National Center for Health Statistics, Advance Report of Final Mortality Statistics 1984; 33:No. 9, 1997.
22. Waters WE. Trends in mortality from nephritis and infections of the kidney in England and Wales. Lancet 1968;1:241–243.
23. Modan B, Moore BP, Paz B. Mortality from renal disease in Israel, some epidemiologic aspects. J Chron Dis 1970;22:727–732.
24. Holland H, Busch R. Chronic pyelonephritis as a cause of end stage renal disease. J Urol 1982;127:642–643.
25. Murray T, Goldberg M. Chronic interstitial nephritis: Etiologic factors. Ann Intern Med 1975;82:453–459.
26. Dontas AS, Kasviki-Charvati P, Papanayiotou DC, Marketos SG. Bacteriuria and survival in old age. N Eng J Med 1981;304:939–943.
27. Sourander LB, Kasanen A. A 5-year follow-up of bacteriuria in the aged. Geront Clin 1972;14:274–281.
28. Dontas AS, Tzonou A, Kasviki-Charvati P, et al. Survival in a residential home: an eleven-year longitudinal study. J Am Geriatr Soc 1991;39:641–649.
29. Freeman RB, Richardson JA, Thurm RH, et al. Long-term therapy for chronic bacteriuria in men. Ann Intern Med 1975;83:133–147.
30. Nicolle LE, Henderson E, Bjornson J, et al. The association of bacteriuria with resident characteristics and survival in elderly institutionalized men. Ann Intern Med 1987;106: 682–686.
31. Abrutyn E, Mossey J, Berlin JA, et al. Does asymptomatic bacteriuria predict mortality and does antimicrobial treatment reduce mortality in elderly ambulatory women? Ann Intern Med 1994;120:827–833.

Suggested Readings

Asscher AW. The challenge of urinary tract infections. New York: Grune and Stratton, 1980.
Brumfitt W, Asscher AW. Urinary tract infection. New York: Oxford University Press, 1973.
Gillespie L, Blakeslee S. You don't have to live with cystitis! New York: Rawson Associates, 1986.
Hanno PM, Staskin DR, Krane RJ, et al., eds. Interstitial cystitis. London: Springer-Verlag, 1990.
Kass EH, Brumfitt W, eds. Infections of the urinary tract. Chicago: University of Chicago Press, 1975.
Kass EH, ed. Progress in pyelonephritis. Philadelphia: Davis,1965.
Kass EH, Svanborg-Edén C, eds. Host-parasite interactions in urinary tract infections. Chicago: University of Chicago Press, 1989.
Kaye D, ed. Urinary tract infections. The Medical Clinics of North America. Philadelphia: WB Saunders, 1991.
Kincaid-Smith P, Fairley KF. Renal infection and renal scarring. Melbourne: Mercedes, 1970.
Mobley HLT, Warren JW, eds. Urinary tract infections. Molecular pathogenesis and clinical management. Washington: ASM Press, 1996.
O'Grady F, Brumfitt W, eds. Urinary tract infection. London: Oxford University Press, 1968.
Quinn EL, Kass EH, eds. Biology of pyelonephritis. Boston: Little Brown, 1960.
Sanford JP. Urinary tract symptoms and infections. Annu Rev Med 1975;26:485–498.
Slade N, Gillespie WA. The urinary tract and the catheter∫infection and other problems. New York: Wiley, 1985.
Stamey TA. Pathogenesis and treatment of urinary tract infections. Baltimore: Williams & Wilkins, 1980.

2

Bacteriuria, Pyuria, Proteinuria, Hematuria, and Pneumaturia

Overview

The quantitative count of uropathogenic microorganisms in the urine provides the clinician and epidemiologist with a useful diagnostic marker for urinary tract infections. As with all laboratory tests, significant bacteriuria needs to be carefully defined and must be clinically meaningful. Pyuria is the hallmark of the inflammatory response. It occurs in a wide variety of conditions, including urinary tract infection. Sterile pyuria needs to be interpreted within a broad differential diagnosis and should not be attributed to urinary tract infection without good reason. Soon after the concept of significant bacteriuria was developed, it was noted that the urine of many entirely asymptomatic people contained large numbers of bacteria that could not be accounted for by contamination. The term asymptomatic bacteriuria was coined to describe this condition. Strictly speaking, asymptomatic bacteriuria cannot be considered an infection unless there is evidence of inflammation and invasion of the structures of the urinary tract. Only about half the individuals found to have asymptomatic bacteriuria have significant pyuria. Nevertheless, asymptomatic bacteriuria has great predictive value for the emergence of symptomatic infections and must be considered an abnormal finding. This chapter describes the microbiologic basis for significant bacteriuria and the clinical criteria for bacteriuria and pyuria in the diagnosis of urinary tract infections. The clinical implications of cytokinuria, proteinuria, hematuria, and pneumaturia are also considered.

The Concept of Significant Bacteriuria

Bladder urine is ordinarily sterile. Small numbers of microorganisms may enter the urine as contaminants during passage of the stream through the distal urethra and over the vaginal introitus. The concept of "significant bacteriuria" was developed to differentiate between growth of microorganisms in the bladder urine from contaminants collected during voiding (1–3). "Bacteriuria" literally means that bacteria are present in the urine. "Significant bacteriuria" implies that the microorganisms are actually multiplying in the urine or are derived from infected tissues. The most practical, noninvasive method to determine the presence of "significant bacteriuria" is to collect a clean (not necessarily midstream), freshly voided specimen of urine and perform a quantitative culture. When this step is done, voided urine from a sterile bladder will contain either no bacteria or a small number of contaminants. Patients with urinary tract infections will usually have counts of $\geq 1 \times 10^5$ cfu/ml of uropathogens (see definition of uropathogens). Contamination with commensal microorganisms is usually associated with counts of $< 10^3$ cfu/ml. In practice, most patients with urinary tract infections will have counts well in excess of 1×10^6 cfu/ml.

Voided urine is usually adequate for culture. Care needs to be taken to avoid contamination with vaginal or periurethral microorganisms. Routine urethral catheterization is not necessary or wise because microorganisms can be introduced into the bladder and cause urinary tract infections. Catheters or suprapubic aspiration may be needed at times to confirm the diagnosis in young children, in patients who cannot void spontaneously, or in patients who are too weak or obese to provide a clean-voided specimen. Methods to collect and culture urine will be described in the next chapter.

The distribution of bacterial colony counts in the voided urine of infected and noninfected patients as determined in large surveys is shown diagrammatically in Figure 2.1. Note that the counts in infected patients are usually $\geq 1 \times 10^5$ cfu/ml. The overlap between infected and noninfected patients is observed in the range of 1×10^3 and 1×10^4 cfu/ml. Under certain circumstances, counts of $< 1 \times 10^5$ cfu/ml are found in patients with urinary tract infections (Table 2.1). In addition, a patient is considered to have "significant bacteriuria" with counts of $< 1 \times 10^5$ cfu/ml, when the same uropathogen is isolated repeatedly or the urine is obtained by suprapubic aspiration (SPA) or urethral catheterization. Under certain circumstances, the urine may be sterile even in the presence of infection (see Table 1.1).

Microbiologic Basis for Significant Bacteriuria

Urinary infections are most often caused by enteric gram-negative bacteria, staphylococci, and enterococci that grow well in urine. The infectious process begins when small numbers of microorganisms enter the bladder urine, adhere to the surface of the bladder mucosa, and resist the wash-out by the urinary stream. After a lag phase of a few hours, the microorganisms begin to grow logarithmically and double about every 30 minutes until they reach a stationary phase (Fig. 2.2). Under ideal conditions, the microorganisms may attain full growth within 5 to 6 hours, but longer periods may be required depending on the inoculum size, growth properties of the urine, and urinary hydrodynamics (Table 2.2). Full growth, at colony counts well in excess of 1×10^8 cfu/ml, usually will be reached within 24 hours. (See "Growth in Urine," Chapter 11 for a more detailed discussion of factors that determine growth of bacteria in urine.)

Isolation of More than One Organism

Most urinary tract infections are caused by a single microorganism. Recovery of more than one microorganism may be a result of contamination during collection or may represent polymicrobic infection. These possibilities can be differentiated by the clinical presentation of the patient. A single organism is almost invariably present in patients with uncomplicated infections. Occasionally, *E. coli*, together with *Staphylococcus saprophyticus* or other

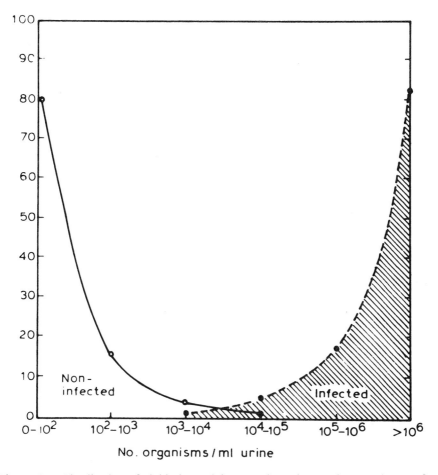

Figure 2.1. Distribution of viable bacterial counts in early morning specimens of urine obtained from large populations of subjects with asymptomatic bacteriuria (l———l) and noninfected controls (i———i). Reproduced with permission from Asscher AW (4).

enteric bacteria, will be recovered from the same specimen in patients with acute cystitis. Patients with complicated infections (associated with stones, renal abscesses, or long-term indwelling urinary catheters) often will have multiple organisms in their urine. As many as four to five or more different species may be recovered from patients on long-term catheter drainage. Bacterial counts of some of the microorganisms may be $< 1 \times 10^5$ cfu/ml because of microbial competition. The diagnostic microbiology laboratory should be alerted to the possibility of polymicrobic bacteriuria. If this is not done, the specimen may be rejected as "contaminated."

Table 2.1. Situations in Which the Criteria for "Significant Bacteriuria" with Uropathogens May Fall Below the Standard Count of $\geq 1 \times 10^5$ cfu/ml.

Water diuresis combined with frequent voiding
First day of a urinary catheter-induced infection
Early stages of the "pyuria-dysuria" syndrome
Slow growing microbes in urine (*Staphylococci,* yeasts)
With suppressive antimicrobial therapy
Renal tuberculosis
Systemic mycoses (blastomycosis, cryptococcosis, histoplasmosis and coccidioido-mycosis)

Criteria for Significant Bacteriuria

The standard definition of significant bacteriuria for a clean-voided urine is $\geq 10^5$ cfu/ml of a uropathogen. This criterion has stood the test of time (5). It is particularly useful for screening and epidemiologic studies and for entering patients into clinical trials. There are several important exceptions. Lower counts are acceptable in males because contaminants are not likely to be present in voided urine. Lower counts are also valid in women with the pyuria-dysuria syndrome, during the first day a urinary drainage system

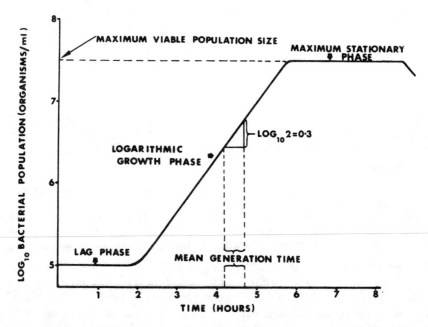

Figure 2.2. Bacterial growth in a liquid medium. Reproduced with permission from Asscher AW (4).

Table 2.2. Factors That Determine the Rate of Growth of Microorganisms in Urine and the Colony Count

Inoculum size
Intrinsic growth properties of the microorganism in urine
Urine pH
Constituents of the urine
Rate of urine flow
Frequency of voiding
Volume of residual volume

becomes contaminated, and in patients who drink large volumes of fluids and void frequently (Table 2.1). Small numbers of uropathogens may be present in the urine of females between recurrent episodes of infection even though the bladder urine is sterile. This condition is not considered to represent significant bacteriuria, but rather reflects persistent colonization of the periurethral zone with the uropathogen destined to produce the next episode of infection (6).

Slow Growing Microorganisms

Certain bacterial species, particularly coagulase-negative staphylococci, grow slowly in urine and may reach counts of only 10^4 to 10^5 cfu/ml (7). This is the appropriate range for "significant bacteriuria" for these organisms. The tubercle bacillus and systemic fungi (blastomycosis, histoplasmosis cryptococcosis, and coccidioidomycosis) grow poorly in urine. The finding of any number of these microorganisms is considered to be significant. Fastidious bacteria such as *Haemophilus influenzae* require special culture media and will not be detected by routine cultures.

Catheterized Patients

Small numbers of microorganisms may be found in the urine within a few days after placement of an indwelling catheter. This is the earliest phase of bacterial growth after the microorganisms are introduced into the bladder. The bacterial count will rapidly increase and will usually reach $> 10^5$ cfu/ml within 24 hours (8).

Screening for Asymptomatic Bacteriuria

Screening programs for asymptomatic bacteriuria are designed for epidemiologic purposes or for defining populations at special risk (pregnant women, diabetics). Asymptomatic bacteriuria should not be diagnosed on the basis of a single urine culture. This may lead to unnecessary diagnostic tests and treatment. In general, a single voided specimen containing $\geq 1 \times 10^5$ cfu/ml of uropathogens is about 80% specific; two consecutive positive specimens are about 90% specific, and three positive consecutive specimens are about 95% specific for significant bacteriuria that can be proven by culture of a catheterized specimen (2,9). Specificity is virtually 100% when the nitrite test is positive and is increased if the same serotype or biotype of the microorganism is recovered repeatedly.

Diagnosis in the Symptomatic Patient

Less diagnostic certainty is needed for patients with urinary tract symptoms and pyuria or those suspected of sepsis arising from the urinary tract. They need to be treated promptly. A significant proportion of patients with urinary tract infections and bacteremia will have bacterial counts in the range of 10^4 to 10^5 cfu/ml (10,11). A single culture is all that is needed before beginning therapy in a symptomatic patient. A presumptive diagnosis can be made based on symptoms, urine microscopy, and dip-stick tests for pyuria and nitrite. Cultures are used for confirming the diagnosis and for susceptibility tests.

Clinical Trials

Some experts recommend less stringent criteria than $\geq 10^5$ cfu/ml for entry of patients into clinical trials and equate low-count bacteriuria, as seen in the pyuria-dysuria syndrome, with urinary tract infections (12). The Food and Drug Administration (FDA) requires $\geq 10^5$ cfu/ml of a uropathogen for entry into clinical trials.

Rationale For Requiring Strict Criteria For Bacteriuria in Studies of New Drugs (13,14)
- Not all clinical investigators have adequate experience in obtaining clean-voided urine specimens and are capable of differentiating low-count bacteriuria from contaminants.
- Drugs are certified for all urinary tract infections regardless of the bacterial count.
- Patients with low-count bacteriuria might respond differently to shorter courses or lower doses than might patients with higher counts.
- It is difficult to define the end-point for cure when low counts are used because uropathogens may continue to colonize the periurethral zone even after the bacteria are eradicated from the bladder.
- Urinary tract infections are common. It is not difficult to identify a sufficient number of patients with $\geq 10^5$ cfu/ml of a uropathogen.

Diagnostic Criteria

These criteria are presented as general guidelines for diagnosis of urinary tract infection. *A positive nitrite test is considered to be highly confirmatory.*

Asymptomatic Females
(Strict criteria are needed to avoid overdiagnosis.)

Field Screening Programs
- Three consecutive clean-voided specimens containing $\geq 10^5$ cfu/ml of the same uropathogen in all (e.g., all *E. coli* or all Pseudomonas). Cultures should be obtained on three separate days.

-or-

- Three consecutive clean-voided specimens containing 10^4 to 10^5 cfu/ml with same uropathogen in all. In this case, all *E. coli* should be of the same serotype or biotype; all Proteus are of the same species; and all staphylococci are of the same phage or biotype type. Cultures should be obtained on three separate days.
- Two consecutive clean-voided specimens containing $\geq 10^5$ cfu/ml of the same uropathogen with a positive nitrite test in at least one.

Office Screening
- Same as field screening programs, except only two consecutive positive cultures or one positive culture with a positive nitrite test are required.

Asymptomatic Males
(Most patients will have counts of $\geq 10^5$ cfu/ml, but less strict criteria can be used because contamination is unlikely.)
- Two consecutive clean-voided specimens containing $>10^4$ cfu/ml with same uropathogen in each or one positive culture with a positive nitrite test. Most infected males will have counts of $\geq 10^5$ cfu/ml.

Symptomatic Males or Females (acute urethritis, cystitis, or pyelonephritis)
(Most patients will have counts of $\geq 10^5$ cfu/ml, but less strict criteria are necessary to avoid underdiagnosis.)

Office or Clinic Practice
- Pyuria-dysuria syndrome—One clean voided specimen with $>10^3$ cfu/ml of a uropathogen combined with pyuria >20 leukocytes/mm^3.
- Acute, uncomplicated infection—One clean voided specimen with $>10^4$ cfu/ml of a uropathogen combined with pyuria >20 leukocytes/mm^3.
- Chronic, complicated infection—One clean voided specimen with $>10^5$ cfu/ml of a uropathogen. Lower counts (10^4 to 10^5 cfu/ml) may be noted at times.

Clinical Trials
(Strict criteria are required to avoid bias.)
- Urinary tract infection—One or two clean voided specimens with $> 10^5$ cfu/ml of a uropathogen combined with pyuria >20 leukocytes/mm^3.

Catheterized or Suprapubic Aspirated Specimens
(Most patients will have counts of $\geq 10^5$ cfu/ml, but less strict criteria may be used because urethral contamination is avoided.)
- $>10^3$ cfu/ml of a uropathogen. Specimens obtained from an indwelling catheter or urine drainage tubing will almost invariably exceed $> 10^5$ cfu/ml except during the first 24 hours of infection.

Key Points About Bacteriologic Criteria for Urinary Tract Infection

- The most common uropathogens in uncomplicated infections are *E. coli* and other *Enterobacteriaceae, Staphylococcus saprophyticus,* and enterococci.
- The most common uropathogens in complicated infections are more resistant strains of *E. coli* and other *Enterobacteriaceae*, Pseudomonas, *Staphylococcus aureus,* coagulase-negative staphylococci (other than *Staphylococcus saprophyticus*), enterococci, and Candida.
- Lactobacilli, streptococci, diphtheroids, Gardnerella, Mycoplasma, and coagulase negative staphylococci are common contaminants.
- Symptomatic patients need to be treated before the results of urine cultures are available. A presumptive diagnosis may be made by microscopic examination of the urine or dip-stick tests for pyuria and nitrite.
- A positive nitrite test is virtually diagnostic of infection.
- Most symptomatic patients will have bacterial counts well in excess of $\geq10^5$ cfu/ml of uropathogens.
- Lower counts of uropathogens are acceptable in females with the pyuria-dysuria syndrome, acute cystitis, and pyelonephritis.
- Lower counts of uropathogens are acceptable with urethral catheterization or suprapubic aspiration.
- Lower counts of uropathogens are considered to be significant in males because contamination is rare.
- Strict criteria ($\geq10^5$ cfu/ml of uropathogens) are required for the diagnosis of asymptomatic bacteriuria to avoid unnecessary treatment.
- Strict criteria ($\geq10^5$ cfu/ml of uropathogens) are required for clinical trials to avoid over-diagnosis and allow an end-point for cure.
- Mycobacteria and systemic fungi do not grow well in urine. Any number of these microorganisms are considered to be significant.

Pyuria

Pyuria is defined as the presence of an abnormal number of inflammatory cells in the urine. Urine normally contains a small number of leukocytes

($< 10/mm^3$ or $< 5/hpf$). Larger numbers indicate that inflammation is present somewhere in the urinary tract or adjacent structures, or that the urine is contaminated with vaginal or preputial secretions. Polymorphonuclear leukocytes are the hallmark of acute inflammation and are the predominant cell type in urinary tract infections. Other inflammatory conditions need to be considered when monocytes, lymphocytes eosinophiles, or basophiles are present.

Clinical Significance of Pyuria

Pyuria needs to be interpreted in relation to all other clinical and laboratory information. *Pyuria should not be automatically equated with urinary tract infections.* Other important causes of pyuria are listed in Table 2.3. The differential diagnosis is broad. Some textbooks list fever, pregnancy, and adrenocortical steroids as nonspecific causes of pyuria, but these notions need to be confirmed. A Wright or Giemsa, and sometimes a Papanicolaou stain, may detect unusual causes of pyuria. Mononuclear cells and eosinophiles suggest interstitial nephritis or eosinophilic cystitis. Polymorphonuclear leukocytes

Table 2.3. Conditions That May be Associated With Sterile Pyuria

Contamination During Collection
    Vaginal secretions (often associated with Lactobacilli)
    Prepuce (foreskin) secretions
Noninfectious Diseases
    Tubulointerstitial nephritis (analgesic nephropathy, β lactam antibiotics)
    Stones and foreign bodies
    Cyclophosphamide therapy
    Renal transplant rejection
    Genitourinary trauma
    Renal or bladder tumors
    Glomerulonephritis
Infectious Diseases
    Chlamydial and Gonococcal urethritis
    Tuberculosis and other mycobacterial infections
    Systemic fungal infections
    Viral cystitis (herpes, adenoviruses, varicella-zoster)
    Leptospirosis, *Hemophilus influenzae*
    Bilharzia (may see eggs)
Infections Adjacent To The Urinary Tract
    Appendicitis
    Diverticulitis
    Prostatitis
Urinary Tract Infections
    Partially treated infection. Pyuria may persist for up to a week following successful treatment of a urinary tract infection.

mixed with epithelial cells and gram positive rods (Lactobacilli) suggest vaginal contamination. The Papanicolaou stain may show neoplastic cells from kidney or bladder tumors.

Illustrative Cases of Sterile Pyuria Unrelated to Urinary Tract Infections

1. A 68-year-old woman came to an emergency department complaining of pain in the right knee. She was afebrile. Her knee was slightly swollen and tender without erythema. The joint fluid contained polymorphonuclear leukocytes, but no bacteria or urate crystals were seen. Urinalysis revealed > 100 WBCs/hpf and a few bacteria. She was thought to have a metastatic infection to the right knee from a urinary tract infection and was treated with a nonsteroidal anti-inflammatory drug and a fluoroquinolone. Cultures of the knee, urine, and blood were sterile. She did not disclose to the emergency room physicians that she had been taking several anti-inflammatory drugs for her knee and that it had been injected with a corticosteroid a few days earlier. Several days later she developed nausea, vomiting, and prostration. She was found to have acute renal failure with a serum creatinine of 5.5. The urine still contained > 100 WBCs/hpf, but the culture was sterile. A renal ultrasound showed no evidence of obstruction. She died a few days later because of an adverse event in the hospital. At autopsy, she was found to have extensive tubulo-interstitial nephritis with extensive infiltration by mononuclear cells. The bladder, ureters, and renal pelvis showed no evidence of inflammation, ruling out ascending pyelonephritis. In retrospect, the pyuria was caused by analgesic nephropathy and the joint pain by long-standing osteoarthritis. Had the cells in the urine been examined more carefully, they would have been found to be mononuclear. This finding might have led to the diagnosis of analgesic nephropathy rather than urinary tract infection.

2. A previously healthy, 20-year-old man was referred because of recurrent urinary tract infections. Six months before admission, he developed "high" fever, left lower quadrant pain, and dysuria. The urine culture was sterile. An intravenous urogram and cystoscopy were normal. He was treated with a combination of intravenous cephalosporin and aminoglycoside antibiotics, became afebrile, and the symptoms disappeared. Three months before admission, the dysuria recurred and he responded to treatment with norfloxacin. Three days before admission, he again developed fever and generalized abdominal pain and was found to have sterile pyuria. Rectal examination revealed tenderness on the right side. A ruptured appendix was found on CT scan of the abdomen. He did well after surgery. This is a classic case of irritation of the bladder by acute appendicitis. The appendicitis was temporarily masked by antimicrobial until it ruptured. The key point of this case is that the presence of sterile pyuria

in a patient with abdominal pain can be caused by diverticulitis or appendicitis.

Measurement of Pyuria

A variety of microscopic and chemical methods are available to detect the presence of pyuria. Many of the same factors that affect the bacterial count will influence the number of cells present in urine (Table 2.2). Pyuria is easy to recognize even without staining (Figures 2.3 and 2.4). Numerous pus cells (> 10–100/hpf) and bacteria generally will be seen on microscopic examination. The leukocyte esterase test is almost always positive. The major source of error is vaginal contamination in adult females. This contamination can be recognized on gram stain by the presence of epithelial cells with adherent gram positive rods (Lactobacilli). Microscopic methods are discussed in greater detail in the next chapter.

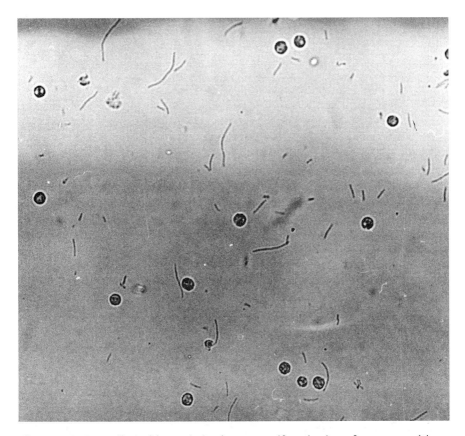

Figure 2.3. Pus cells and bacteria in the uncentrifuged urine of a woman with acute cystitis in a wet mount preparation magnified 100×.

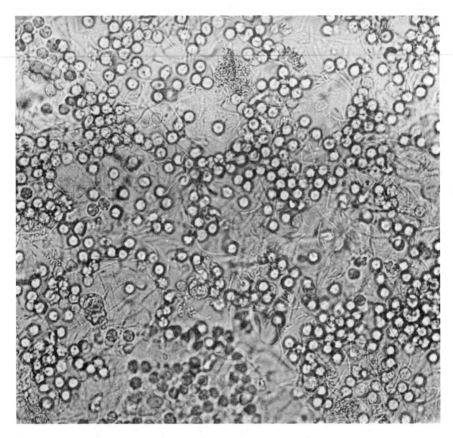

Figure 2.4. Pus cells and bacteria in the centrifuged urine of the same specimen shown in Figure 2.3 with the same magnification.

The Counting Chamber Method

The hemocytometer chamber count is the "gold standard" to measure pyuria (15,16). Dukes used this method in his pioneering studies of the indwelling catheter as the cause of postoperative fever in patients undergoing colorectal surgery (17). A drop of Kova stain added to the urine makes it easier to visualize cellular elements (Kova Stain, ICL Scientific Euclid, California). Chamber counts are not needed when innumerable cells or none at all are seen in the sediment. The lower limit of normal is generally ≥ 10 WBC/mm^3. I prefer a threshold of ≥ 20 WBC/mm^3 in young adult women to avoid false positives caused by vaginal contamination (18). Pyuria of ≥ 20 WBC/mm^3 was present in almost 20% of asymptomatic college women and those with vaginal symptoms (Figure 2.5). Pyuria in the asymptomatic women was associated closely with vaginal leukorrhea. The magnitude of

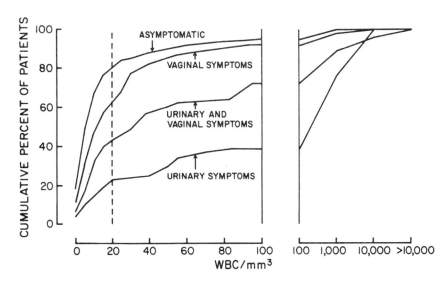

Figure 2.5. Relation between the presence or absence of urinary and vaginal symptoms and the leukocyte count in the urine of 639 female university students. Reproduced with permission from Kunin, White and Tong (18).

pyuria was well in excess of 20 WBC/mm³ in most women with urinary symptoms. We also found a direct relationship between the bacterial and WBC counts in the urine (Fig. 2.6).

Microscopic Examination of the Sediment of Centrifuged Urine

This procedure is commonly used to evaluate patients for urinary tract infections. Even though it lacks precision, it provides immediate and useful information about bacteriuria as well as pyuria. The reproducibility of this method varies with volume of urine examined, the force and duration of centrifugation, the volume in which the cells are resuspended, the size of the high-powered field examined, and observer error. These variables are difficult to control. There may be as much as a tenfold variation in the cell count by varying resuspension volume (19). In addition, the survival of leukocytes in urine is decreased by high pH, low osmolality, and elevated temperature (20). The criterion for pyuria is > 5 leukocytes/hpf (400 ×).

Microscopic Examination of the Uncentrifuged Urine

This method may be used when a hemocytometer is not available. The finding of 1 WBC/low-powered microscopic field (100 ×) indicates the presence of 3 WBC/mm³ (21). "Infected" urine will usually contain 30 WBCs per low powered field, or 1 to 2 WBCs/hpf (400 ×).

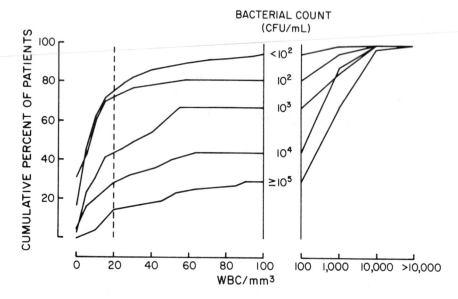

Figure 2.6. Relation between the bacterial and leukocyte counts in urine of 639 female university students. Reproduced with permission from Kunin, White and Tong (18).

Volumetric Measurement of White Blood Cell Excretion

An excretion rate of 400,000 or more leukocytes/hour has been shown to correlate well with the presence of urinary tract infection. This rate corresponds to about ≥ 10 WBC/mm^3 (22).

Cell Morphology

The morphology or staining characteristics of polymorphonuclear leukocytes in urine are not helpful. "Glitter cells" are leukocytes with highly motile granules that give a sparkling appearance. This effect depends on the tonicity of the urine and will vary considerably depending on the time of day the urine is collected and on fluid intake. Lightly staining cells described by Sternheimer and Malbin (23) are nonspecific.

Provocative Tests

Tests to "unmask" the presence of pyelonephritis in patients in whom there is minimal pyuria or other signs of infection have been described (24, 25). An intravenous injection of prednisolone or bacterial pyrogen is given and quantitative rates of excretion of WBCs are determined. These tests should be reserved for research purposes and must be undertaken with considerable caution. Injection of bacterial pyrogens can lead to severe reactions. Urinary tract infections may be exacerbated by prednisolone.

The Dip-Stick Leukocyte-Esterase Test (LE Test)

Neutrophils contain several esterases that are not present in serum, urine, or kidney tissues. They are unrelated to lysosomal or other enzymes released by injured tissue or to muramidase. The molecular weights of the esterases range from 30,000 to 70,000 daltons. The leukocyte esterase test provides a rapid and reliable method to detect pyuria. The test consists of a filter-paper pad containing indoxyl carboxylic acid ester. Leukocyte esterase(s) converts this substrate into an indoxyl moiety. This is then oxidized in room air to form insoluble indigo (Figure 2.7). The test is considered to be positive if the paper turns any degree of blue a minute after being dipped in urine.

The LE test compares well to the chamber count method. Using a cut-off of ≥ 10 WBC/mm^3, the sensitivity is about 90% and the specificity is about 95% (26–28). The test is not influenced by most drugs, proteinuria, and pH of the urine. One advantage of the test is that lysed cells give a positive reaction. The test may not be interpretable when the strips are discolored by blood, rifampin (which stains orange), or by bilirubin or nitrofurantoin (which stain yellow). Ascorbic acid may inhibit the oxidation of indoxyl. The leukocyte esterase test is very useful for screening patients for pyuria. It is particularly helpful when negative because a negative test virtually rules out the presence of infection.

Some investigators have needlessly criticized the LE test because of its purportedly poor sensitivity or specificity to detect urinary tract infections in unselected patients (29). These criticisms are unfortunate because pyuria can be caused by a variety of unrelated conditions (30) (Table 2.3). Bacteriuria is the major hallmark of urinary tract infection, not pyuria.

The leukocyte esterase test can also be used to detect peritonitis in patients on chronic ambulatory peritoneal dialysis (31) and in patients with meningitis. It cannot be applied to examination of purulent sputum because saliva gives a rapidly positive test.

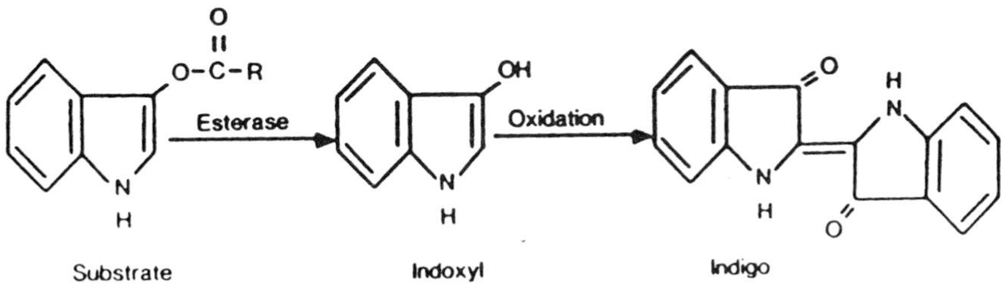

Figure 2.7. The chemical basis of the action of leukocyte esterase on the substrate in the dip-stick to produce blue indigo in ambient air.

Cytokineuria

Cytokines are well-known mediators of inflammation. Elevated levels of interleukin-6 (IL-6), IL-2, IL-2 inhibitor, and IL-8 have been observed in the urine of patients with urinary tract infections (32–34). IL-8 is of particular interest because it is a potent chemoattractant and activator of neutrophils. It is produced by a variety of cells, including monocytes, endothelial cells, and mesangial cells upon stimulation by endotoxin, IL-1, and tumor necrosis factor alpha. In one study (34), elevated urinary levels of IL-8 were found in virtually all patients with urinary tract infections irrespective of whether the invading microorganism contained endotoxin. IL-8 cytokineuria correlated well with the number of leukocytes in the urine. IL-8 appears to be produced in the urinary tract because higher levels are found in the urine than in the blood. Measurement of IL-8 in the urine may prove to be a useful tool to differentiate infection from colonization. It does not help localize the site infection to the upper or lower tract.

Proteinuria

Small amounts of albumin are normally present in urine. The upper limits of normal are about 100 to 150 mg per 24 hours. Larger amounts, usually in excess of 300 mg per 24 hours, do not necessarily indicate the presence of renal disease, but they may occur as a physiologic response to prolonged standing or exercise. Orthostatic proteinuria is characterized by its intermittent nature and increased excretion of protein after recumbency and standing in the lordotic position. The condition has been found benign in several long-term follow-up studies (35).

Proteins may originate from the blood (albumin, transport proteins, lysozyme, and immunoglobulins) or be released during injury from renal tubular cells (Tamm-Horsfall protein, lysosomal enzymes, and alkaline phosphatase). "Selective" proteinuria is characterized by the presence of albumin as the predominant protein in the urine. In "nonselective" proteinuria, albumin is accompanied by larger proteins, such as complement, globulins, and lipoproteins. "Selective" proteinuria tends to occur in people with orthostatic proteinuria, with mild to moderate forms of renal disease, and during the early phase of diabetic nephropathy. "Nonselective" proteinuria is seen more often in people with severe renal disease and in irreversible forms of the nephrotic syndrome.

Proteinuria is not ordinarily found in patients with urinary tract infections and is not associated with asymptomatic bacteriuria (9). It is often present during the end-stages of chronic pyelonephritis and with reflux nephropathy. Massive excretion of protein may be seen in patients with reflux nephropathy.

Hematuria

Gross or microscopic hematuria is relatively common in patients with acute urinary tract infections. If the hematuria persists, another etiology should be sought. Other causes of hematuria include urinary calculi, tumors, trauma, bleeding disorders, polycystic kidney disease, bilharzia and radiation, cyclophosphamide, and viral cystitis.

Key Points About Pyuria, Proteinuria, and Hematuria

- Pyuria and hematuria commonly occur in association with urinary tract infections.
- The hallmark of urinary tract infections is significant bacteriuria, not pyuria.
- Look for another cause if the urine is sterile.
- The leukocyte esterase test correlates well with microscopic examination of the urine, but is more sensitive because it will detect lysed cells.
- The chamber count is the "gold standard" for pyuria, but it need not be done if many or no WBCs are seen on microscopic examination.
- We prefer a cut off of ≥ 20 WBC/mm^3 rather than the more standard ≥ 10 WBC/mm^3 in adult females because of potential contamination by vaginal secretions.
- Most patients with urinary tract infections will have counts of >20 WBC/mm^3.
- There is a direct relationship between the magnitude of pyuria and the bacterial count in patients with urinary tract infection.
- Pyuria and microscopic hematuria may persist for up to a week after eradication of infection.
- Proteinuria is not a sign of urinary tract infection.

Pneumaturia

Pneumaturia is a rare condition in which gas is present in the bladder urine. The patient will report flatus-like sound during urination. The urine may be frothy. Radiologic examination may reveal collections of gas within the bladder or bladder wall (emphysematous cystitis). The differential diagnosis includes vesico-vaginal and vesico-enteric fistulae, gas derived from the fermentation of glucose in diabetics, and emphysematous cystitis. The patient's history and gram stain of the urine are very helpful in differentiating among these possibilities. Vesico-vaginal fistulas are usually complications of gynecologic surgery; vesicoenteric fistulas may be seen in patients with regional ileitis, diverticulitis, and after abdominal surgery. The gram stain of the urine is very helpful. Mixed flora suggests the presence of a vesico-enteric fistula. Thin gram positive rods suggest Lactobacilli from a vesico-vaginal fistula; thick, club-shaped gram positive bacteria suggest Clostridia. In patients suspected of fistulae, the site can be determined by instillation of contrast material into the bladder, bowel, or vagina.

Pneumaturia in diabetic patients is usually caused by enteric bacteria and yeasts. Less common microorganisms include staphylococci, streptococci, and Nocardia (36–38). The gas consists of hydrogen, carbon dioxide, and nitrogen produced by fermentation of glucose. It will disappear after appropriate antimicrobial therapy.

References

1. Marple CD. The frequency and character of urinary tract infections in an unselected group of women. Ann Intern Med 1941;14:2220–2239.
2. Kass EH. Asymptomatic infections of the urinary tract. Trans Assoc Am Physicians 1956;69:56–63.
3. Boshell BR, Sanford JP. A screening method for the evaluation of urinary tract infection in female patients without catheterization. Ann Intern Med 1958;48:1040–1045.
4. Asscher AW. The challenge of urinary tract infections. New York: Grune and Stratton,1980.
5. Platt R. Quantitative definition of bacteriuria. Am J Med 1983;75:44–52.
6. Stamey TA, Timothy M, Miller M, et al. Recurrent urinary infections in adult women. Calif Med 1971;115:1–19.
7. Stamey TA, Mihara G. Observations on the growth of urethral and vaginal bacteria in sterile urine. J Urol 1980;124:461–463.
8. Stark R, Maki D. Bacteriuria in the catheterized patient. What quantitative level of bacteriuria is relevant? N Engl J Med 1984;311:560–564.
9. Kunin CM, Deutscher R, Paquin AJ. Urinary tract infection in school children: epidemiologic, clinical, and laboratory study. Medicine (Baltimore) 1964;43:91–130.
10. Beccia D, Crowley M, Gleckman R. Lessons learned from a patient. Changing concepts rather than facts. JAMA 1976;236:1268.
11. Strand CL, Bryant JK, Sutton KH. Septicemia secondary to urinary tract infection with colony counts less than 50,000 cfu/ml. Am J Clin Pathol 1985;83:619–622.
12. Rubin RH, Shapiro ED, Andriole VT, et al. Evaluation of new anti-infective drugs for the treatment of urinary tract infections. Clin Infect Dis 1992;15(suppl 1):S216-S227.
13. Kunin CM. Guidelines for the evaluation of new anti-infective drugs for the treatment of urinary tract infections. Clin Infect Dis 1992;15:1041–1044.
14. Washington JA. Bacterial cultures for cystitis. Ann Intern Med 1990;112:387–388.
15. Addis T. The number of formed elements in the urinary sediment of normal individuals. J Clin Invest 1926;2:409–415.
16. Block EB, Nyun K. The importance of counting pus cells in the urine. South Med J 1916;9:972–973.
17. Dukes C. Urinary infections after excision of the rectum: their cause and prevention. Proc Royal Soc Med 1928;22:1–11.
18. Kunin CM, White LVA, Tong HH. A reassessment of the importance of "low-count" bacteriuria in young women with acute urinary symptoms. Ann Intern Med 1993;119: 454–460.
19. Gadeholt H. Quantitative estimation of urinary sediment, with special regard to sources of error. Br Med J 1964;1:1547–1549.
20. Trigger DR, Smith JWG. Survival of urinary leukocytes. J Clin Pathol 1966;19:443–447.
21. Musher DM, Thorsteinsson SB, Airola VM. Quantitative urinalysis. Diagnosing urinary tract infection in men. JAMA 1976;236:2069–2072.
22. Little PJ. A comparison of the urinary white cell concentration with the white cell excretion rate. Br J Urol 1964;36:360–363.
23. Sternheimer R, Malbin B. Clinical recognition of pyelonephritis with a new stain for urinary sediment. Am J Med 1951;11:312–323.
24. Little PJ, DeWardener HE. The use of prednisolone phosphate in the diagnosis of pyelonephritis in man. Lancet 1962;1:1145–1149.
25. Katz YJ, Bourdo SR, Moore RS. Effect of pyrogen and adrenal steroids in pyelonephritis. Lancet 1962;2:1140–1144.

26. Kusumi RK, Grover PJ, Kunin CM. Rapid detection of pyuria by leukocyte esterase activity. JAMA 1981;245:1653.
27. Gillenwater JY. Detection of urinary leukocytes by chemstrip-l. J Urol 1981;125:383–384.
28. Bailey RR, Blake E. A simple test for detecting pyuria. N Z Med J 1981,682:269–270.
29. Lachs MS, Nachamkin I, Edelstein PH, et al. Spectrum bias in the evaluation of diagnostic tests: lessons from the rapid dipstick test for urinary tract infection. Ann Intern Med 1992;117:135–140.
30. White LV, Kunin CM. Leukocyte esterase tests detect pyuria, not bacteriuria. Ann Intern Med 1993;118:230.
31. Chan LK, Oliver DO. Simple method for early detection of peritonitis in patients on continuous ambulatory peritoneal dialysis. Lancet 1979;2:1336–1337.
32. Ohta K, Takano N, Seno A, et al. Detection and clinical usefulness of urinary interleukin-6 in the diseases of the kidney and the urinary tract. Clin Nephrol 1992;38:185–189.
33. Hedges S, Anderson P, Lidin-Janson G, et al. Interleukin-6 response to deliberate colonization of the human urinary tract with gram-negative bacteria. Infect Immun 1991;59:421–427.
34. Ko YC, Mukaida N, Ishiyama S, et al. Elevated interleukin-8 levels in the urine of patients with urinary tract infections. Infect Immun 1993;61:1307–1314.
35. Glassock RJ. Postural (orthostatic) Proteinuria: no cause for concern. N Engl J Med 1981;305:639–641.
36. Lyon DC. Primary pneumaturia. Br J Surg 1969;56:315–316.
37. Spring M, Hymes JJ. Pneumaturia: report of a case in a diabetic with review of the literature. Diabetes 1952;1:378–382.
38. Synhaivsky A, Malek RS. Isolated pneumaturia. Am J Med 1985;78:617–620.

3

Diagnostic Methods

Overview

This chapter deals with the practical aspects of methods to collect urine, perform cultures and microscopic examinations, interpret antimicrobial susceptibility tests, localize infection, and evaluate renal function. It is assumed that the reader is familiar with the concepts of significant bacteriuria and pyuria, uropathogens, and the clinical syndromes of urinary tract infections presented in previous chapters. The laboratory diagnosis of urinary tract infections is quite straight forward. Urine is readily available, chemical reagent strips provide rapid information about the pH, presence of leukocytes, nitrite, protein, and red blood cells, and microscopic examination usually reveals the invading microorganism. Quantitative cultures and susceptibility tests provide useful information. Uncomplicated infections ordinarily can be differentiated from complicated infections on clinical grounds. Special tests to localize infection to the upper or lower tract are rarely necessary. Chronic prostatitis can be distinguished from prostadynia by differential cultures of urine and expressed prostatic secretions. The most common defect in renal function is transient decrease in the ability to concentrate urine. Renal failure is rare in acute pyelonephritis but, when present, should alert the clinician to consider underlying obstruction, reflux nephropathy, or other causes of renal disease.

Collection of Urine

The objective is to collect a specimen that resembles bladder urine as closely as possible. Reliable urine specimens usually can be obtained for culture of voided urine. Urethral catheterization should be avoided whenever possible, but may be needed for patients who cannot void spontaneously, are immobilized, too ill, or too obese to provide a clean sample. Suprapubic bladder puncture (SPA) is particularly helpful in newborns and infants.

Voided urine is rarely sterile even in the absence of infection. Urine from men may contain small numbers of commensal gram positive bacteria that colonize the fossa navicularis (coagulase-negative staphylococci, streptococci, and diphtheroids). Urine obtained from females is often contaminated with vaginal fluid and periurethral microorganisms. Lactobacilli adherent to vaginal epithelial cells are commonly seen on gram stain of the urinary sediment in females. The periurethral zone of some women, particularly those prone to recurrent infections, may be colonized with small numbers of gram negative uropathogens. The quantitative bacterial count helps to distinguish colonization from infection by ignoring the small numbers of commensal microorganisms and determining the number of uropathogens present in the urine.

Timing of Collections

Bacterial counts will be highest in the first voided morning urine after overnight incubation in the bladder. First void specimens also increase the sensitivity of the nitrite test and are optimal for self-screening. In practice, the best time to collect a urine specimen is when the patient is able to provide an adequate sample. It may be necessary at times to force fluids to help the patient void. Large volumes of water can dilute the urine and reduce the colony count. If forcing fluids is necessary, this should be noted in the record to aid interpretation of the bacterial count.

Transport

Enteric bacteria grow well in urine kept at room temperature and can reach high densities within several hours. Prolonged storage of urine at room temperature also promotes lysis of casts and cells. Urine specimens should be delivered to the laboratory without delay and should be cultured within 1 hour after voiding or be refrigerated. Several additives are available that preserve bacteria for up to several days without refrigeration. These include boric acid, sodium chloride-polyvinyl pyrrolidone, or a mixture of boric acid-glycerol-sodium formate. Commercial transport media available include the Vacutainer® Urine Collection Kit (Becton, Dickinson Microbiology Systems, Cockeysville, MD), and the Sterile Midstream Urine Systems Tube (Sage Products, Inc. Cary, IL), Boricon® (Medical Wire and Equipment). The Flora-Stat Urine Transport System (Wadley Biosciences Corp./Lymphokine Partners Ltd., Dallas, TX) contains a proprietary mixture that deactivates antibiotics and stabilizes the microbial count. These systems add to the cost of urine cultures and should not be needed in a well-run clinic or hospital.

Collection for Culture

It is generally recommended that urine for culture be obtained by a clean-voided, mid-stream specimen in females and a midstream specimen from males. The value of these procedures has been questioned by many investigators, for good reasons (1–3). Adequate specimens can be obtained from uncircumcised boys and most men without special precautions (4,5). It seems reasonable to instruct uncircumcised males to retract the foreskin and rinse the glans and try to collect a mid-stream specimen, but this is not essential. Cleansing of the vulva is not necessary in prepubertal girls (6). They should be instructed to straddle the toilet seat backwards, spread the labia away from the urethral meatus, and void into a clean container. Methods to obtain urine from infants using strap-on devices and suprapubic aspiration are discussed in Chapter 4. It is not necessary to collect urine in a sterile container as long as it is "dish washer" clean.

The major problem is in collecting clean specimens from adult women. Urine is readily contaminated as it flows over the vagina, around the labia, and through pubic hair. Small numbers of enteric bacteria can be caught in the urine flow, and the urine can be contaminated with small amounts of vaginal fluid. It may be particularly difficult to obtain a valid clean-voided urine from women in busy clinical settings. The patient is usually given a commercial kit and told to collect a midstream specimen. The toilets are often too small to move about, commercial kits are often hard to open, the small cotton swabs are useless, and the plastic holders and lids can be difficult to manage. It is too much to expect women to start and stop their urinary stream under such conditions. Cleansing should be done with nonmedicated soap. The soap in the kits may contain chlorhexidine, which can lower the bacterial count or povidone iodine and therefore give a false-positive test for occult blood (7). The following instructions should make it less difficult for the patient to provide an adequate specimen of urine.

Instructions to Obtain a Clean-Catch Urine From an Ambulatory Woman

The patient should be provided with clear and detailed instructions. She should be asked whether she needs fluids to stimulate voiding and be allowed to drink fully before proceeding further. It is essential that she have privacy and not be hurried. She should be provided with a culture kit that will enable her to carefully wash and dry the periurethral area and wide-mouth cup in which to void. A dilute solution of soap is all that is needed for cleansing, and an adequate number of clean cotton sponges should be available. If a commercial culture kit is used, it should be pretested by the nursing staff to be sure that it can adequately cleanse the periurethral area in a sanitary and esthetic manner. An alternative approach is to provide a paper plate or a closed plastic food container with the necessary supplies (Fig. 3.1). Each kit should contain at least four large cotton sponges dampened with liquid soap and four

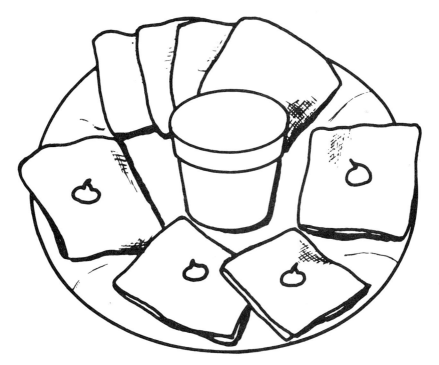

Figure 3.1. Paper plate with sterile collection cup and 4 × 4 cotton sponges used for obtaining clean-voided urine from females. The sponges are moistened with plain tap water; four of them have soap solution added. A closed plastic food container can be used for the same purpose.

sponges dampened with warm tap water. Additional dry sponges should be available in the toilet in a clean container. The kit should contain a sterile urine cup with an easily detachable cap. The patient should be cautioned not to place her fingers into the cup.

Instructions to the Adult Female Patient to Collect a Clean-voided Specimen

1. Remove your underpants completely so they will not get soiled.
2. Sit comfortably on the seat. Swing one knee to the side as far as you can.
3. Spread your genitals with one hand, and continue to hold yourself spread while you clean and collect the specimen.
4. Before you collect the urine sample, wash between the folds of your genitals around the area from which you pass urine. Begin with the soaped pads and then remove excess soap with the moistened pads. Pat yourself dry with clean pads. Wash slowly, but not hard.
5. Put the sponges back in the kit. Do not put them in the toilet.
6. Hold the cup by the outside and pass your urine into the cup.
7. PLEASE ASK QUESTIONS IF YOU ARE IN DOUBT ABOUT ANY STEP IN THE PROCEDURE.

Collection at Home

It is not uncommon for a patient to call her physician reporting a sudden onset of frequent, painful urination and suprapubic pressure. She will ask to be treated immediately and have a prescription called into her local pharmacy. This situation can be dealt with by either asking the patient to come to the office as soon as possible, or by instructing her to collect a urine specimen at home before taking a drug prescribed by telephone (if indicated). She should be told to clean her labia and periurethral area with a soaped wash cloth, rinse the wash cloth with tap water, dry herself with a clean cloth and void, as previously instructed, into a clean, but not necessarily sterile, jar that has a screw-top lid. The specimen should be placed in a small bag and refrigerated until she can bring it to the office for analysis. Patients who are known to have recurrent infections may be given a small supply of a suitable antimicrobial drug to be taken as soon as new symptoms develop. It may be helpful to provide the concerned patient with a packet of reagent strips to test her urine for pyuria, hematuria, and nitrite and call in the results.

Urethral Catheterization

Urethral catheterization is not recommended as a routine method for collecting urine because of the risk of producing infection. Care needs to be taken to avoid introducing microorganisms. The following aseptic procedure is recommended.

Tools for Urethral Catheterization

Sterile Tray Containing

Waterproof pad	Forceps (optional)
Fenestrated drape	Urethral catheter
Gloves	Lubricant
Sponges (5 to 8)	Specimen cup with cap
Antiseptic solution	Collecting basin for urine
Label	Laboratory slip

If Indwelling Catheter is to be Used

Foley catheter	10-ml syringe of sterile water
Drainage bag and tubing	

Procedure for Urethral Catheterization

Important Steps	Key Points
Place patient in supine position with legs spread apart.	
Drape patient with draw sheet.	
Wash hands.	
Open tray.	Use antiseptic technique.
Expose perineal area.	
Place waterproof pad under buttocks.	Touch only the corners.
Don gloves.	
Place fenestrated drape in such a fashion that the metal region is visible.	
Saturate sponges with antiseptic solution.	
Open lubricant and place in accessible area.	
FEMALES	
Separate labia with thumb and index finger.	Do not use this hand on sterile tray.
Continue to separate labia until catheter is inserted.	
Cleanse the labia with sponges.	Use a clean sponge with each stroke.
Cleanse the meatus.	
MALES	
Hold the penis with one hand, cleanse glans with the other. Retract the foreskin if necessary.	
CATHETER	
Lubricate about 4 inches from the tip to shaft.	
Place distal end of the catheter in receptacle to collect urine.	
Insert catheter into meatus.	Insert catheter until urine flows.
Never force the catheter.	Insert about 3 inches in the female and 6 inches in males.

Catch some urine in specimen cup.
Collect remaining urine in basin.
Do not contaminate distal end of catheter.
Send labeled specimen to laboratory with slip.

Insertion of an Indwelling Catheter

Insert catheter 1 inch beyond the balloon.	This will provide adequate room for inflation.
Inflate the balloon with amount designated on the catheter.	
Connect the catheter to the drainage bag.	
Tape the catheter to inner aspect of the thigh.	Allow some slack to guard against trauma to urethra.
Velcro anchoring devices are helpful.	
Position the drainage bag to avoid kinks.	Place at foot of bed.
Dry patient and make comfortable.	

Notes on Urethral Catheterization
- If the catheter enters the vagina by mistake during insertion, leave it in place as a guide and insert a fresh, sterile catheter into the urethra. Then remove the catheter from the vagina and discard it.
- If the catheter is to be left in place for many days in the male, the proximal end should be taped to the abdomen and not to the leg to prevent necrosis or ischemia at the penile scrotal junction.
- It is generally advised to not remove more than 1000 ml of urine at a time to guard against rapid decompression of the bladder and hemorrhage. This is a rare complication and is usually not a problem.

Suprapubic Needle Aspiration

Suprapubic aspiration of urine from the bladder (SPA) is considered to be the "gold standard" for obtaining urine for culture. The procedure avoids urethral contaminants. With good antiseptic technique, there should not be any skin contaminants. The method is particularly useful in small children when it is difficult to obtain an adequate specimen. The patient must have a full bladder before aspiration is attempted. The bacterial count may be lower than with voided specimens because hydration dilutes the urine. Any number of bacteria found in the SPA is considered to be significant, but the counts will usually be $\geq 10^3$ cfu/ml. In most series (5, 8–11), about half to two-thirds of specimens obtained by SPA will contain $\geq 10^5$ cfu/ml. The major complication of SPA is a hematoma at the site of aspiration (12). Fortunately, this complication is rare.

Procedure

Before a suprapubic needle aspiration is done, the patient should force fluids until the bladder is full. The site of the needle puncture is the midline between the symphysis pubis and the umbilicus and directly over the palpable bladder. The full bladder in the male is usually palpable because of its greater muscle tone. A full bladder may not be felt in females. Infants should have a dry diaper to be certain that they have not voided recently. The operator should determine that suprapubic pressure directly over the bladder produces an unmistakable urge to urinate. After determining the approximate site for needle puncture, the local area may be shaved and the skin cleansed with an alcohol sponge (Fig. 3.2). A cutaneous wheal is raised with a 25-gauge needle containing a local anesthetic. A 3.5 inch, 20-gauge needle is introduced through the anesthetized skin; the progress of the needle is arrested just below the skin within the anesthetized area. Then, with a quick plunging action, similar to giving an intramuscular injection, the needle is advanced into the bladder. Most patients experience more discomfort from the initial anesthetization of the skin than when the needle is advanced into the bladder. After the needle has been introduced, a 20-ml syringe is used to aspirate about 5 ml of urine for culture and 15 ml of urine for centrifugation and urinalysis. The obturator is reintroduced into the needle, and the instrument is withdrawn. A small strip-dressing is placed over the needle site in the skin. If urine is not

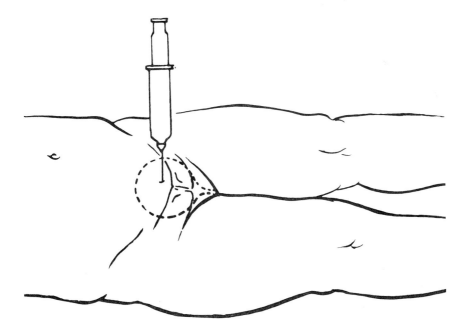

Figure 3.2. Site of insertion of the needle when obtaining urine from a small child by suprapubic aspiration. Reproduced with permission from Nelson and Peters (9).

obtained with complete introduction of the needle, the patient's bladder is not full or may be located deep within the retropubic area.

Tools for Suprapubic Needle Aspiration

Antiseptic solution	Culture tubes
Sterile 4 × 4 sponges	Unopened bottle of local anesthetic
0.5 inch, 25 gauge needle and syringe	3.5 inch, 20 gauge needle and 20 ml syringe
Laboratory slip	Label
Sterile rubber gloves	Strip-bandage

Performance of a Suprapubic Aspiration

Important Steps	Key Points
Provide privacy for the patient.	
Place the patient on a flat surface in the supine position.	
Cleanse the area above the pubic symphysis with an antiseptic solution.	
Let the solution dry.	
Locate the symphysis pubis with one finger.	
Insert the needle 2 cm above the symphysis in the midline.	
Aspirate urine through needle.	
	Hold the syringe at a 10° angle toward the bladder.
	Insert the needle until a perceptible resistance is felt.
	Rotate the needle if bevel abuts the bladder wall.
Remove the needle.	
Swab the area with antiseptic solution.	
Apply a strip-bandage.	
Squirt the urine into the culture tube.	
Label specimen and send to laboratory with a slip.	

Notes on Suprapubic Aspiration
- Be certain that the diaper is dry when attempting to perform the procedure on an infant.
- Do not apply excessive pressure. This may draw the bladder mucosa against the bevel of the needle and obstruct flow.
- The procedure should be done rapidly before the patient is stimulated to void spontaneously.

Key Points About Collection on Urine Specimens for Culture

- The clean-voided urine is recommended for adult females. It does not have to be midstream.
- No special preparation is needed to collect specimens for prepubertal girls.
- No special preparation is ordinarily needed for males, but the foreskin should be retracted.
- Urethral catheterization and suprapubic aspiration may be needed in young children and adults who are suspected to have infection and cannot provide a clean-voided specimen.

General Examination of the Urine

Macroscopic examination is not reliable unless the urine is grossly bloody. A cloudy appearance is usually caused by crystals rather than bacteria or pus cells. Yellow-orange urate salts may appear in acid urine. Crystals of phosphates salts are common in alkaline urine. A foul odor is suggestive of infection but may be caused by vaginitis or consumption of foods such as asparagus. The specific gravity is not helpful. An alkaline pH over 8.0 is suggestive of a urease-producing microorganism such as Proteus or Providencia, but may also be caused by a vegetarian diet. Large populations of the world subsist on a virtually total vegetarian diet and tend to have an alkaline urine (Fig. 3.3). The

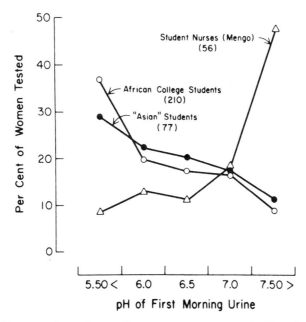

Figure 3.3. First morning urinary pH among young women in Uganda. African and "Asian" (East Indian origin) students ate a well-balanced diet containing abundant meat. Student nurses ate a typical Bugandan vegetarian diet. (Unpublished data by the author.)

hydrogen ion content of the urine is caused principally by sulfur-containing amino acids in animal proteins.

Urine Culture Methods

The standard methods for quantitative urine cultures are the pour plate and surface streak plate methods. All other methods are derivative and need to be validated by the standard methods.

Pour Plate Method

Urine is serially diluted in broth or buffer solution. A fresh pipette is used to add 0.1 ml of each dilution to a sterile Petri dish. Approximately 10 ml of molten agar (MacConkey or Trypticase Soy), maintained at 45°C in a water bath, is poured into the dish. The plate is gently swirled, the agar is allowed to harden, and the inverted plate is placed in a 37°C incubator and held for about 18 to 24 hours. The number of colonies on each plate are then counted. The final count in cfu/ml equals the number of colonies on the plate $\times$ 10 $\times$ the dilution factor. For example, one colony on a plate diluted to $1 \times 10^4 = 10^5$ cfu/ml.

It is not ordinarily necessary to perform serial tenfold dilutions because the counts provide overlapping information on serial plates. A simplified method may be used as follows:

- Add 0.1 ml of undiluted urine to a plate. Each colony represents 10 cfu/ml. *(This plate may be used to detect low count bacteriuria.)*
- Add 0.1 ml of undiluted urine to 9.9 ml of diluent. Vortex and then add 0.1 ml to a plate. Each colony represents 1000 cfu/ml. *(This plate is sufficient for most purposes.)*
- Add 0.1 ml of the above dilution to 9.9 ml of diluent. Vortex and then add 0.1 ml to a plate. Each colony represents 100,000 cfu/ml. *(This plate may be used to isolate single colonies from urine containing very large numbers of bacteria.)*

The entire procedure should take only a few minutes.

The Streak Plate Method

The streak plate method is much simpler to perform than the agar dilution method and provides reliable results. MacConkey (MAC) or eosin-methylene blue (EMB) are commonly used as selective media for gram negative enteric bacteria. Lactose fermentation is detected readily by the blue or red color of the colonies. Most strains of *E. coli* ferment lactose, whereas Klebsiella, Enterobacter, Proteus, and Pseudomonas do not. A second plate containing 5% sheep blood agar is used to culture gram positive bacteria, including staphylococci and enterococci. Some laboratories prefer to use cysteine-lactose-electrolyte-deficient agar (CLED) for urine cultures. CLED is a differential, nonselective medium. It allows the detection of lactose-fermenting gram negative enteric bacteria and inhibits the swarming of Proteus and other motile bacteria. Disposable plastic calibrated loops are used to deliver a fixed amount of urine to the plate. An 0.001 ml loop is dipped into the urine and streaked onto an agar plate. Some laboratories will streak down the middle of the plate and cross streak to isolate colonies. Others use a horizontal rotation device to apply the inoculum in a swirl-like pattern. A four quadrant streak method is shown in Figure 3.4. One colony on the plate is equivalent to 1,000 cfu/ml. It may be desirable at times to increase the sensitivity of the test by using a 0.01 ml loop. One colony is equivalent to 100 cfu/ml.

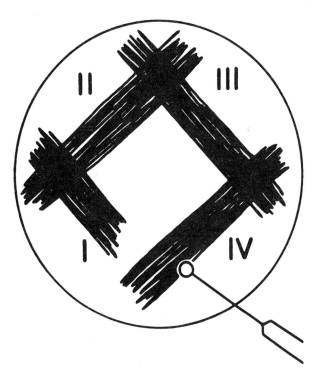

Figure 3.4. A method to streak urine on a culture plate. Redrawn from Hirsch and Blay (13).

Simple Culture Techniques

Several relatively simple and inexpensive methods have been developed for use in office practice and screening. They offer the advantage of providing results within 24 hours and avoid the large mark-ups of hospital and commercial laboratories. Some of these devices are no longer commercially available, but they may be resurrected in the future, and the principles are interesting.

Dip-Slide Method

This method is based on the principle that the amount of urine that adheres to agar is determined by surface tension (14). The technique uses a glass slide or a grid-marked plastic plate attached to the cap of a clear plastic storage tube. Different media are placed on each side. These may be combinations of nutrient and EMB agar or MAC and CLED agar. The slide is dipped briefly into the urine specimen (Fig. 3.5). It is then held vertically to drain excess urine, screwed back into the sterile container, and placed in an incubator or left at room temperature until brought to the laboratory. The bacterial count is determined by comparing the density of the colonies with a reference standard (Fig. 3.6). It may be difficult to isolate a single colony when there is confluent growth. These devices are particularly useful in office practice and for self-screening. Dip-slides and similar devices may be obtained, such as Uricult™ (Orion Laboratories, Helsinki, Finland, distributed by Medical Technology Corporation, Hackensack, NJ), the Oxoid dipslide (Flow Labora-

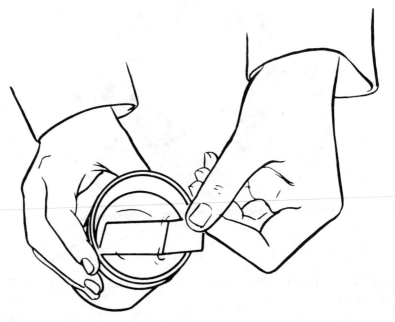

Figure 3.5. Using the dip-slide for culture.

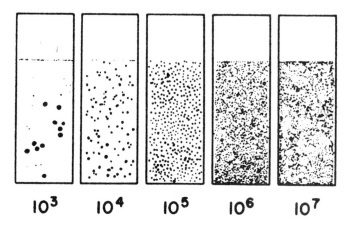

10^3 10^4 10^5 10^6 10^7

Figure 3.6. Interpretation of the dip-slide by colony density.

tories, Rockville, MD), Dipinoc™, (Stayne Diagnostics, East Rutherford, NJ), and Dip N Count™ (Starplex Scientific, Ontario, Canada).

The Tube and Cup Methods
These devices are based on the same principles as the dip-slide. They consist of either a tube internally coated with indicator culture medium, Bactur-cult™ (Wampole Laboratories, Cranbury, NJ), or media placed at the base of a flat cup. The urine is poured in and out of the device, leaving a thin film on the surface. The bacterial count is determined by comparing the density of the colonies with a reference standard (Figs. 3.7 and 3.8). These devices

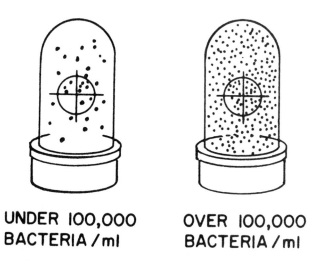

UNDER 100,000   OVER 100,000
BACTERIA / ml   BACTERIA / ml

Figure 3.7. The tube culture demonstrating the density of bacterial growth. Note that counting is recommended on a discrete area of the tube.

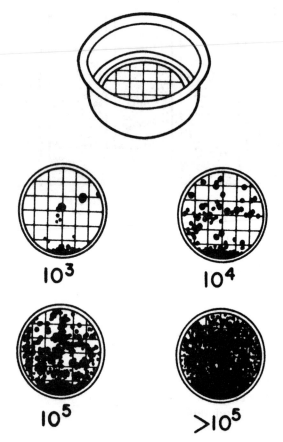

Figure 3.8. Illustration of the agar-cup quantitative culture method. Only one medium is employed. Cups are incubated on their sides after pouring the urine out.

provide about the same information as dip-slides but are limited to one culture medium. The same results could be obtained simply by pouring urine in and out of regular MAC, EMB, CLED, or blood agar plates, draining away the excess urine, and placing the plates face down on absorbent paper for a few minutes before incubation.

Filter Paper Method

The inoculum is delivered by means of a filter paper strip that has been dipped in the urine to the surface of trypticase soy agar contained in a small plastic plate (Testuria™) (15) (Fig. 3.9). The paper is of standard porosity and therefore delivers the same quantity of urine to each plate. The device is sealed by its cover and incubated at 37°C for 10 to 24 hours. More than

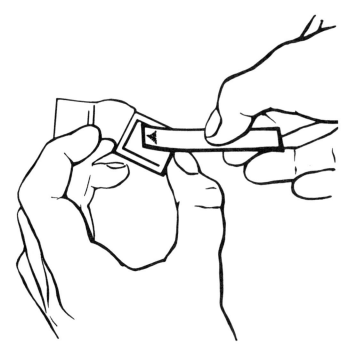

Figure 3.9. The filter paper inoculation method.

25 colonies on the plate are equivalent to $\geq 10^5$ cfu/ml of urine. Because most aerobic bacteria will grow on the medium, identification requires subculture into appropriate diagnostic media. Positive and false-negative results are probably no more than 5% if rigid adherence to proper criteria is maintained. The cost of this test is relatively low. A small incubator is required.

The Pad Culture Method

The pad culture method Microstix®-3 Reagent Strip Test (Miles, Inc. Diagnostic Division, Cockeysville, MD) consists of a plastic dip-strip containing a nitrite indicator and two small pads containing dehydrated culture media (Fig. 3.10). One pad contains an inhibitor of gram-positive organisms; the other supports growth of both gram-positive and gram-negative bacteria. The media pads contain colorless tetrazolium which, when reduced in the presence of bacterial multiplication, produces discrete red spots on the pad. The strips are placed in a sterile plastic packet and incubated for 18 to 24 hours at 37°C. The density of the reduced tetrazolium spots indicates the number of bacteria originally inoculated onto the pad. The disadvantage of this system is that the spots are not bacterial

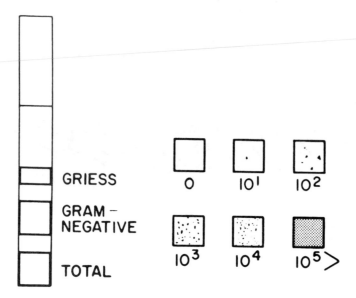

Figure 3.10. The pad culture and Griess' (nitrite) test dip-stick. The density of reduced tetrazolium precipitates shown on the right is used to quantitate bacteriuria.

colonies. Subcultures cannot be obtained for identification and susceptibility tests.

Automated Methods to Detect Bacteriuria

A variety of automated tests have been developed to provide rapid information to identify and quantitate microorganisms and provide antimicrobial susceptibility. They are based on the principles outlined in Table 3.1. A more detailed description of these tests is available in the review by Eisenstadt and Washington (16).

Table 3.1. Automated Methods to Detect Bacteriuria

Method	Principle
Photometry	Measures light scatter over time
Bioluminescence	Assays ATP with luciferin/luciferase
Electrical Impedance	Altered by rapidly growing organisms
Limulus	Endotoxin coagulates amoebocyte lysate
Microcalimetry	Measures heat production with growth
Particle Size	Adaptation of the Coulter counter™
Radiometry	Release of $^{14}CO_2$ from substrate

Nonculture Methods to Detect Urinary Tract Infections

Macro-Staining Filtration Devices

Semiautomated rapid screening tests use a filtration device to capture bacteria onto a pad (17). The pad is stained with safranin and compared to a standard. The Bac-T-Screen™ (Becton Dickinson; Viteck Systems, Inc., Hazelwood, MO) uses a semiautomated device to prepare the specimens. In the procedure, 1 ml of urine is mixed with 3 ml of diluent containing 14.5% acetic acid to lyse the cellular material. The mixture is suctioned through a filter card. Three ml of safranin and 3 ml of 2.4% acetic acid decolorizer are then passed through the apparatus. The color intensity is compared to a guide on the filter guide. A positive test is said to correspond to $\geq 10^5$ cfu/ml. Pigments in the urine may interfere with interpretation of the appearance of color and clogging of the filter may be caused by urinary debris. The Filtracheck-UTI™ (Meridan Diagnostics, Inc., Cincinnati, OH) uses a disposable colorimetric-electrostatic filtration system. Only a few drops of urine are needed. These tests are used as a screening procedure for clinical microbiology laboratories that process large numbers of urine specimens. Positive results need to be confirmed by culture.

Microscopic Examination

Microscopic examination of the urine is the most rapid and inexpensive means to diagnose urinary tract infections and determine the response to therapy. It provides useful information concerning the likely invaders and whether cultures and susceptibility tests might be needed. The urine may be examined with or without staining and with or without centrifugation, depending on the expertise of the examiner. Unstained specimens are useful for rapid diagnosis; Gram stains provide more reliable information about the potential pathogen.

Unstained Specimens

The most rapid method is to place a drop of urine on a microscope slide, add a cover slip, and examine the specimen under high dry magnification (400 ×) under reduced light (condenser down) or with a phase contrast microscope. In florid cases of urinary tract infections, numerous bacteria and pus cells may be seen. It is preferable to examine the sediment of a centrifuged specimen. Centrifugation concentrates the microorganisms and pus cells about 10 fold. A drop of Kova™ stain or methylene blue helps to identify leukocytes. The specimen is centrifuged at 2,000 rpm for 3 to 5 minutes in a desk top machine. The supernatant is poured off, and the sediment is shaken and added to glass slide with a cover slide or composite device. The criterion for a positive sediment is the presence of many (preferably more than 20) obvious bacteria (Figs. 2.3 and 2.4). Motility is not helpful. The correlation between microscopic examination of the sediment with the colony count is shown in Figure 3.11.

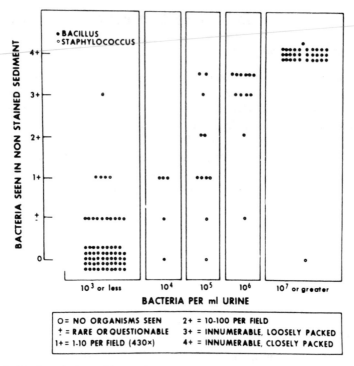

Figure 3.11. Correlation of bacteria visualized in the unstained urinary sediment with quantitative bacterial counts. Reproduced with permission from Kunin CM (18).

Heavy pyuria can mask bacteria in the sediment. The presence of large epithelial cells indicates that the specimen is contaminated with vaginal fluid. Fresh urine should be used to avoid interference by crystals that may appear on standing or refrigeration. If crystals are present, the urine should be warmed until they dissolve. The advantages of this method is that it is simple and rapid and can be combined with inspection for pyuria casts and crystals. The disadvantages are that it cannot detect bacterial counts of $< 10^5$ cfu/ml. Lactobacilli may be mistaken for gram negative bacilli, and gram positive cocci are very difficult to visualize without staining.

The Gram Stain

The Gram stain method takes more time than wet mount preparations, but it offers the advantage of being able to distinguish gram negative and positive bacteria, yeasts, and fastidious microorganisms such as *Haemophilus influenzae*. The test can be performed much more rapidly than is generally taught. After the specimen is dried and fixed with heat, each of the reagents are added and washed away immediately. There is no need for timing. Cell nuclei appear pink in a properly decolorized specimen. Vaginal contamination is detected by the presence of large gram positive rods (Lactobacilli) adherent to epithelial cells. Large numbers of gram negative cocco-bacilli adherent to epithelial cells (clue cells) suggest bacterial vaginosis. The criteria for a positive gram stain (corresponding to about $\geq 10^5$ cfu/ml) are 1 or more microorganisms per hpf (1000 ×) for uncentrifuged specimens and 5 to 10 bacteria per hpf for centrifuged specimens. The standardized cytospin centrifuge method provides more precise results. Well-mixed urine (0.2 ml) is spun at 2,000 rpm for 5 minutes in a capped chamber. The slides are heat fixed and Gram stained. The presence of the same organism in six or more fields is interpreted as being positive. This method is reported to have a sensitivity of 98% and specificity of 90% (16).

Chemical Tests for Bacteriuria

Several chemical tests have been developed to permit rapid diagnosis of significant bacteriuria. The ideal test should have the following characteristics:

- Can be self-administered
- Can be performed on voided urine without special preparation
- Results can be obtained rapidly (within a few minutes)
- Inexpensive
- Highly sensitive (few false negatives)
- High specific (few false positives)

Nitrite (Greiss) Test

This test is based on the concept that dietary nitrate is converted to nitrite by the enzyme nitrate reductase. This enzyme is synthesized by *Enterobacteriaceae* and some gram positive bacteria. A dip-strip containing the reagents turns pink within 30 seconds after being exposed to nitrite in urine. The test is highly specific and virtually diagnostic for significant bacteriuria unless confounded by blood, dyes, or urobilinogen. A negative test does not rule out infection because it takes about 4 to 6 hours for bacteria to convert nitrate to nitrite in bladder urine. This accounts for its poor sensitivity when used with random specimens of urine. The ideal time to use the test is with a first morning voided specimen. It is available as a separate test for self screening or in combination with the leukocyte esterase test.

The nitrite test is ideal for self screening (19). We evaluated this test in almost 1,000 women. They were asked to test their first voided specimen for 3 consecutive days. The urine was saved and brought to the laboratory for a confirmatory test and quantitative culture. There were no false positives with self-read tests. Forty cases of significant bacteriuria were detected. The prevalence of bacteriuria was 4%, which was expected in this population. Two-thirds of cases were positive on the first test. A second test improved the sensitivity to 80%, and a third test to 90%. We employed the same method to screen pre-school girls in a community-wide program (20). The mothers performed the test to their child's first voided specimen. Again, there were no false positives and the prevalence of significant bacteriuria was about 1%, as expected. In follow-up studies, the test, when used on 3 consecutive days each month, detected 81.8% of recurrent episodes of significant bacteriuria (21).

Other Tests

- **The leukocyte esterase (LE) test.** This test detects pyuria only. Pyuria is commonly associated with urinary tract infections, but may also be caused by inflammation, tumors, and vaginal contamination. The LE provides presumptive evidence for infection, but needs to be confirmed by microscopic examination or culture of the urine for bacteria.
- **The catalase test.** This is based on the principle that most uropathogens, other than enterococci, contain the enzyme catalase. The test is commercially available in a kit (Uriscreen™ catalase detection system, Analytab Products, Plainview, NY). The test tube contains proprietary reagents with a blue dye. The urine is added to the tube, followed by a few drops of 10% hydrogen peroxide. A positive test consists of the appearance within 2 minutes of a layer or ring of foam on the surface of the urine. The test is highly sensitive but lacks specificity because catalase is present in leukocytes, erythrocytes, and cellular debris. The test cannot differentiate between urinary infection and other causes of inflammation.
- **Glucose oxidase test.** This test is based on the principle that the small amounts of glucose (2 to 10 mg/100 ml) normally present in urine are metabolized by bacteria during prolonged incubation in the bladder. Absence of glucose is detected by a sensitive dip-stick. The test can only be applied to a first morning specimen. The test cannot be used in patients with diabetes mellitus (22).
- **The Limulus gelation test.** This test detects minute amounts of endotoxin. It is said to be able to accurately detect significant bacteriuria and can be automated (23).

Key Points about Microscopic and Chemical Tests for Urinary Tract Infection

- Microscopic examination of fresh urine is the most rapid, least expensive means to make the diagnosis. The gram stain is preferred because it can distinguish gram positive and gram negative bacteria, yeasts, Lactobacilli adherent to epithelial cells, and "clue" cells suggestive of bacterial vaginosis.
- The nitrite test is highly specific but has poor sensitivity unless performed on a first voided morning urine.
- The leukocyte esterase test is highly sensitive and specific for pyuria and is a useful screening test. Although pyuria is common in patients with urinary tract infections, it is not diagnostic for infection because pyuria can be produced by other inflammatory conditions and vaginal contamination.
- The catalase test is sensitive but does not distinguish bacteriuria from pyuria or hematuria.

Antimicrobial Susceptibility Tests

Most patients with urinary tract infections need to be treated before the results of culture and susceptibility tests are available. The likelihood that a microorganism will be susceptible to a specific drug can be predicted on clinical and epidemiologic grounds, by laboratory studies, and can be confirmed by the response of the patient to treatment. Acute, uncomplicated urinary tract infections are usually caused by *E. coli* and *Staphylococcus saprophyticus* and rarely by other uropathogens. These microorganisms are often resistant to drugs commonly used in the community (such as ampicillin, amoxicillin, and first generation cephalosporins). They are more likely to be susceptible to trimethoprim, nitrofurantoin, and the quinolones. Chronic or complicated infections are usually caused by microorganisms that are resistant to multiple drugs.

The choice of drug for treatment of urinary tract infections depends on the susceptibility of the microorganism, ability to achieve adequate concentrations in the urine and tissues, rate of emergence of resistant strains, ease of administration, relative safety, and cost (see Chapter 12, Management of Urinary Tract Infections). Susceptibility tests are not always needed to manage acute uncomplicated infections, but they are helpful guides for treatment of recurrent uncomplicated and chronic, complicated infection. Generally, an excellent correlation exists between laboratory susceptibility tests and clinical efficacy. Nevertheless, there are times when the patient will respond to treatment even though the laboratory reports that the microorganism is resistant. This is because the cut-offs for susceptibility tests are based on achievable blood levels rather than concentrations that can be achieved in urine.

The "In Vivo" Susceptibility Test

Microorganisms should be virtually eliminated from the urine within a day or two after treatment with an effective drug. This can be determined by microscopic examination of the urine or culture. The drug is considered to be effective if the microorganisms disappear from the urine. The clinician must recognize failure if the microorganisms persist in the urine and change to another drug. This procedure is known as the *in vivo* susceptibility test. It is particularly useful in patients who continue to have symptoms and pyuria for several days after initiation of therapy. They often will have a sterile urine, and there is no need to change therapy.

Selection of Drugs to be Tested in the Laboratory

Most hospital and commercial laboratories employ panels of drugs that are predominantly active against gram negative or gram positive bacteria. The drugs to be tested should correspond to the hospital formulary. A representative of each class of an oral drug is usually sufficient (e.g., an aminopenicillin, tetracycline, trimethoprim, cephalosporin, nitrofurantoin, aminoglycoside, and a quinolone). I prefer to test trimethoprim alone rather than in combination with sulfamethoxazole because trimethoprim is the more active ingredient and has fewer side effects than the combination. The panel should include drugs active against enterococci and staphylococci as well as gram negative enteric bacteria. Susceptibility testing to sulfonamides is optional. Sulfonamides are used only for a first or second episode of uncomplicated infection. Susceptibility tests are not available for methenamine mandelate or hippurate. These drugs are effective only in an acid urine and there is no practical method for routine testing. Chloramphenicol should be reserved for unusual circumstances because of its potential to produce irreversible aplastic anemia. It should not be routinely tested. Carbenicillin is included among the agents tested for oral therapy because the indanyl derivative is active against Pseudomonas.

Types of Susceptibility Tests

Three general types of susceptibility tests are available. These include the broth tube dilution, the microtiter plate dilution, and the disk diffusion methods. All are semiquantitative and provide reliable results if properly conducted and interpreted. Results may be reported by minimum inhibitory concentration (MIC) or as sensitive, intermediate, or resistant. The breakpoints for susceptibility are based on achievable concentrations in the blood. Drugs with intermediate susceptibility are often effective for urinary tract infections because of the high concentrations achieved in urine. A detailed description of these tests is beyond the scope of this book. The reader is referred to earlier editions of this book and manuals of medical microbiology.

The Direct Susceptibility Test

Antimicrobial susceptibility can be rapidly determined by inoculating urine freshly obtained from a patient on agar plates or in microtiter wells. The method is unofficial, but quite valuable. The procedure is performed as follows. A urine specimen is obtained and the sediment is examined. The urine will contain a sufficient inoculum if 20 to 40 or more bacteria are readily visualized at about 400 $\times$ magnification. A cotton swab is dipped into the urine and evenly streaked on the surface of a Mueller-Hinton agar plate. Appropriate susceptibility disks are then added. The plate is examined at 8 to 12 hours, depending upon the inoculum size. Zones of inhibition are interpreted as with the Kirby-Bauer method or NCCLS guidelines. This test was found to be useful in a busy urologic clinic and compared favorably with more standard methods (Perez and Gillenwater, personal communication). The test can also be applied to the microtiter method. The direct susceptibility test has been validated by several groups of investigators (24–26). It is most reliable when a single microorganism is present.

> **Key Points about Antimicrobial Susceptibility Tests**
>
> - Susceptibility tests are not needed to manage the first few episodes of uncomplicated infection provided that the drug selected is likely to be effective based on epidemiologic information.
> - The patient's response to therapy is an excellent guide to success or failure. The urine should be sterile within 1 to 2 days after starting treatment.
> - Susceptibility tests are valuable for patients with recurrent or complicated infection.
> - Direct susceptibility tests are reliable when the infection is caused by a single microorganism.

Localization of Infections of the Urinary Tract

Virtually all parts of the urinary tract are in close proximity to the urinary stream. The entire system is in risk of infection when the urine is colonized by microorganisms. Some patients may only have "bladder bacteriuria," whereas others may have extensive tissue invasion. Localization tests are designed to distinguish between these possibilities.

There is somewhat of an obsession with methods to localize infection to the "lower" or "upper" tracts. I call this the nephrologic bias. The implication is that if an infection is "lower" (bladder), it is insignificant; if it is "upper" (kidney), it is important. This bias is unfortunate and misleading because the prognosis of urinary tract infections, as stated repeatedly in this book, depends not on the presumed location of infection, but rather on whether the patient has uncomplicated or complicated infection. *Localization studies are rarely needed as a guide to therapy and should be considered as interesting research tools to study the natural history of urinary infections and evaluate chemotherapeutic drugs.*

Localization studies may be divided into several types (Table 3.2). The only way to directly determine whether the kidney is infected is to culture a biopsy specimen. This is rarely accomplished during life. All other tests are indirect. The clinical "gold" standard for acute and chronic pyelonephritis is the history, physical examination, presence of fever, leukocytosis, bacteremia, and radiologic examination. The laboratory "gold" standards are ureteral catheterization and the bladder washout. All other methods are derivative.

Clinical

The clinical history of the patients offers excellent information. Patients with complicated infections (obstruction, foreign bodies, catheters, diabetes, renal transplantation, and neurologic disease) and infections with urease-producing microorganisms (Proteus, Providencia, Morganella) will predictably have infection of the kidney and other tissues of the urinary tract. It does not matter much whether patients with uncomplicated infections

Table 3.2. Methods Used To "Localize" Urinary Tract Infections

Indicator	Indicates Renal or Tissue Involvement
Clinical	Pyelonephritis, perinephric abscess, cystitis, prostatitis, and urethritis or complicated infection. Presence of urease-producing bacteria.
Response to Therapy	Relapse within a few days after receiving single dose therapy.
Functional	Transient loss of concentrating ability.
Urinalysis	Pus cell casts suggest pyelonephritis. Bits of tissue indicate renal papillary necrosis.
Differential Culture	Localization of prostatic infections. Ureteral catheterization and bladder wash-out methods to distinguish lower from upper tract infection.
Serologic	Four fold or > rise, or high titers to the antigens of the infecting microorganism, or a rise in titers to the common *Enterobacteriaceae* antigen. High titers of C reactive protein, antibody to Tamm-Horsfall protein, elevated sedimentation rate.
Antibody-Coated Bacteria	Suggests invasion of the kidney, prostate or other tissues accompanied by an antibody response.
Radionuclide Scanning	Dynamic changes in distribution of radionuclides in the kidney.
Enzymuria	Lactic dehydrogenase isoenzymes in urine.
Microglobulins	Beta 2 microglobulin in urine.

have upper or lower tract involvement. Their long-term prognosis is excellent, and response to therapy is usually excellent.

Response to Therapy

Patients with recurrent infections or who delay seeking medical management tend to have upper tract infection (27). Those who relapse early after treatment, particularly when given a single dose of an effective agent, are more likely to have "upper tract" infection (27, 28).

Functional (Urine Concentrating Ability)

A transient decrease in renal concentrating ability often occurs in patients with upper tract infections. Concentrating ability returns to normal after successful antimicrobial therapy unless there is extensive damage to the renal medulla. Indomethacin and sodium meclofenamate reverse the concentrating defect in experimental enterococcal infections in rats, suggesting that prostaglandins play an important role (29). There is no need to test for a concentration defect if the patient has concentrated urine in a first-morning voided sample. The specific gravity should be 1.020 to 1.030 and the urinary osmolality should be 700 to 1200 mOsm/kg after an overnight fast. If the urine does not become concentrated overnight, a vasopressin stimulation test (snuff or intramuscular injection) may be warranted. Dehydration or vasopressin stimulation are contraindicated in patients with azotemia (elevated BUN or serum creatinine). These patients are already known to have renal disease.

Differential Culture

Ureteral Catheterization Method (Stamey, Govan, and Palmer [10])

The ureteral catheterization method is based on the supposition that if the kidney is infected, microorganisms will be present in urine obtained from the ureters. Microorganisms present in the bladder are washed out prior to ureteral catheterization.

The technical problem is to pass ureteral catheters through infected bladder urine and be sure that the subsequent ureteral urine cultures represent uncontaminated samples of renal urine. The cystoscope is introduced into the bladder of a patient who has been previously hydrated, and a culture is obtained through the open stopcock of the cystoscope (labeled CB). The bladder is then washed repeatedly with 1 or 2 liters of sterile irrigating fluid. Number 5 French polyethylene ureteral catheters are introduced with the catheterizing element into the cystoscope, but passed only as far as the bladder. At this time, a few ounces of irrigating fluid are allowed to enter the bladder to facilitate catheterization of the ureteral orifices; the stopcock controlling the inflow of irrigating fluid is then turned off. The irrigating fluid passing from the bladder out through the ureteral catheters is collected for culture by holding the ends of both catheters over the open end of a sterile culture tube. This culture (labeled WB1) indicates the number of bacteria per ml carried within the lumina of the catheters as they are advanced to the midureter. These bacteria represent the maximal contamination possible in the first kidney culture if the total volume of urine collected from the kidney is equal to the volume of irrigating fluid displaced from the ureteral catheter (approximately 1.0 ml for a #5 French polyethylene catheter).

The ureteral catheters are placed in the moderator, and consecutive urine cultures are obtained in paired, simultaneous samples from each kidney (LK, RK, LK2, RK2); the first 5 to 10 ml to pass through each ureteral catheter are discarded. The specific gravity, urine creatinine concentration, and usually urine osmolality are determined on several pairs of renal samples because the major functional defect in pyelonephritis is a failure to reabsorb water in the medulla of the kidney. Because a water diuresis, when compared with an antidiuresis, tends to mask this functional defect in concentrating ability, some patients have one or two urine samples collected before water diuresis. A positive test is the finding of significantly larger numbers of bacteria in the samples obtained from the ureter than in the washed bladder perfusate.

The Bladder Washout Method (Fairley [30])

This method avoids cystoscopy and ureteral catheterization. It is considered to be the most suitable laboratory method by which all other localization tests are measured. It is based on the concept that if bacteria are present only in bladder urine or lightly adherent to the bladder mucosa, they can be washed away with water and the residual organisms can be killed by neomycin. If bacteria are present in the "upper tract," they should enter the bladder soon after the washout.

A catheter is inserted into the bladder through the urethra and left in place. Next, 50 ml of a solution of neomycin (0.1%) and two ampoules containing fibrinolysin and deoxyribonuclease (Elase Parke-Davis, Ann Arbor, MI) are introduced into the bladder through the catheter and left in place for 30 minutes. The enzymes remove the fibrinous exudate from the bladder wall, and the neomycin sterilizes the bladder contents. The bladder is then washed out with 2 liters of sterile water. Urine specimens are obtained from the initial catheterization, immediately after bladder washout, and at 0 to 10, 10 to 20, and 20 to 30 minutes after washout. Patients with infection localized to the bladder will have sterile urine during all collection periods after the washout. Patients with renal (upper tract) infection will have microorganisms (usually in the range of 10^3 to 10^4 cfu/ml) in each of the post-washout samples.

This method compares favorably with that of Stamey, Govan, and Palmer (10) in localizing infection to the upper or lower tracts. It has the advantage of not requiring expert urological aid. One drawback is that it can not localize the infection to an individual kidney. Some patients with bladder bacteriuria may be cured by the washout procedure.

Localization of Infection to the Prostate (Meares and Stamey [31])

This method is designed to obtain a sample of prostatic fluid for culture. It is used to differentiate between prostadynia and bacterial prostatitis. The urine must be sterile. For bacteriologic localization, the voided urine (VB) and expressed prostatic secretions (EPS) are partitioned into segments: the first-voided 5 to 10 ml (VB1); the midstream aliquot (VB2); the pure prostatic secretion expressed by prostatic massage (EPS); and the first-voided 5 to 10 ml immediately after prostatic massage (VB3) are quantitatively cultured (Fig. 3.12).

The patient must be well hydrated with a full bladder to ensure proper collections. The foreskin is fully retracted. The glans is cleaned with a detergent soap. All of the soap is removed with a wet sponge, and the glans is then dried carefully with a sterile sponge. The bladder urine is collected by holding a sterile culture tube directly in front of the urethral meatus. As the patient continues to void, the physician quickly removes the VB1 culture tube from the stream of urine. When the patient has voided approximately 200 ml (about one-half of the bladder urine), a second sterile culture tube (VB2)

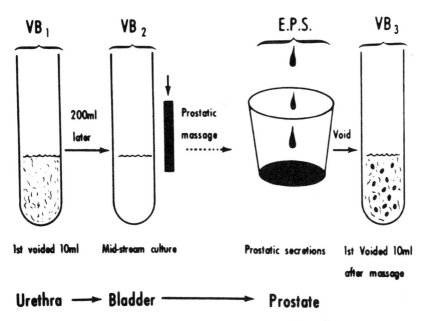

Figure 3.12. Partition of voided urine in the male into four aliquot parts to localize infection to urethra, bladder, or prostate. Reproduced with permission from Meares and Stamey (31).

is inserted into the stream of urine to obtain a 5 to 10 ml sample. The patient is instructed to stop voiding. He then bends forward, maintains the foreskin in a retracted state with one hand, and holds a wide-mouth sterile container near the meatus with the other hand. As the physician massages the prostate gland, drops of prostatic fluid (EPS) fall directly into the specimen container held by the patient. Immediately after massage, the patient voids again, and the VB3 is collected in a manner similar to that for the VB1. Throughout the collections, contamination of the specimens must be prevented in the uncircumcised male; if the foreskin slips over the meatus during the collections, the glans must be cleaned again. It is equally important to remove all the detergent before collecting any of these specimens. If the patient is circumcised, it is not necessary to cleanse the glans before collecting the cultures. A positive test requires that the bacterial counts are significantly higher in the EPS than in the VB2. The VB3 contains a mixture of EPS and urine and should also have higher counts than the VB2.

Localization of Infection to the Prostate Using Semen Cultures (Mobley [32])
The glans is washed after the foreskin, if present, is retracted. The ejaculate is cultured quantitatively in the same manner as expressed prostatic secretions (EPS). The test is valid only in patients with sterile urine. It is important not to be mislead by the presence of staphylococci and other gram

positive bacteria in the semen unless pus cells are also present (33). These bacteria are commensal microorganisms normally present in the urethra. The semen should contain the same uropathogens found in most urinary tract infections. The leukocyte esterase cannot be used to evaluate inflammation because sterile semen will give a positive test. About half of the culture positive semen specimens will have antibody-coated bacteria (34).

Specific Serologic Methods

Pyelonephritis resembles other infectious diseases in that there is a prompt antibody response. As expected IgM antibody to bacterial antigens appears before IgG. A variety of antigens have been used to assess the immune response. These include whole bacteria agglutination, indirect hemagglutination test with antigen-coated erythrocytes, and ELISA. Most of the tests measure antibody response to a panel of O, K, or H, or the common *Enterobacteriaceae* antigen. Antigens derived from the invading microorganism are particularly useful. Antibodies to virtually all of the *E. coli* O antigens are acquired early in life from the gastrointestinal tract and there may be cross-reactions with blood group or other antigens present in food (35). Significant serologic rises (usually fourfold or greater) provide strong evidence of tissue invasion (36,37).

Nonspecific Serologic Methods

So-called "nonspecific phase reactants" appear in the blood in the presence of inflammation, regardless of their type or location in the body. Acute rheumatic fever is classically accompanied by a rise in C-reactive protein (CRP) in the serum and an elevated erythrocyte sedimentation rate (ESR). These tests are also elevated in patients with acute pyelonephritis. Swedish investigators are particularly fond of measuring phase reactants to diagnose pyelonephritis in young children and determine their response to therapy (38). The tests are simple and inexpensive, but nonspecific. They are outmoded for research purposes by radionuclide studies that specifically localize infection to the kidney.

Antibodies to Tamm-Horsfall Protein

Tamm-Horsfall protein (THP) is a fibrillar glycoprotein that is normally shed in small amounts into the urine, from renal tubular cells. Low levels of antibody can be detected in healthy individuals. Antibodies to this protein are elevated in some patients with infection and obstruction of the urinary tract (39). Antibodies to Tamm-Horsfall protein are not helpful to detect reflux in children (40). Some investigators have found elevated levels of anti-THP in girls with acute pyelonephritis, but not in those with cystitis (41).

Antibody-Coated Bacteria (ACB) Test

The principle of this ingenuous test is that microorganisms elicit a local antibody response and coat the surface of the bacteria at the site of infection (42). Some of the antibody-coated bacteria (ACB) are shed into the urine where they are detected by fluorescein-conjugated immunoglobulins raised against human antibodies in other species. Specific immunoglobulin classes may be identified on the ACB with sera directed against human IgG, IgA, and IgM. Because unbound antibodies do not coat bacteria in urine, it is assumed that the ACB must have risen from infected tissues. The presence of ACB in the urine correlates reasonably well with the bladder washout method and can be used as a surrogate test to localize infection to the kidneys or the prostate. The test cannot be used for Candida or staphylococci because these microorganisms bind the Fc region of immunoglobulins and produce nonspecific fluorescence. The ACB test is positive in bacterial prostatitis as well as pyelonephritis. It does not strictly localize infection to the upper tract, but indicates tissue invasion in some part of the tract.

The ACB test is often positive in patients with long-term indwelling urinary catheters, diabetes, and other complicated infections. The test has been extensively used in clinical trials to distinguish patients who might best respond to single dose therapy (28). The ACB test is a reasonably good predictor of patients who will require prolonged courses of antimicrobial therapy. For example, in a multicenter trial of single-dose therapy with amoxicillin, the cure rate was 89.5% in patients who were ACB negative compared to 33.3% in those who were ACB positive (43). Despite these excellent results, the ACB test is rarely used in clinical practice today because of the need to treat patients promptly before laboratory results are available, the costs of the test, and because 3-day therapy is currently much more popular than single dose therapy. Another potential use of the test is to define patients who might require further uroradiologic evaluation. This has proven to be disappointing because most females with recurrent infections do not have important or correctable urologic abnormalities.

As more experience has been gained with the antibody-coated bacteria test, it has become apparent that it may not be as useful as initially promised (44). The test is not sufficiently sensitive or specific to be used in children (45).

Radionuclide Methods

Radionuclide scans have become much more sensitive and specific in recent years. They allow virtually direct visualization of the infected kidney and have for the most part replaced other localizing methods. These tests are relatively expensive and are indicated only for difficult diagnostic problems, for children with severe grades of vesicoureteral reflux, and for research purposes.

Enzymuria and β2 Microglobulins

Excretion into the urine of excess amounts of high-molecular-weight en-zymes, such as β glucuronidase, N acetyl β glucosaminidase, and the lactic dehydrogenase (LDH), suggest the presence of renal damage. Enzymuria is nonspecific because elevated levels may be produced by virtually any cause of renal damage, including ischemia, nephrotoxic drugs, neoplasms, trans-plant rejection, and pyelonephritis. Some investigators have reported that urinary excretion of LDH isoenzyme 5 correlates well with the bladder washout method and the ACB test (45,46). Because LDH 5 can originate from leukocytes as well as renal tissue, a positive test may simply reflect the presence of pyuria unless the leukocytes are removed (47).

Beta 2 microglobulins are small proteins with a molecular weight of 11,800 Daltons. The clearance and excretion of these proteins are reported to be increased in patients with "upper tract" infection (48). The test is non-specific because urinary excretion is also increased in the presence of shock, nephrotoxic agents, fever, and underlying renal disease.

Key Points about Localization of Infection

- Clinical assessment of uncomplicated versus complicated infection is more useful than any laboratory test to guide therapy, assess the need for uroradiologic studies, and de-termine prognosis.
- The "gold standards" for localization studies are the ureteral catheterization and the bladder washout methods. The bladder washout method is preferred for research pur-poses because it is less invasive.
- Bacterial prostatitis may be distinguished from prostadynia by culture of the expressed prostatic secretions or semen. Coagulase negative staphylococci are common contami-nants of the male urethra and do not indicate infection unless they are accompanied by pus cells.
- A specific antibody response occurs in pyelonephritis. The most specific antigens are obtained from the invading microorganism.
- Nonspecific acute phase reactants (CRP, ESR) are elevated in pyelonephritis but are also elevated in many other inflammatory states.
- The antibody-coated bacteria (ACB) test correlates reasonably well with other localiz-ing tests, but is time consuming, adds extra expense, is not useful in children, and does not predict the need for urologic studies. It should be reserved for research purposes.
- Radionuclide and other scanning methods provide excellent visualization of acute pyelonephritis and residual scars. They are expensive and should be reserved for diag-nostic problems.
- Enzymuria (lactic dehydrogenase isoenzyme 5) and excretion of β microglobulins in urine suggest the presence of upper tract infection, but are not needed for routine use.

Creatinine Clearance

The blood urea nitrogen and serum creatinine are usually not elevated in patients with acute pyelonephritis. Increased blood levels are warning signs of dehydration, urinary obstruction, or underlying renal disease. Azotemia, proteinuria, and hypertension are late findings in chronic pyelonephritis. It may be difficult to distinguish the small shrunken kidneys of chronic pyelonephritis from other causes of end-stage renal disease, such as glomerulonephritis, diabetic nephropathy, and arteriolar nephrosclerosis. Hypertension and massive proteinuria may be seen in patients with severe grades of vesico-ureteral reflux.

The creatinine clearance is a useful method to measure glomerular filtration rate and global renal function. The test is based upon the principle that endogenous serum creatinine derived from muscle is constant throughout the day. Most of the creatinine is cleared from the blood by glomerular filtration and not reabsorbed. Urinary excretion is not significantly affected by the rate of urine flow. It is exceedingly important to obtain a complete urine collection. A 24-hour urine collection is not necessary because the limiting factor is not the duration of collection, but the accuracy of the urine collection over time. The patient should be well hydrated before beginning the test. I prefer to collect three consecutive 2 hour collections during the day rather than 24 hour collections because the collections can be supervised more closely and the urine can be sent directly to the laboratory. The three values should be in close agreement.

Instructions for the Patient for Three Consecutive 2-hour Collections
On awakening, completely empty your bladder into the commode, and discard the urine. Record the time. Your bladder is now empty, and all urine that forms from this time on should be collected for the test. Drink two large glasses of fluid immediately after voiding and every hour during the 6 hour test. Carefully collect all urine passed in the first 2 hours in bottle No. 1. Pass your next specimen as close as possible to the end of the second 2-hour time into bottle 2. Pass the last 2-hour specimen into bottle No. 3. You may void only once, if you wish, provided that the time you void is at the end of each 2-hour period. A blood sample will be taken during the 6-hour collection period.

Instructions for the Physician, Nurse, or Technician
Measure the volume of urine in each 2-hour collection bottle to the nearest 5 ml. Save 10 ml of urine from each bottle in a stoppered test tube and send it to the laboratory along with a tube of clotted blood for measurement of serum creatinine.

Creatinine clearance for each 2-hour period is calculated by the formula:

$$Cl\ creat = \frac{U \times V}{P} = \left[\frac{mg/ml\ urine \times ml\ urine/min}{mg/ml\ plasma} \right]$$

The three clearances are averaged. Major differences in the values usually mean that collection has been faulty, and the test should be repeated. The duration of each collection may be increased as best suits the individual case. If the timing is changed, the volume of urine collected should be divided by the appropriate number of minutes of collection to determine the value of V in the formula. Normal values for creatinine clearance are generally 90 to 140 ml per minute for men and 85 to 125 ml per minute for women. The creatinine clearance value obtained by voided urine samples is not valid if the patient has a significant residual urine (more than 30 to 50 ml). Catheter-collected specimens will be required for such patients.

Because the amount of creatinine excreted per day varies with body size (particularly muscle mass), it is customary to correct the clearance as follows:

$$\text{Corrected clearance for meter square body surface} = \text{observed clearance} \times \frac{1.73}{\text{surface area (M}^2)}$$

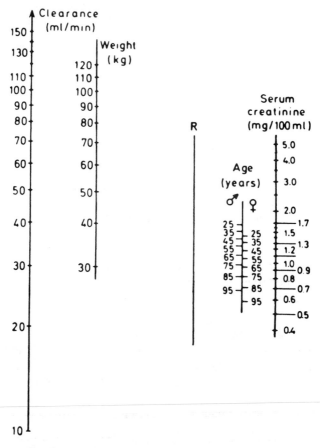

Figure 3.13. Nomogram for rapid evaluation of endogenous creatinine clearance (reproduced with permission from Siersbaek-Nielsen et al. [50]). Instructions: With a ruler, join weight to age. Keep the ruler at the crossing point of the line marked R. Then move the right hand side of the ruler to the appropriate value for serum creatinine and read the clearance from the left side of the nomogram.

Estimation of the Creatinine Clearance from the Serum Creatinine

For clinical purposes, it is usually not necessary to perform a creatinine clearance. Several formulae and nomograms (Fig. 3.13) have been developed that are adequate. The Cockcroft-Gault formula for estimating creatinine clearance is well established and compares favorably with more elegant inulin, iothalamate, ^{51}CrEDTA, and ^{99m}Tc-DPTA clearance tests (49).

For Adults:

$$Cl\ creat = \frac{(140 - \text{age in years})}{\text{serum creatinine mg/dl}} \times \frac{\text{weight kg*}}{72}$$

*For females deduct 15%. An estimate of lean body weight should be used in obese subjects.

Children require different methods because renal function is more closely related to surface area than body weight.

For Young Children:

$$Cl\ creat = \frac{0.55 \times \text{length in centimeters}}{\text{Serum Creatinine}}$$

References

1. Norden CW, Kass EH. Bacteriuria of pregnancy—a critical appraisal. Annu Rev Med 1968;19:431–470.
2. Morris RW, Watts MR, Reeves DS. Perineal cleansing before midstream urine, a necessary ritual? Lancet 1979;2:158–159.
3. Immergut MA, Gilbert EC, Frensilli FJ, et al. The myth of the clean catch urine. Urology 1981;17:339–340.
4. Lohr JA, Donowitz LG, Dudley SM. Bacterial contamination rates for non-clean-catch and clean-catch midstream urine collections in boys. J Pediatr 1986;109:659–660.
5. Lipsky BA, Inui TS, Plorde JJ, et al. Is the clean-catch midstream void procedure necessary for obtaining urine culture specimens from men? Am J Med 1984;76:257–262.
6. Lohr JA, Donowitz LG, Dudley SM. Bacterial contamination rates in voided urine collections in girls. J Pediatr 1989;114:91–93.
7. Said R. Contamination of urine with povidone-iodine: cause of false-positive test for occult blood in urine. JAMA 1979;242:748–749.
8. Bailey RR, Little PJ. Suprapubic bladder aspiration in diagnosis of urinary tract infection. Br Med J 1969;1:293–294.
9. Nelson JD, Peters PC. Suprapubic aspiration of urine in premature and term infants. J Pediatr 1968;36:132–134.
10. Stamey TA, Govan DE, Palmer JM. The localization and treatment of urinary tract infections: the role of bactericidal urine levels as opposed to serum levels. Medicine 1965;44:1–36.
11. Gower PE, Roberts AP. Qualitative assessment of midstream urine cultures in the detection of bacteriuria. Clin Nephrol 1975;3:10–13.
12. Carlson KP, Pullon DH. Bladder hemorrhage following transcutaneous bladder aspiration. Pediatrics 1977;60:765–766.
13. Hirsch H, Bray E. A comparison of different methods of quantitative bacteriologic urinalysis. In: Kass EH, ed. Progress in pyelonephritis. Philadelphia: FA Davis, 1955:550.

14. Arneil GC, McAllister TA, Kay P. Measurement of bacteriuria by plane dipslide culture. Lancet 1973;1:94–95.
15. Dodge WF, West EF, Fras PA, et al. Detection of bacteriuria in children. J Pediatr 1969;74: 107–110.
16. Eisenstadt J, Washington JA. Diagnostic microbiology for bacteria and yeasts causing urinary tract infections. In: Mobley HLT, Warren JW, eds. Urinary tract infections: molecular pathogenesis and clinical management. Washington, DC: ASM Press,1996:29–66.
17. Wallis C, Melnick JL, Longoria CJ. Colorimetric method for rapid determination of bacteriuria. J Clin Microbiol 1981;14:342–346.
18. Kunin CM. The quantitative significance of bacteria visualized in the urinary sediment. N Engl J Med 1961;265:589.
19. Kunin CM, DeGroot JE. Self-screening for significant bacteriuria. JAMA 1975;231:1349–1353.
20. Kunin CM, DeGroot JE, Uehling D, et al. Detection of urinary tract infections in three to five year old girls by mothers using a nitrite indicator strip. J Pediatr 1976;57:829–835.
21. Kunin CM, DeGroot JE. Sensitivity of a nitrite indicator strip method in detecting bacteriuria in preschool girls. Pediatrics 1977;60:244–245.
22. Alwall N, Lohi A. Factors affecting the reliability of screening tests for bacteriuria. I. Nitrate Test (Urnitest), Uriglox and Dipslide (Inculator). Acta Med Scand 1973;193:499–503.
23. Jorgensen JH, Alexander GA. Rapid detection of significant bacteriuria by use of an automated Limulus amoebocyte lysate assay. J Clin Microbiol 1982;16:587–589.
24. Tilton RE, Tilton RC. Automated direct antimicrobial susceptibility testing of microscopically screened urine cultures. J Clin Microbiol 1980;11:157–161.
25. Oakes AR, Badger R, Grove DI. Comparison of direct and standardized testing of infected urine for antimicrobial susceptibilities by disk diffusion. J Clin Microbiol 1994;32:40–45.
26. Johnson JR, Tiu FS, Stamm WE. Direct antimicrobial susceptibility testing for acute urinary tract infections. J Clin Microbiol 1995;33:2316–2323.
27. Ronald AR, Boutros P, Mourtada H. Bacteriuria localization and response to single-dose therapy in women. JAMA 1976,235:1854–1856.
28. Fang LST, Tolkoff-Rubin NE, Rubin RH. Localization and antibiotic management of urinary tract infection. Annu Rev Med 1979;30:225–239.
29. Levison SP, Levison ME. Effect of indomethacin and sodium meclofenamate on the renal concentrating defect in experimental enterococcal pyelonephritis in rats. J Lab Clin Med 1976;88:958–964.
30. Fairley KF, Bond AAG, Brown AB, et al. Simple test to determine the site of urinary-tract infections. Lancet 1967;2:7513–7514.
31. Meares EM, Stamey TA. Bacteriologic localization patterns in bacterial prostatitis and urethritis. Invest Urol 1968,5:492–518.
32. Mobley DR. Semen cultures in the diagnosis of bacterial prostatitis. J Urol 1975;114:83–85.
33. Nickel JC, Costerton JW. Coagulase-negative Staphylococcus in chronic prostatitis. J Urol 1992;147:398–401.
34. Riedasch G, Ritz E, Mohring K, et al. Antibody-coated bacteria in the ejaculate: a possible test for prostatitis. J Urol 1977;118:787–788.
35. Kunin CM. Distribution of antibodies against various nonenteropathic *E. coli* groups: relation to age, sex, and breast feeding. Arch Intern Med 1962;110:676–686.
36. Hanson LA, Ahlstedt S, Fasth A, et al. Antigens of *Escherichia coli*, human antibody response, and the pathogenesis of urinary tract infections. J Infect Dis 1977;136:(suppl) S144-S149.
37. Clark H, Ronald AR, Turck M. Serum antibody response in renal versus bladder bacteriuria. J Infect Dis 1971;123:539–543.
38. Jodal U, Hanson LA. Sequential determination of C-reactive protein in acute childhood pyelonephritis. Acta Paediatr Scand 1976;65:319–322.
39. Marier R, Fong E, Jansen M, et al. Antibody to Tamm-Horsfall protein in patients with urinary tract obstruction and vesicoureteral reflux. J Infect Dis 1978;138:781–790.
40. Fasth A, Hanson LA, Asscher AW. Autoantibodies to Tamm-Horsfall protein in detection of vesicoureteric reflux and kidney scarring. Arch Dis Child 1977;52:560–562.
41. Hanson LA, Fasth A, Jodal U. Autoantibodies to Tamm-Horsfall protein, a tool for diagnosing the level of urinary-tract infection. Lancet 1976,1:226–228.
42. Thomas V, Shelokov A, Forland M. Antibody-coated bacteria in the urine and the site of urinary-tract infection. N Engl J Med 1974;290:588–590.

43. Rubin RH, Fang LST, Jones SR, et al. Single dose amoxicillin therapy for urinary tract infection. Multicenter trial using antibody coated bacteria localization technique. JAMA 1980;244:561–564.
44. Greenberg RN, Sanders CV, Lewis AC, et al. Single-dose cefaclor therapy of urinary tract infection. Am J Med 1981;71:841–845.
45. Lorentz WB Jr, Resnick MI. Comparison of urinary lactic dehydrogenase with antibody-coated bacteria in the urine sediment as means of localizing the site of urinary tract infection. Pediatrics 1979;64:672–677.
46. Appelmelk BJ, MacLaren DM. Localization of urinary-tract infection with urinary lactic dehydrogenase isoenzyme 5. Lancet 1981;2:1417–1418.
47. Malik GM, Canawati HN, Keyser AJ, et al. Correlation of urinary lactic dehydrogenase with polymorphonuclear leukocytes in urinary tract infections in patients with spinal cord injuries. J Infect Dis 1983;147:161.
48. Schardijn G, Statius van Eps LW, Swaak AJG. Urinary beta 2 microglobulin in upper and lower urinary tract infections. Lancet 1979;1:805–807.
49. Cockcroft DW, Gault MH. Prediction of creatinine clearance from serum creatinine. Nephron 1976;16:31–41.
50. Siersbæk-Nielsen K, Mølholm Hansen J, Kampmann J, et al. Rapid evaluation of creatinine clearance. Lancet 1971;1:1133–1134.

4

Urinary Tract Infections in Children

Overview

The care for the child with urinary tract infections requires special knowledge and skills. Urinary infections in children resemble those in adults in regard to the invading microorganisms, pathogenesis of infection, principles of laboratory diagnosis, and antimicrobial therapy. But there are important differences in host susceptibility, epidemiology, and the clinical expression of infection. The differentiation between uncomplicated and complicated infections is paramount for all age groups. Children with normal urinary tracts suffer considerable morbidity from recurrent infections, but rarely develop renal damage. The major exception is overwhelming infection in the newborn caused by virulent strains of *E. coli* and other microorganisms. More virulent strains are required to invade the healthy host. Children with obstructive uropathy and severe grades of vesico-ureteral reflux are at increased risk of pyelonephritis. Less virulent strains can produce severe damage in the structurally compromised host.

Congenital abnormalities, particularly vesicoureteral reflux, play a very important role in childhood infections and will be discussed in the next chapter. Other important conditions include dysfunctional voiding, hydronephrosis, and posterior urethral valves in boys. The role of spina bifida and other neurologic diseases is important because of the remarkable improvement in care provided by intermittent catheterization. The clinician needs to consider mechanical factors such as whirlpool baths when an otherwise healthy child is found to be infected with Pseudomonas or factitious infection when unusual or multiple microorganisms are isolated.

Our current knowledge of urinary tract infections in children is based on several major advances. These are (1) the use of the quantitative bacterial count to detect significant bacteriuria in large populations, (2) the development of noninvasive ultrasound and scintillation scanning devices to detect anatomical abnormalities, (3) an appreciation of the role of vesicoureteral reflux and reflux nephropathy in producing renal damage, (4) advances in pediatric urology, and (5) long-term studies of the natural history of the disease. This chapter will focus on the clinical, microbiologic, and epidemiologic expression of urinary tract infections in children and management. More detailed discussions of pathogenesis and therapy will be considered in greater detail in later chapters.

Epidemiology

Population surveys using the quantitative bacterial count to detect significant bacteriuria have been of great value in defining the prevalence of urinary tract infections among children and adults (Fig. 1.1). A summary of the findings in large surveys is presented in Table 4.1.

Table 4.1. Prevalence of Urinary Tract Infections in Children According to Age and Sex*

Age Group	Males (%)	Females (%)	References
Newborns and infants	1.5–3.6	0.4–1.0	(1–8)
1–5 years	0.0–0.4	0.7–2.7	(9–14)
School children	0.04–0.2	0.7–2.3	(15–19)
Diabetic school children	–	1.0–2.0	(20–22)

In a large, prospective study among school children in Virginia, we found the prevalence of significant bacteriuria among girls to be 1.2% and 0.04% in boys; a ratio of 30:1 (23). Similar prevalence rates have been found by other investigators in the United States, Sweden, and the United Kingdom.

URINARY TRACT INFECTION IN SCHOOL GIRLS

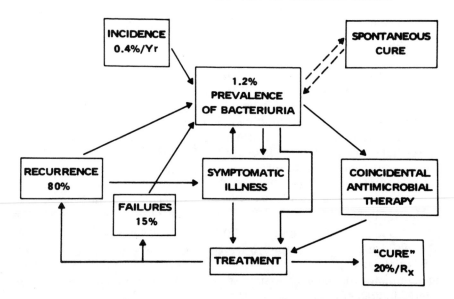

Figure 4.1. The epidemiologic dynamics of bacteriuria in school girls. Redrawn from Kunin CM, Deutscher R, Paquin A (15).

The actual risk of a girl acquiring bacteriuria during the school years is much greater than the prevalence of 1.2% because this rate represents only those found to be colonized at one point in time. It is estimated that 5% to 6% of girls will have had at least one episode of bacteriuria between the times of entering the first grade and graduating from high school. This must be the minimum frequency since it is based on school surveys conducted only once yearly and does not account for girls who developed symptomatic episodes between surveys and received effective treatment. The epidemiologic dynamics of bacteriuria in school girls are summarized in Figure 4.1. Note the annual incidence is about 0.4% per year and the annual rate of recurrence of about 80%. Based on these findings it seems reasonable to assume that symptomatic infections that may occur when young women become sexually active may be expressions of asymptomatic bacteriuria that originated during childhood. This notion is supported by the finding that about 50% of girls, known to have had bacteriuria as school girls, developed symptomatic infection about the time they married or were pregnant.

Demographic and Other Characteristics

Race

The prevalence of asymptomatic bacteriuria among black school girls aged 5 to 14 years was 0.5% compared to 1.2% for the same age group in Caucasians. In the 15- to 19-year age group, the rates were 3.5% in black girls and 1.4% in Caucasians (15).

Familial Susceptibility

Urinary tract infections are so common in females that it is difficult to distinguish increased susceptibility from "background noise." We found no difference in history of urinary tract infections among family members of bacteriuric and nonbacteriuric schoolgirls, but we were struck by what appeared to be clusters of cases in some families. Fennell et al. (24) found that 14% of female siblings also had urinary tract infections. Stansfeld (25) did not find any enhanced susceptibility in families.

Socio-economic Class

No association has been found between socio-economic class and urinary tract infections (15).

Urinary Infections in Mothers During Pregnancy

There are two studies that have examined the frequency of bacteriuria among children of mothers who had urinary tract infections during pregnancy.

Gower et al. (26) found no cases among 25 infants whose mothers had bacteriuria in the last trimester. Gillenwater et al. (27) described bacteriuria in 7 of 65 children born to women who had bacteriuria in the past, as compared to 0 of 24 without evidence of previous infection.

Breast Feeding

Breast feeding may have a protective role, but needs to be confirmed (28) (see "Breast Feeding" in Chapter 6).

Personal Habits

The high prevalence of urinary infections in girls and the short length of their urethras raises the question as to whether personal habits, such as use of diapers, wiping, bubble baths, masturbation, or constipation, may play a role. These factors are extremely difficult to evaluate without controlled studies. Bubble baths may produce an irritative vulvitis but have not been shown to produce urinary tract infections. The role of pinworms in producing urinary infection is also difficult to evaluate from the studies reported in the literature (29).

Enuresis

Most children are toilet trained at age 3 or 4, but some normal children will continue to wet their bed for many years. A variety of clinical conditions may produce uncontrolled voiding. These include the uninhibited bladder, nocturnal enuresis, giggle incontinence, the daytime frequency syndrome, and the lazy bladder syndrome (30). Only some of these children will have an associated urinary tract infection. A characteristic sign of the uninhibited bladder, frequently observed in girls, is squatting and sitting on the heel to compress and obstruct the urethra.

Constipation and Diarrhea

Correction of constipation in children has been reported to decrease the frequency of urinary tract infections, but this report is based on anecdotal evidence (31). An association with diarrheal diseases has been reported, but the causal relationships are unclear (32). Children with urinary tract dysfunction from a variety of causes often have associated constipation. Removal of large fecal impactions may relieve some of the urinary symptoms. The rectal impaction acts like a space-occupying mass. At times there may be an association between constipation, vesicoureteral reflux, and dysfunctional voiding. It is doubtful, however, that constipation causes urinary tract infections.

Fever

Sometimes the only suggestive evidence of urinary tract infection is fever of unknown or uncertain origin. It must be emphasized, however, that fever may be caused by a variety of causes. In one study, fever was associated with urinary infection in only 1 of 82 acutely febrile children who came to an emergency room (33). In another study (34), the frequency of significant bacteriuria among acutely ill, febrile children younger than 5 years of age was only 1.7%.

Environmental Factors

Hot whirlpool tubs are well known to become colonized with *Pseudomonas aeruginosa* and to produce cutaneous folliculitis. Three cases of Pseudomonas urinary infection, one in an adult male and two in young girls (13 and 15 years old), have been traced to hot tubs (35). The male had ejaculated into the water jets. The girls were not recently sexually active. This report is of great interest because it implies that the ascending route of infection can occur in both sexes.

Renal Disease

The prevalence of bacteriuria in 30 children with the nephrotic syndrome was reported by McVicar et al. (36). Seven episodes were recorded in 5 children over a 4-year period. Four of the children were girls and one was a boy. Urinary infections did not appear to alter the course of the disease. The most common microorganism was *Proteus mirabilis*. None of the children had undergone genitourinary instrumentation. This series is too small to allow further interpretation.

Nutrition

A study of bacteriuria among 200 malnourished and 118 well-nourished Peruvian children showed no significant difference in prevalence of infection (37).

Season

Urinary tract infections caused by gram negative enteric bacteria occur about equally throughout the year. The frequency of infections with *Staphylococcus saprophyticus* is increased during the summer and early autumn. The reservoir and mode of acquisition of infection with this microorganism is not clear.

Diabetes

Diabetics are uniquely susceptible to pyelonephritis. The more severe forms, such as emphysematous pyelonephritis, medullary (papillary) necrosis, and perinephric abscess, are much more common in adults than in children. This may be due to the appearance of microvascular complications as the disease progresses. The frequency of urinary infection among diabetic children is the same as in the general population (20–22).

Catheter-associated Infections

Intermittent catheterization is a major advance in the management of children with myelomeningocoele and other disorders of bladder function. Urinary tract infections occur commonly in these children, but they are less hazardous when bladder is emptied by catheterization. A report by Uehling et al. (38) is representative of many large series. The number of children who had numerous symptomatic urinary tract infections decreased after the initiation of catheterization, but colonization of the urine was observed in at least one-half of the patients thereafter. Most of the infections could be controlled by intermittent or prophylactic therapy. Despite intermittent episodes of bacteriuria, most children maintained normal concentrating ability, and episodes of sepsis were rare.

Hospital-acquired Infections

Most nosocomial urinary tract infections occur in association with indwelling urinary catheters. In a prospective study, Lohr et al. (39) identified 60 patients with hospital-acquired urinary infections. The distribution of infections was about equal in males and females and proportionate to the black population. Fever was the only symptom among children in the newborn intensive care unit. Only one patient had an associated bacteremia. It was caused by a coagulase-negative staphylococcus acquired from a central venous catheter. Mortality could not be directly attributed to urinary tract infections in this series.

Factitious and Self-induced

Several cases have been described in which patients have introduced contaminated material into their bladder to produce urinary tract infection. Reich et al. (40) described a 15-year-old boy who introduced feces and foodstuff into his bladder presumably through a syringe. A case of Munchausen syndrome, by proxy, was described by Meadow (41). A 6-year-old girl was evaluated for recurrent infection because of the repeated passage of foulsmelling, bloody urine. Only after exhaustive investigation, including 12 hospital admissions, 7 major radiographic procedures, 6 examinations under anesthesia, catheterizations, and numerous courses of therapy, was it discovered that her mother was substituting or adding her own menstrual discharge or urine to that of the child's.

Sexually Abused Children

Urinary tract infections are not common after sexual abuse. Reinhart (42) obtained urine cultures from 170 sexually abused children, including 132 girls. No case of significant bacteriuria was found. In a similar study, 20% of girls complained of one or more genitourinary symptoms, but only 2 of 53 victims were found to have urinary tract infections, compared to 0 of 53 controls (43).

Microbiology

The Normal Flora of the Introitus and Urethra in Girls

The urethra and periurethral zones are distinctive ecologic niches or microenvironments. The composition of the microbes in these regions differ considerably from those of the feces and skin. Healthy male and female infants are heavily colonized with *E. coli* and enterococci during the first few weeks of life (44). Thereafter, anaerobes account for 95% of the periurethral flora of healthy girls (45). The urethral flora of 2- to 15-year-old girls contains an average of 6.5 different bacterial species equally divided among anaerobes and aerobes (46). The most common aerobes include *Lactobacillus spp., Corynebacterium spp.,* Coagulase-negative staphylococci, and a variety of streptococci. Gram negative aerobic bacilli are rarely present. The anaerobes consist of a wide variety of gram positive cocci and gram negative bacilli.

The Invading Microorganisms

The microorganisms that cause uncomplicated and complicated urinary infections in children are virtually identical to those in other age groups (Chapter 1, Tables 1.3 and 1.4). *Escherichia coli* accounts for most uncomplicated infections in children. *E. coli* and group B streptococci are important causes of sepsis and pyelonephritis in the newborn. *Staphylococcus saprophyticus* is less frequent in children than in young adult women (47). Other less common microorganisms include *Staphylococcus aureus,* Salmonella (48), and Shigella (49,50). Both nontypeable and group B strains of *Hemophilus influenzae* as well as *Hemophilus parainfluenzae* (51–56) may cause urinary infections in children. Hemophilus species require special media for isolation and are usually detected by gram stain in children with "sterile" pyuria. Other unusual organisms include Campylobacter (57), *Mycobacterium tuberculosis,* and atypical mycobacteria. Adenovirus types 11 and 21 produce hemorrhage cystitis in boys (Chapter 7). *Pseudomonas aeruginosa* urinary tract infections may occur in association with whirlpool baths (see previous section) and in complicated infections.

The Quantitative Bacterial Count in Children

The cut-off point for significant bacteriuria of $\geq 10^5$ cfu/ml for voided urine has been well validated in children (58). Lower counts may occur in children who drink large volumes of fluid and void frequently. The same microorganism should be recovered on repeated cultures. So-called "low-count" bacteriuria that is seen in the urethral syndrome in adult women is rare in childhood. In a large epidemiologic study of asymptomatic bacteriuria among schoolgirls, we found that girls with bacterial counts of 10,000 to 50,000 colonies per ml were not at higher risk of acquiring significant bacteriuria during the following year than were girls with lower counts (59). Any number of bacteria found obtained by SPA or by urethral catheterization are usually considered to be "significant." About one-third to one-half of specimens obtained by SPA will contain $< 10^5$ cfu/ml.

Periurethral Colonization

Periurethral colonization with *E. coli* is relatively uncommon in otherwise healthy girls. The wide variety of electrophretic types of *E. coli* found in the periurethral zone suggests that the clonal composition is frequently changing (60). This fits with the observation that most recurrent infections in girls are caused by a new serotype of *E. coli* or a new bacterial species. Periurethral colonization with *E. coli* usually precedes the onset of infection. Nevertheless, the mere presence of a virulent strain of *E. coli* in the periurethral zone does not necessarily indicate that the child will become infected (61). Strains of *E. coli* expressing the *pap*+ gene for P fimbriae appear to be particularly virulent. Young children who develop their first urinary tract infection tend to carry P fimbriated strains in their large intestine and are more likely to be infected with these strains (62). Virulence factors for *E. coli* and other microorganisms are described in Chapter 10, The Invading Microorganisms.

Characteristics of Girls With Recurrent Urinary Tract Infections

There appears to be a special population of girls who are more prone than others to develop recurrent urinary infections. These girls exhibit the following features:

- There is a high rate of recurrence even after a prolonged course of prophylaxis (63).
- Recurrent infection is more likely to be caused by reinfection with a new microorganism than by failure or relapse with the same microorganism (15,64).
- The rectum and periurethral zone of girls with recurrent infection is colonized with enteric gram-negative bacteria during periods when they are free of infection (44,45).
- The rate of recurrent infections decreases after intermittent courses of antimicrobial therapy (23).
- There is no association between recurrent infections and the presence of vesico-ureteral reflux (15).

Clinical Syndromes

The clinical expression of urinary tract infections in children depends on age, sex, the invading microorganism, and the presence of underlying abnormalities of the voiding mechanism (Table 4.2).

Table 4.2. Clinical Syndromes in Children with Urinary Tract Infections

Disseminated bacterial infection and pyelonephritis in the newborn
    More frequent occurrence in males
    Nursery outbreaks
Urinary tract infection in uncircumcised males
Hemorrhagic cystitis caused by adenoviruses, predominantly in males
Uncomplicated urinary tract infection, mostly in females
    Asymptomatic bacteriuria
    Cystitis syndromes
    Acute pyelonephritis
Special situations
    Pseudomonas infections associated with whirlpool baths
    Infections caused by enteric pathogens (Salmonella and Shigella)
    Association with diabetes
    Renal transplantation
Complicated urinary tract infections superimposed on congenital abnormalities
    Vesicoureteral reflux
    Hydronephrosis (uretero-pelvic obstruction)
    Posterior urethral valves in boys
    Neurologic disorders (meningomyelocoele)
    Urinary calculi
    Sickle cell anemia
    Polycystic kidneys
Urinary tract infections associated with voiding disorders
Nosocomial urinary tract infections
    Instrumentation of the urinary tract
    The urinary catheter
    Complications of surgery
Factitious and self-induced infection

Newborns and Infants

Pyelonephritis in the newborn is often associated with bacteremia and sepsis. Older infants are either asymptomatic or are noted to be irritable, strain with voiding, or have unexplained fever and pyuria. Urinary tract infections are much more common among infant boys than girls (Table 4.1). The highest rates are among children in newborn intensive care units. The most severe infections are associated with bacteremia and meningitis. There are several reports of outbreaks of urinary infections among newborns in nurseries, caused by virulent strains of *E. coli*. Kenny et al. (65) described an outbreak caused by *E. coli* O4, and Sweet and Wolinsky (66) described a nursery epidemic among premature infants over a 5-month period. The suspect strain was an antibiotic multi-resistant *E. coli* O4:H5. It was present in the throat and stool of several of the cases. Three infants died and 5 others were found to have urinary tract infections with this organism. One of the fatal cases developed meningitis. No underlying renal disease was found in the three fatal cases.

A clinical study of 100 infants, aged 5 days to 8 months, hospitalized because of acute urinary tract infection, is very instructive (67). Male infants accounted for 75% of patients in the first 3 months of life; thereafter females predominated (Fig. 4.2). Symptoms included fever, irritability, vomiting, and diarrhea. Blood cultures were positive in 21.9% of cases with the same organism isolated from the urine by suprapubic puncture. *E. coli* accounted for 88% of infections; the remainder were caused by other gram negative bacteria (8%), group D streptococci (4%), and *Staphylococcus aureus* (1%). Bacteremia and sepsis occurred mostly in male infants less than 2 months of age. Reflux was present in 18 of 86 patients (20.9%), and in 9 patients it was grade 3 or 4. Hydronephrosis was found in 3 patients (3.5%). Abnormalities were more common in girls than in boys, 45% versus 7% respectively.

Preschool

Urinary tract infections in preschool children are about 10 to 20 times more common in girls than in boys. Most will either be asymptomatic or present

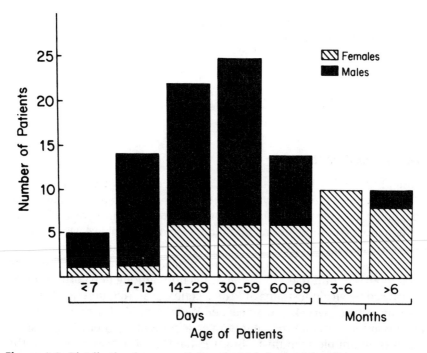

Figure 4.2. Distribution by age and sex of 100 infants with urinary tract infections. Reproduced with permission from Ginsburg CM, McCracken GH (67).

with nonspecific complaints. They may be irritable or listless and complain of difficulty or pain on voiding. The mother may note a foul odor to the urine. This is an important finding that should be pursued. Dip-stick tests for pyuria and nitrite and microscopic examination of the urine for bacteria are simple and inexpensive and are recommended in the evaluation of children with unexplained fever. Careful questioning of older children or parents often reveals either a past history of infection or unrecognized symptoms.

Warning Signs and Symptoms of an Underlying Urologic or Neurologic Abnormality*

Worrisome Signs
- Lumbosacral spine abnormalities
  Hairy patches, Lipomata, Cutaneous dimples or tracts, Bony irregularities
- Reduced anal sphincter tone
- Fixed low urinary specific gravity

Symptoms
- Day and night frequency and bedwetting
- Painful urination
- Rectal pain
- Penile pain or discharge
- Vaginal pain or discharge
- Straining to urinate

*Courtesy of Dr. Stephen Koff

School Girls

Urinary tract infections in school children are often asymptomatic. The symptomatic child may report just not feeling well accompanied by pain on urination and urgent and frequent voiding. A questionnaire administered to parents of girls with and without bacteriuria revealed that bacteriuric girls were more likely to have a prior history of kidney infection, bed wetting after the age of 5 years, attacks of pain in the loin, passing cloudy or smelly urine on more than one occasion, and urgency of urination (68).

Long-term Studies of Asymptomatic Bacteriuria In Girls

There has been considerable interest in the potential to discover urinary tract infections in childhood in the hope that detection of urologic abnormalities and treatment of infection might prevent renal damage later in life.

In a case control study, girls found to have persistent significant bacteriuria were followed for up to 18 years (27). The cases were first detected in a screening program conducted in communities in Virginia. Sixty girls (48 white and 12 black) found to have significant bacteriuria were matched to 38 controls for age; these controls were randomly drawn from the same population that participated in the screening program. The controls never had significant bacteriuria during annual surveys. During the follow-up years, urine cultures were performed on each group at 6-month intervals and intravenous pyelograms were obtained on two occasions. The overall findings are shown in Table 4.3. Hospitalization for complications of urinary tract infection (including 5 for acute pyelonephritis) was required in 10 cases and only 1 control. One case required 19 admissions for control of infection and other complications. Blood pressure, however, did not differ significantly between groups. The serum creatinine was significantly higher among the cases but was within the normal range for all, except for one case with bilateral atrophic pyelonephritis. It is clear from this study that detection of asymptomatic bacteriuria in school girls is a strong predictor of morbidity from symptomatic urinary tract infections later in life and that asymptomatic bacteriuria is associated with important underlying urologic abnormalities in many of the girls. The key finding, however, was that virtually all the girls with significant underlying lesions eventually became symptomatic. This point will be emphasized in considering whether large scale screening programs are justified.

Should Asymptomatic Bacteriuria in Girls Be Treated?

Several long-term controlled studies have been conducted to determine the long-term prognosis of girls with asymptomatic bacteriuria and whether treatment might be worthwhile (Table 4.4). The important finding was that the long-term prognosis was excellent in girls, without major underlying urologic lesions, regardless of whether or not they were treated. In Sweden, Hansson and his associates elected not to treat asymptomatic girls with renal scarring

Table 4.3. Long-term Follow-up of School Girls Found to Have Significant Bacteriuria on Annual Surveys Compared to Matched Controls.

	Bacteriurics (60)		Controls (38)	
	No.	%	No.	%
Symptomatic Infections				
One or more episodes	42	70.0	14	39.5
More than five episodes	13	21.7	1	2.6
With pregnancy	23/36	63.8	4/15	26.7
Uroradiologic Studies				
Renal scars or caliectasis	16	26.7	None	
Reflux requiring repair	5	8.3	None	
Complications				
Hospitalized for urinary infection	10	16.7	1	2.6
Required urologic surgery	9	15.0	None	
Nephrectomy	2	3.3	None	
Decreased renal function	1	1.7	None	
Urinary Tract Infection				
In children of the cohort	7/65	10.8	0/24	0.0

From Gillenwater JY, Harrison RB, Kunin CM (27).

Table 4.4. Long-term Follow-up Studies of School Girls Found to Have Asymptomatic Bacteriuria

Author	Year	Cases No.	Follow-up Years	Renal Damage
Savage et al.* (70)	1975	63	2	No progression
Welch et al. (71)	1976	40	6.5	No progression
Lindberg et al.* (72)	1978	116	5	No progression
Cardiff-Oxford* (73)	1978	208	4	No progression
Gillenwater et al.† (27)	1979	60	9–18	See Table 4.3
Newcastle (74)	1981	56	10–12	Minor defects

*Treatment trials.
†Comparison study with normal controls.

unless they became symptomatic (69). Untreated girls did just as well as those who were treated. The investigators propose that persistent bacteriuria with an established strain might be beneficial by protecting against invasion by more virulent strains.

Is Mass Screening of Girls for Asymptomatic Bacteriuria Worthwhile?

A great deal of information has been learned about the natural history of urinary tract infections from community screening programs of asymptomatic school children. It is clear, however, that although detection is not difficult, treatment does not affect long-term prognosis (Table 4.5). Furthermore, the yield of important correctable abnormalities is low and often too

Table 4.5. Arguments For and Against Mass Screening of School Girls for Asymptomatic Bacteriuria

Arguments in Favor of Screening
   The yield of screening programs is relatively high (1.2% point prevalence in girls).
   Dip-stick tests for pyuria (leukocyte esterase) and nitrate are highly sensitive and
      specific; confirmatory urine cultures can be reserved for those with positive tests.
   Noninvasive tests such as ultrasonography can detect the presence of important
      structural abnormalities.
   Early detection may lead to improved management.
   Over 50% of girls found to have bacteriuria during school surveys will develop
      symptomatic infections with marriage and pregnancy.
Arguments in Against Screening
   Urinary tract infections are benign and do not lead to hypertension or decreased renal
      function unless associated with major structural abnormalities.
   Most of the renal damage is associated with vesicoureteral reflux that occurred earlier
      in life; progression is rare, and the value of corrective surgery is uncertain.
   Treatment is effective for a short period but does not prevent recurrent infections.
   Most girls with urinary tract infections will become symptomatic and eventually will be
      detected by their physicians.

late. Major urologic abnormalities need to be detected within the first year of life before they produce irreversible damage. This notion is supported by the following observations. Stansfeld (25) found that the age of onset of symptoms among 156 children with pyelonephritis was under 1 year in 90 children and under 1 month in 20. Smallpiece (75) reported that 55% of 343 cases of symptomatic urinary tract infections in childhood had developed their first infection before the age of 3 years and 70% were diagnosed by that time. Similar results were obtained in a study of urinary tract infections in a general practice by Mond et al. (76). Important urologic abnormalities can be detected early, even in the absence of infection, by ultrasonography during pregnancy and the neonatal period. Even with this technology, considerable debate exists as to the need to correct many of the lesions found on ultrasonography (see next chapter).

Urinary Tract Infections in Boys

Urinary tract infections are much more common among boys than girls during the first few months of life. Infections in females predominate thereafter. The high rates in neonatal boys may reflect their greater susceptibility to bacterial infections and the presence of a foreskin. The invading bacteria appear to be more virulent in otherwise healthy boys. This concept is substantiated by the finding that P fimbriated and hemolysin producing *E. coli* are more frequent among boys than girls with "lower" urinary tract infection (77). Structural abnormalities of the urinary tract go undetected in boys because of the lack of warning signs of infection. This is the reason for recommending that urinary tract infections in boys be fully investigated.

Microorganisms

Several groups, mostly European, have reported a disproportionately high frequency of Proteus infections in males, which they attributed to colonization of the prepuce (78). In the United States, studies conducted by Wiswell and his associates (79) found that the most common microorganisms isolated from the urine were *E. coli*, followed by Klebsiella in both circumcised and uncircumcised boys. The glans of uncircumcised boys contained significantly greater numbers of enteric, gram negative bacteria (*E. coli*, Klebsiella-enterobacter, *Proteus mirabilis*, and Pseudomonas). *Staphylococcus aureus* was recovered more frequently from circumcised boys at 2 weeks, but this did not lead to infection.

Circumcision

Wiswell and his associates have shown in a series of studies (79) that the incidence of urinary tract infection during the first year of life in uncircumcised boys is significantly greater than in females and circumcised males. In a 4-year study conducted at Brooke Army Medical Center, the rate of infection during the first year of life among 1905 infant females was 0.42%. The rate among 1575 circumcised males was 0.0%, and among 444 uncircumcised males was 1.8%. Winberg et al. (80) were so favorably impressed by this and other studies that they concluded that the prepuce was a mistake of nature. They estimate that circumcision of the newborn male will reduce the frequency of urinary tract infections by about 90%.

The advantages of circumcision must be balanced by the risk. For example, an infant developed overwhelming infection with a group A beta hemolytic streptococcus after circumcision (81), and there have been isolated cases of sepsis and meningitis related to circumcision. It is critical that the operation be performed by competent physicians using aseptic methods. In a very large study of 136,086 boys born in U.S. Army hospitals, complications occurred in 0.19% of circumcised boys (79). These complications included bleeding, bacteremia, surgical trauma, and urinary infections. However, 32 of the uncircumcised boys with urinary tract infection had concomitant bacteremia, 3 had meningitis, 2 had renal failure, and 2 died.

Key Points About Urinary Tract Infections in Boys

- Neonatal and infant boys are at higher risk of developing pyelonephritis than girls.
- Uroradiologic evaluation is recommended in all boys with urinary tract infections.
- The yield of important urologic abnormalities is greatest during the first year of life.
- Circumcision has been shown to decrease the occurrence of urinary tract infections by 90%.
- The long-term prognosis is excellent in boys who do not have major urologic abnormalities.

Diagnosis

Methods to collect specimens, perform microscopic examinations, perform dip-stick tests, and collect urine culture are described in detail in Chapter 3. A brief review of the procedures and additional considerations for children are presented in this section.

Voided Specimens

It may be difficult to obtain a clean voided urine specimen in young children. Some physicians and nurses are adept at catching a spontaneous urinary stream, almost in midair, from an infant or very young child. Strap-on collection cups positioned over the perineum are often used to collect voided specimens. These devices must be used with considerable care because they are readily soiled by vaginal and fecal contamination. To avoid this problem, urine should be collected as soon as possible after voiding. Strap-on devices are better at helping to rule out infection. The diagnosis of urinary tract infection needs to be confirmed by collecting a free-flowing sample of urine or by suprapubic bladder aspiration or catheterization.

It is much less difficult to collect a voided urine from a toilet-trained boy or girl. It is now well established that cleaning of the vulva in prepubertal girls is not necessary. They should be instructed to straddle the toilet seat backwards, spread the labia away from the urethral meatus, and void into a sterile container. Cleaning of the urethral meatus is not needed in circumcised or uncircumcised boys.

Suprapubic Aspiration (SPA) and Catheterization

The gold standard for urine culture in the young child is suprapubic aspiration (SPA) (Fig. 3.2). SPA is particularly useful in small children from whom it is difficult to obtain an adequate specimen. The diaper should be dry before the procedure. A wet diaper indicates that the bladder was recently emptied. Suprapubic aspiration has the advantage of bypassing urethral contaminants. Skin contaminants can be avoided with good antiseptic technique. The major complication of SPA is formation of a hematoma at the site of aspiration. Fortunately, this complication is rare. Urethral catheterization should be attempted only by skilled personnel.

Dip-stick Tests

Dip-stick tests that detect pyuria by the leukocyte esterase test and nitrite are particularly useful in children. The nitrite test has excellent specificity and good sensitivity when performed on first morning urine specimens. Home testing is useful, particularly for children with recurrent infections.

The Gram Stain

Significant bacteriuria can be readily detected by microscopic examination of the urine. The gram stain is particularly useful in children with "sterile pyuria" to detect rare, but important, cases of urinary tract infections caused by fastidious microorganisms such as Hemophilus influenzae and Hemophilus parainfluenzae. A viral or noninfectious cause of cystitis should be suspected when pus cells are present and the gram stain is negative for bacteria.

Key Points About Collection of Urine and Diagnosis of Urinary Tract Infection in Children

- Collection of spontaneously voided, free flowing urine from infants is least invasive.
- There is no need to wash the perineum in prepupertal girls or retract the foreskin in boys.
- The cut-off point for significant bacteriuria is generally $\geq 10^5$ cfu/ml for voided specimens.
- Lower bacterial counts with voided specimens are considered to be significant when the same microorganism (usually E. coli) is recovered repeatedly in a child with fever and pyuria. Lower counts may be seen with infections caused by staphylococci.

- The diagnosis of asymptomatic bacteriuria must be confirmed by at least 1 and preferably 2 consecutive positive cultures with $\geq 10^5$ cfu/ml with the same microorganism.
- Symptomatic patients are considered to have urinary tract infections based on the presence of pyuria and a single positive culture.
- Gram stain of the urine should be performed in children with "sterile" pyuria to look for fastidious microorganisms (such as Hemophilus species).
- Suprapubic aspiration of the bladder (SPA) is the gold standard. Be sure the diaper is dry.
- Any number of bacteria is considered significant when urine is collected by SPA or catheterization, but bacterial counts should be expected to exceed 10^4 cfu/ml.
- Dip-stick tests for pyuria (leukocytes esterase) and nitrite are valuable tools to detect infection and for follow-up. The nitrite test is more sensitive when used to test first morning specimens.

Management

A detailed discussion of treatment of urinary tract infections is presented in the last chapter of this book. Most of the studies of the treatment of urinary tract infection are conducted in adults and may not be applicable to children. Selected aspects of the treatment of urinary infection in children are therefore provided in this section.

Uncomplicated Infection

The goal of management in patients with uncomplicated infection is to eradicate the infection and reduce the morbidity of recurrence caused by relapse or reinfection. It is not difficult to eradicate bacteria with a drug to which the organism is susceptible. The major problem is managing recurrent infections. Within a year after treatment, about 80% of young girls will have a recurrent infection. Most of these will be caused by reinfection with a new strain of *E. coli* or a new bacterial species (15,64). Relapses with the same organism will occur usually within a few weeks after treatment and are caused mainly by an inadequate duration of therapy. Each course of treatment will fractionally extract about 20% of patients into long-term remission (Fig. 4.3). Thus, by close follow-up and repeated effective treatment of each recurrent episode, most girls will eventually do well.

Long-term, bed-time prophylaxis is reserved for a relatively small proportion of the population who have frequent, closely spaced symptomatic episodes. The duration of prophylaxis is arbitrary. Most physicians use prophylaxis for about 3 to 6 months. A longer period is difficult to achieve because of problems with compliance. Most patients will develop recurrent infections once prophylaxis is stopped, but a proportion will go into long-term remission as with intermittent therapy (82) (Fig. 4.4). Prophylaxis can be remarkably effective in decreasing anxiety on the part of the patient and

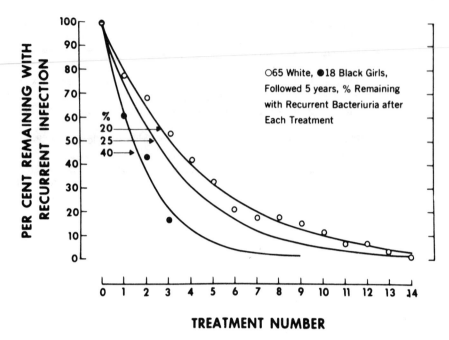

Figure 4.3. Rates of extraction of school girls into remission after short courses of specific chemotherapy directed toward each episode of recurrence. Rates are presented for removal of 20%, 25%, and 40% for each treatment. The observed percentage of the population that required further treatment is superimposed on the theoretical projections for white and black girls followed for 5 years. Reproduced with permission from Kunin (23).

her mother. The use of long-term prophylaxis in patients with vesico-ureteral reflux has not, to my knowledge, been subjected to the scrutiny of a controlled clinical trial (see next chapter).

Complicated Infection

The goal in management of patients with complicated infection is to correct or ameliorate the underlying anatomical or physiological problems and use antimicrobial agents to eradicate infection. At times, it might not be possible to eradicate infection completely, and long-term prophylactic or suppressive therapy may be necessary. One must be careful to distinguish between suppressive therapy that is effective in reducing the population of bacteria from ineffective therapy which has no such effect. It is important to recognize failure. Prolonged use of an ineffective drug will not help the patient and may increase the risk of side effects and superinfection with resistant microorganisms.

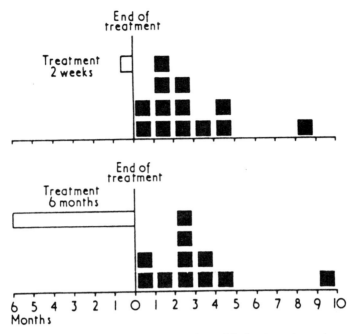

Figure 4.4. Time of relapse after treatment of 24 girls for 2 weeks and prophylaxis of 21 girls for 6 months with trimethoprim/sulfamethoxazole. Each black box represents a girl with recurrent infection. Reproduced with permission from Stansfield (82).

Duration of Therapy

Short courses of therapy, varying from a single dose to several days, are remarkably effective in treatment of acute, uncomplicated infections in adult women, but longer courses are recommended in children (83–86). In both children and adults, single dose therapy is inferior to 3 days of treatment, and 3 days is as effective as 7 to 10 days (84).

Choice of Drug

The choice of drug depends on the susceptibility of the organism, ease of administration, and relative cost. The most popular agents for oral therapy are trimethoprim/sulfamethoxazole (TMP/SMZ), aminopenicillins (ampicillin or amoxicillin), cephalosporins, nitrofurantoin, and sulfonamides. Amoxicillin plus clavulanic acid is usually not effective against ampicillin-resistant strains of *E. coli*. I prefer to use trimethoprim alone because it is as effective as trimethoprim/sulfamethoxazole and has fewer side effects. Sulfonamides have not been shown to delay the emergence of resistance to trimethoprim. Tetracyclines and quinolones are not recommended for use in young children.

Children with acute pyelonephritis are managed best in a hospital setting where they can receive adequate replacement of fluids and parenteral antibiotics. A wide variety of effective agents are available, including ampicillin, aminoglycosides, and the new beta lactam compounds. Choice of drug depends almost entirely on the expectation of susceptibility or resistance. In general, a child who has not received ampicillin previously should have a susceptible organism, but this drug has been used so widely that resistant strains may have been acquired from another family member or contact. A useful series of recommendations for treatment may be found in the reviews by Eichenwald (85) and McCracken (86).

Uroradiologic Studies

Radiologic studies should be reserved for children during the first few years of life, for boys, for patients with pyelonephritis, and for difficult diagnostic problems. There is no need to conduct routine uroradiologic studies in school age girls. The yield of correctable lesions is low even in girls with frequent, recurrent infections. A screening ultrasound is usually sufficient. Routine cystoscopy should not be done in older girls with episodic urinary tract infections unless important structural lesions are detected by ultrasonography or intravenous urograms. Many young women delay seeing physicians for treatment of urinary tract infections because of traumatic experiences with cystoscopy as a child. Ultrasonography is now greatly improved and is often sufficient to detect important structural lesions and suggest the need for CT scans and scintillography.

Recommendations for Uroradiologic Studies in Children

Groups at Highest Risk
- During the first three years of life (when most of the renal damage occurs).
- Boys of all ages (underlying lesions may be missed because of low frequency of infection).

Procedures
- Screen by ultrasound looking for dilated upper tracts and dysfunctional voiding.
- Follow-up positives by voiding cystourethrography or radionuclide cystography.
- Cystoscopic evaluation is important in boys to detect posterior urethral valves.

Optional
- Radionuclide scans, intravenous urograms, retrograde studies only when indicated.

Not Recommended
- Repeat studies in children shown to have normal urinary tracts or low grades of reflux.
- Cystoscopy in children with normal urinary tracts or low grades of reflux.
- Cystoscopy to determine the effect of antimicrobial therapy.
- Urethral dilatation in the absence of clearly defined obstruction.

References

1. Lincoln K, Winberg J. Studies of urinary tract infections in infancy and childhood. II. Quantitative estimation of bacteriuria in unselected neonates with special reference to the occurrence of asymptomatic infections. Acta Paediatr 1964;53:307–316.
2. Randolph MF, Greenfield M. The incidence of asymptomatic bacteriuria and pyuria in infancy. J Pediatr 1964;65:57–66.
3. Littlewood JM, Kite P, Kite BA. Incidence of neonatal urinary tract infection. Arch Dis Child 1969;44:617–620.
4. Abbott GD. Neonatal bacteriuria: A prospective study in 1460 infants. Br Med J 1972;1:267–269.
5. Edelmann CM, Ogwo JE, Fine BP, et al. The prevalence of bacteriuria in full-term and premature newborn infants. J Pediatr 1973;82:125–132.
6. Davies JM, Gibson GL, Littlewood JM. Prevalence of bacteriuria in infants and preschool children. Lancet 1974;2:7–9.
7. Maherzi M, Gougnard JP, Torrado A. Urinary tract infection in high-risk newborn infants. Pediatrics 1978;62:521–523.
8. Gower PE, Husband P, Coleman JC, et al. Urinary tract infection in two selected neonatal populations. Arch Dis Child 1970;45:259–263.
9. Saxena SR, Collis A, Laurance BM. Bacteriuria in preschool children. Lancet 1974;2: 517–518.
10. Savage DC, Wilson MI, Ross EM, et al. Asymptomatic bacteriuria in girl entrants to Dundee primary schools. Br Med J 1969;3:75–80.
11. Mair MI. High incidence of 'asymptomatic' urinary tract infection in infant schoolgirls. Scott Med J 1973;18:51–55.
12. Johnson A, Heap GJ, Hurley BP. A survey of bacteriuria, proteinuria, and glycosuria in five-year-old schoolchildren in Canberra. Med J Aust 1974;2:122–124.
13. Davies JM, Gibson GL, Littlewood JM. Prevalence of bacteriuria in infants and preschool children. Lancet 1974;2:7–9.
14. Kunin CM, DeGroot JE, Uehling D, et al. Detection of urinary tract infections in three to five year old girls by mothers using a nitrite indicator strip. J Pediatr 1976;57:829–835.
15. Kunin CM, Deutscher R, Paquin AJ. Urinary tract infection in school children: epidemiologic, clinical, and laboratory study. Medicine 1964;43:91–130.
16. Meadow SR, White RH, Johnston NM. Prevalence of symptomless urinary tract disease in Birmingham schoolchildren. I. Pyuria and Bacteriuria. Br Med J 1969;3:81–84.
17. Lindberg U, Claesson I, Hanson LA, et al. Asymptomatic bacteriuria in schoolgirls. Acta Paediatr Scand 1975;64:425–431.
18. Newcastle Asymptomatic Bacteriuria Research Group: Asymptomatic bacteriuria in schoolchildren in Newcastle upon Tyne. Arch Dis Child 1975;50:90–102.
19. Edwards B, White R, Maxted H, et al. Screening methods for covert bacteriuria in schoolgirls. Br Med J 1975;2:463–467.
20. Etzwiler DD. Incidence of urinary-tract infections among juvenile diabetics. JAMA 1965;191:81–83.
21. Pometta D, Rees SB, Younger D, et al. Asymptomatic bacteriuria in diabetes mellitus. N Engl J Med 1967;276:1118–1121.
22. Lindberg U, Bergstrom AL, Carlsson E, et al. Urinary tract infection in children with type I diabetes. Acta Paediatr Scand 1985;74:85–88.
23. Kunin CM. A ten-year study of bacteriuria in school girls: final report of bacteriologic, urologic and epidemiologic findings. J Infect Dis 1970;122:382–393.
24. Fennell RS, Wilson SG, Garin EH, et al. Bacteriuria in families of girls with recurrent bacteriuria. Clin Pediatr 1977;16:1132–1135.
25. Stansfeld JM. Clinical Observations relating to incidence and aetiology of urinary-tract infections in children. Br Med J 1966;1:631–635.
26. Gower PE, Haswell B, Sidaway MME, et al. Follow-up of 164 patients with bacteriuria of pregnancy. Lancet 1968;1:990–994.
27. Gillenwater JY, Harrison RB, Kunin CM. Natural history of bacteriuria in schoolgirls. N Engl J Med 1979;301:396–399.
28. Pisacane A, Graziano L, Mazzarella G, et al. Breast-feeding and urinary tract infection. J Pediatr 1992;120:88–89.

29. Kropp KA, Cichocki GA, Bansal NK. *Enterobius vermicularis* (pinworms), introital bacteriology and recurrent urinary tract infection in children. J Urol 1978;120:480.

30. Koff SA, Byard MA. The daytime urinary frequency syndrome of childhood. J Urol 1988; 140:1280–1281.

31. Neumann PZ, deDomenico IF, Nogrady MB. Constipation and urinary tract infection. J Pediatr 1973;52:241.

32. Lima NL, Guerrant RL, Kaiser DL, et al. A restrospective cohort study of nosocomial diarrhea as a risk factor for nosocomial infection. J Infect Dis 1990;161:948–952.

33. North AF. Bacteriuria in children with acute febrile illnesses. J Pediatr 1963;63:408–411.

34. Bauchner H, Philipp B, Dashefsky B, et al. Prevalence of bacteriuria in febrile children. Pediatr Infect Dis J 1987;6:239–242.

35. Salmen P, Dwyer DM, Vorse H, et al. Whirlpool-associated *Pseudomonas aeruginosa* urinary tract infections. JAMA 1983;250:2025–2026.

36. McVicar M, Policastro A, Gort D, et al. Asymptomatic bacteriuria and the nephrotic syndrome in children. Nephron 1973;11:325–332.

37. Freyre EA, Rondon O, Bedoya J, et al. The incidence of bacteriuria and pyuria in Peruvian children with malnutrition. J Pediatr 1973;83:57–61.

38. Uehling DT, Smith J, Meyer J, et al. Impact of an intermittent catheterization program on children with myelomeningocele. Pediatrics 1985;76:892–895.

39. Lohr JA, Donowitz LG, Sadler III JE. Hospital-acquired urinary tract infection. Pediatrics 1989;83:193–199.

40. Reich P, Lazarus JM, Kelly MJ, et al. Factitious feculent urine in an adolescent boy. JAMA 1977;238:420–421.

41. Meadow R. Munchausen syndrome by proxy. The hinterland of child abuse. Lancet 1977;ii:343–344.

42. Reinhart MA. Urinary tract infection in sexually abused children. Clin Pediatr (Phila) 1987;26:470–472.

43. Klevan JL, DeJong AR. Urinary tract symptoms and urinary tract infection following sexual abuse. JAMA 1990;144:242–244.

44. Bollgren I, Nord CE, Pettersson L, et al. Periurethral anaerobic microflora in girls highly susceptible to urinary tract infections. J Urol 1981;125:715–720.

45. Bollgren J, Winberg J. The periurethral aerobic flora in girls highly susceptible to urinary infections. Acta Paediatr Scand 1976;65:81–87.

46. Marrie TJ, Swantee CA, Hartlen M. Aerobic and anaerobic urethral flora in healthy females in various physiological age groups and of females with urinary tract infections. J Clin Microbiol 1980;11:654–659.

47. Hovelius B, Mardh P-A. *Staphylococcus saprophyticus* as a common cause of urinary tract infections. Rev Infect Dis 1984,6:328–337.

48. Ross SA, Townes PL, Hopkins TB. *Salmonella enteritidis*. A rare cause of pyelonephritis in children. Clin Pediatr 1986;25:325–326.

49. Ekwall E, Ljungh A, Selander B. Asymptomatic urinary tract infection caused by *Shigella sonnei*. Scand J Infect Dis 1984;16:121–122.

50. Papasian CJ, Enna-Kifer S, Garrison B. Symptomatic *Shigella sonnei* urinary tract infection. J Clin Microbiol 1995;33:2222–2223.

51. Albritton WL, Brunton JL, Meier M, et al. *Haemophilus influenzae*: Comparison of respiratory tract isolates with genitourinary tract isolates. J Clin Microbiol 1982;16:826–831.

52. Back E, Carlsson B, Hylander B. Urinary tract infection from *Haemophilus parainfluenza*. Nephron 1981;29:117–118.

53. Blaylock BL, Baber S. Urinary tract infection caused by *Haemophilus parainfluenzae*. Am J Clin Pathol 1980;73:285–287.

54. Granoff DM, Roskes S. Urinary tract infection due to *Hemophilus influenzae* type b. J Pediatr 1974;84:414–416.

55. Schuit KE. Isolation of Hemophilus in urine cultures from children. J Pediatr 1979;95:565–566.

56. Chesney PJ. Acute epididymo-orchitis due to *Haemophilus influenzae* type b. J Pediatr 1977;91:685.

57. Feder HM Jr, Rasoulpour M, Rodriquez AJ. Campylobacter urinary tract infection. Value of the urine gram's stain. JAMA 1986;256:2389.

58. Pryles CV. The diagnosis of urinary tract infection. J Pediatr 1960;26:441–451.

59. Walten MG Jr, Kunin CM. Significance of borderline counts in screening programs for bacteriuria. J Pediatr 1971;78:246–249.

60. Schlager TA, Hendley JO, Lohr JA, et al. Effect of periurethral colonization on the risk of urinary tract infection in healthy girls after their first urinary tract infection. Pediatr Infect Dis J 1993;12:988–993.
61. Schlager TA, Whittam TS, Hendley JO, et al. Comparison of expression of virulence factors by *Escherichia coli* causing cystitis and E. coli colonizing the periurethra of health girls. J Infect Dis 1995;172;772–777.
62. Plos K, Connell H, Jodal U, et al. Intestinal carriage of P fimbriated *Escherichia coli* and the susceptibility to urinary tract infections in young children. J Infect Dis 1995;171:625–631.
63. Stansfeld JM. Duration of treatment for urinary tract infections in children. Br Med J 1975;3:65–66.
64. Bergström T, Lincoln K, Ørskov F, et al. Studies of urinary tract infections in infancy and childhood VIII. Reinfection vs. relapse in recurrent urinary tract infections. Evaluation by means of identification of infecting organisms. J Pediatr 1967;71:13–20.
65. Kenny JF, Medearis DN, Klein SW, et al. An outbreak of urinary tract infections and septicemia due to *Escherichia coli* in male infants. J Pediatr 1966;68:530–541.
66. Sweet AY, Wolinsky E. An outbreak of urinary tract and other infections due to *E. coli.* Pediatrics 1964;33:865–871.
67. Ginsburg CM, McCracken GH. Urinary tract infections in young infants. Pediatrics 1982;69:409–412.
68. Parsons V, Patel HR, Stodell A, et al. Symptoms by questionnaire and signs by dipstream culture of urinary tract infection in schoolgirls of South-East London. Clin Nephrol 1974;2:179–185.
69. Hansson S, Jodal U, Noren L, et al. Untreated bacteriuria in asymptomatic girls with renal scarring. Pediatrics 1989;84:964–968.
70. Savage DL, Adler K, Howie G, et al. Controlled trial of therapy in covert bacteriuria of childhood. Lancet 1975;i:358–361.
71. Welch TR, Forbes PA, Drummond KM, et al. Recurrent urinary tract infection in girls. Arch Dis Child 1976;51:114–119.
72. Lindberg U, Claesson I, Hanson LA, et al. Asymptomatic bacteriuria in schoolgirls. J Pediatr 1978,92:194–199.
73. Cardiff-Oxford Bacteriuria study group. Sequelae of covert bacteriuria in schoolgirls. Lancet 1978;1:889–893.
74. Newcastle covert bacteriuria research group. Covert bacteriuria in schoolgirls in Newcastle upon Tyne. A five year follow-up. Arch Dis Child 1981;56:585–592.
75. Smallpiece V. Urinary tract infection in childhood and its relevance to disease in adult life. St. Louis: Mosby, 1969.
76. Mond NC, Gruneberg RN, Smellie JM. Study of childhood urinary tract infection in general practice. Br Med J 1970;1:602–605.
77. Westerlund B, Siitonen A, Elo J, et al. Properties of *Escherichia coli* isolates from urinary tract infections in boys. J Infect Dis 1988;158:996–1002.
78. Hallet RJ, Pead L, Maskell R. Urinary infection in boys. Lancet 1976;2:1107–1110.
79. Wiswell TE. Prepuce presence portends prevalence of potentially perilous periurethral pathogens. J Urol 1992;148:739–742.
80. Winberg J, Bollgren I, Gothefors L, et al. The prepuce: a mistake of nature? Lancet 1989;1:598–599.
81. Cleary TG, Kohl S. Overwhelming infection with group B b-Hemolytic Streptococcus associated with circumcision. Pediatrics 1979;64:301–303.
82. Stansfeld JM. Duration of treatment for urinary tract infections in children. Br Med J 1975;3:65–66.
83. Moffatt M, Embree J, Grimm P, et al. Short-course antibiotic therapy for urinary tract infections in children. A methodological review of the literature. Am J Dis Child 1988;142:57–61.
84. Madrigal G, Odio CM, Mohs E, et al. Single dose antibiotic therapy is not as effective as conventional regimens for management of acute urinary tract infections in children. Pediatr Infect Dis J 1988;7:316–319.
85. Eichenwald HF. Some aspects of the diagnosis and management of urinary tract infection in children and adolescents. Pediatr Infect Dis J 1986;5:760–765.
86. McCracken GH Jr. Diagnosis and management of acute urinary tract infections in infants and children. Pediatr Infect Dis J 1987;6:107–112.

Vesicoureteral Reflux and Reflux Nephropathy

Overview

Vesicoureteral reflux and other congenital abnormalities are important causes of kidney disease in childhood. Until recently, these lesions were detected mostly in children who had urinary tract infection, failure to thrive, or renal failure. Improvements in uroradiologic technology now permit congenital abnormalities to be detected *in utero* or during the neonatal period when the child is at greatest risk of renal damage. [99m]technesium DMSA scans help confirm the diagnosis of pyelonephritis and visualize renal cortical scars. These and other advances have improved our understanding of the natural history of vesicoureteral reflux. It is now known that vesicoureteral reflux occurs early in life, precedes urinary tract infection, and can produce severe damage even in the absence of infection. Other important congenital abnormalities include hydronephrosis and hydroureter with ureteropelvic junction obstruction, and posterior urethral valves in boys. Urinary tract infections in children with spina bifida and other neurologic diseases are now better controlled by intermittent catheterization. Considerable controversy remains concerning the role of medical versus surgical therapy in children with vesicoureteral reflux, the need for long-term prophylaxis, and the role of dysfunctional voiding. These and other important issues will be considered in this chapter.

Vesicoureteral Reflux

Primary vesicoureteral reflux is a congenital condition characterized by retrograde flow of urine from the bladder to one or both ureters. It was first described at the turn of the last century (1,2) and was known to occur frequently in rabbits and other rodents. Its differentiation from "chronic atrophic pyelonephritis" was not fully appreciated until Hodson and Edwards in 1960 (3) established the frequent association between vesicoureteral reflux and focal scars in children and noted the progression of the scars over time. Other important pioneers in this field were Hutch, Miller, and Hinman (4), McGovern, Marshall, and Paquin (5) and Stephens (6). Reflux is often transient and relatively benign and may only leave a fixed renal cortical scar. In the more severe forms, it can cause severe renal damage, hypertension, and occasionally massive proteinuria (reflux nephropathy). When both kidneys are involved, it can result in end-stage renal failure. Reflux most likely accounts for congenital aplastic kidneys that occur during fetal development.

Anatomic Findings

The ureter normally enters the bladder obliquely through a submucosal segment. Unlike veins, the ureter does not possess leaflets to prevent reflux of urine into the ureter during bladder contraction. Instead, during voiding, the ureteral meatus and submucosal segment are compressed and closed by the uretero-trigonal longitudinal muscles. The length of the intramural ureter and its submucosal segment are critical to maintain competence. The main factor that determines the effectiveness of the valve mechanism is the ratio of the submucosal tunnel length to the ureteral diameter (Fig. 5.1). Active

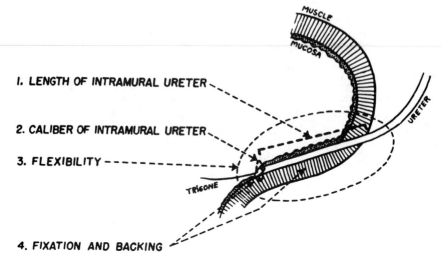

1. **LENGTH OF INTRAMURAL URETER**

2. **CALIBER OF INTRAMURAL URETER**

3. **FLEXIBILITY**

4. **FIXATION AND BACKING**

5. **INTRAVESICAL PRESSURE**

Figure 5.1. Diagrammatic summary of the mechanisms of the vesicoureteral junction. Reproduced with permission from McGovern JH, Marshall VF and Paquin AJ Jr (5).

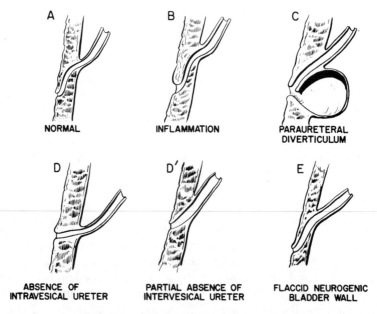

Figure 5.2. Intravesical position of the ureter in the normal person and in patients with vesicoureteral reflux. Redrawn with permission from King LR, et al. (7).

ureteral peristalsis during the flow of urine also tends to drive urine into the bladder. The valve mechanism is defective in individuals with vesicoureteral reflux because of failure of the longitudinal muscle to adequately constrict the submucosal ureter. In patients with reflux, the ureter usually enters the bladder trigone lateral to its normal position without adequate submucosal length (Fig. 5.2). The degree of lateral displacement of the ureteral orifice, as well as the shape, degree of patulousness and the length of the submucosal tunnel, can be visualized by cystoscopy. Vesicoureteral reflux is most pronounced in newborns and infants. As the child grows, the submucosal tunnel elongates and the ratio between the submucosal tunnel length and ureteral diameter decreases. The valve then becomes competent. Reflux tends to disappear with growth and development unless the mechanism is severely deranged.

Vesicoureteral reflux is graded somewhat differently by various groups. A simple scheme is shown in Figure 5.3. The International Reflux Study

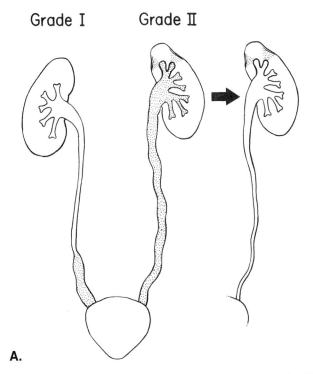

Grade I   Grade II

A.

Figure 5.3. Types of renal scarring associated with vesicoureteral reflux. **A.** In grade I reflux, urine enters the ureter only and does not produce renal scars. In grade II reflux, urine enters the renal pelvis and produces focal scars in the upper pole associated with blunting of the calices. Over time the reflux disappears, but the scars remain.

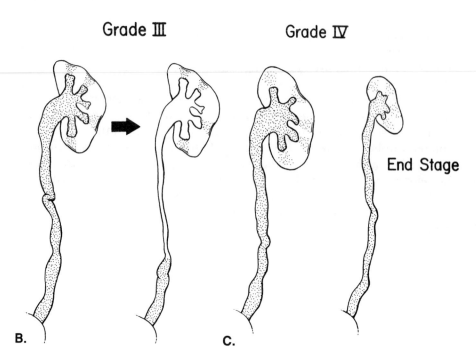

Grade III   Grade IV

End Stage

B.   **C.**

Figure 5.3 (continued). B. In grade III reflux, urine enters the hydronephrotic ureter and dilates the renal pelvis. There are several blunted calices associated with focal scars, generally at the polar regions of the kidney. Over time the reflux lessens, but the scars remain. **C.** In grade IV reflux, urine enters the grossly hydronephrotic ureter and markedly dilates the renal pelvis, giving the impression of severe "back pressure." The calices are blunted and there are multiple focal scars. Drawings are based on the work of Winberg J, Larson H and Bergstrom T (8) and Smellie JM and Norman C (9).

Group classification (10) is shown in Figure 5.4. Renal damage depends on the extent of the defect. Mild grades of reflux almost never produce renal damage (Figs. 5.3A,B). More severe grades may leave a small cortical scar in the polar regions of the kidney. Note, in the figure, the focal nature of the scars, their polar location, and segmental relation to a distorted or clubbed calyx. The most severe form of gross reflux results in a small atrophic, nonfunctioning kidney (Fig. 5.3C).

The natural history of vesicoureteral reflux in childhood is shown in Figure 5.5 (11). Note that each stage tends to lessen with time. Gross reflux is the most severe form and is more likely to lead to progressive renal damage.

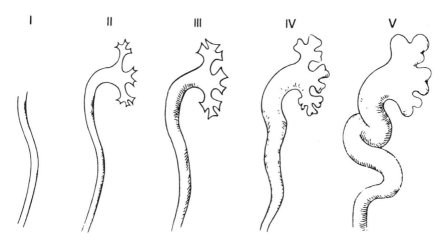

Figure 5.4. Grades of reflux according to the International Reflux Study classification. I. Reflux into ureter only. II. Reflux into the ureter, pelvis and calices with dilatation, but normal caliceal fornices. III. Reflux with mild or moderate dilatation and/or tortuosity of ureter and mild or moderate dilatation of renal pelvis, but no or slight blunting of fornices. IV. Reflux is associated with moderate dilatation and/or tortuosity of ureter, moderate dilatation of renal pelvis, and calices. Complete obliteration of sharp angle of fornices but maintenance of papillary impressions in majority of calices. V. Reflux produces gross dilatation and tortuosity of the ureter and gross dilatation of renal pelvis and calices. Papillary impressions are no longer visible in majority of calices. Reproduced with permission from International Reflux Study Committee (10).

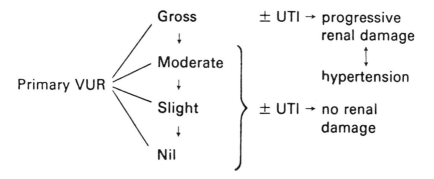

Figure 5.5. Diagram showing the natural history of primary vesicoureteral reflux (VUR). Gross VUR is the form that leads to progressive renal damage. This may occur in the absence of infection. VUR tend to improve with puberty and may disappear completely. Those patients who have renal damage are prone to develop hypertension. Reproduced with permission from Bailey RR (11).

Intrarenal Reflux

The focal nature of the scars associated with vesicoureteral reflux cannot be satisfactorily explained simply by back flow of urine. Pressure from the column of refluxing urine would be expected to be distributed uniformly throughout the renal pelvis and produce diffuse hydronephrosis. Hydronephrosis occurs in patients with uretero-pelvic junction obstruction or benign prostatic hypertrophy, but not with vesicoureteral reflux, except in its most severe form early in life. An attractive hypothesis to explain the focal lesions is based on the observation that certain regions of the kidney are more susceptible to back pressure. Radiologic cystograms in infants reveal that contrast material enters certain renal segments (12). This phenomenon is termed pyelotubular back flow or intrarenal reflux (Fig. 5.6).

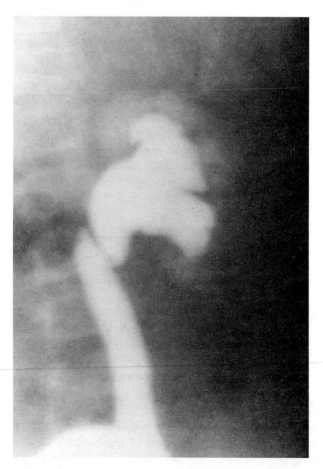

Figure 5.6. Intrarenal reflux in a week-old baby boy with bilateral high grade vesicoureteral reflux. (Courtesy of Dr. Stephen A. Koff)

Renal scars tend to be located in the affected regions and are more severe in young children. Similar observations have been made in miniature pigs (13).

The human kidney is formed by fusion of about 14 subunits. The average kidney contains between 8 to 10 papillae. Most of the papillae are cone shaped and drain only one lobe. Others are fused from several lobes and are compound. Intralobar fusion is maximal in the polar regions of the kidney. These regions tend to be drained by compound papillae. Papillae can thus be divided morphologically into two groups as shown in Figure 5.7. The first group has a convex surface in which the openings are narrow, slit-like orifices. These papillae do not permit intrarenal backflow even under conditions of high renal pelvic pressure. The second type are larger and drain compound lobes. They have a more complex structure with flat, concave, or deeply cleft-like profiles. The papillary duct openings are circular, open-mouthed orifices. These papillae allow contrast material to flow into the kidney, producing intrarenal reflux. They tend to be located in the polar regions, particularly in the upper pole.

Based on these observations, Ransley and Risdon (14) have proposed a "big bang" theory to account for focal renal scars. They postulated that three components are essential for scars to develop. These are 1) vesicoureteral reflux, 2) intrarenal reflux, and 3) superimposed urinary tract infection. It is now clear that severe renal damage may occur in the absence of infection, but superimposed infection can produce further damage (Table 5.1).

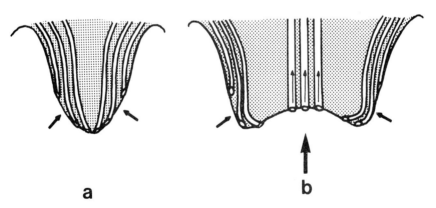

a   **b**

Figure 5.7. Renal papillary factors in intrarenal reflux. *a.* Convex papilla (non refluxing papilla). Crescentic or slit-like openings of collecting ducts obliquely enter the papilla. *b.* Concave or flat papilla (refluxing papilla). Round collecting ducts open at right angles into flat papilla. Redrawn with permission from Ransley PG (14).

Table 5.1. Evidence That Vesicoureteral Reflux Can Produce Renal Damage Without Infection

Reflux occurs *in utero* and neonates in the absence of infection.
The severity of the renal scar is associated closely with the extent of reflux.
The scars often are located in polar regions of the kidney where intrarenal reflux occurs.
Most of the renal damage occurs within the first few years of life and rarely is progressive.
Reflux tends to disappear with time, but the scars often remain.
Renal scars may be found in children with reflux in the absence of pyelonephritis.
Renal scars can be produced in pigs and monkeys in the absence of infection.
Uncomplicated pyelonephritis in adults rarely results in renal scars.
Adults rarely develop reflux except with paraplegia, tuberculosis, or bilharziasis.

Diagnostic Methods

The voiding cystourethrogram is the "gold standard" to demonstrate vesicoureteral reflux. It is performed by instilling iodinated contrast material into the bladder by means of a catheter until bladder capacity is reached. Then, the child voids, the flow of contrast material is visualized by fluoroscopy, and radiographs are obtained (15) (Fig. 5.8). Radionuclide cystography is similar except that ^{99m}technetium pertechnetate is instilled followed by continuous monitoring with a gamma scintillation camera (Fig. 5.9). Voiding cystourethrography with radiocontrast material is said to be more accurate in characterizing and grading reflux. Radionuclide cystography uses a lower radiation dose, permits continuous monitoring, and is useful for screening.

There is considerable debate in the literature concerning the best method to screen for reflux in a child with urinary tract infection. Some groups perform voiding cystourethrograms on all children with urinary tract infections. Others recommend ultrasonography as the initial imaging procedure and reserve voiding cystourethrography for children with abnormal sonograms (16).

A major advance is the use of ^{99m}technetium dimercaptosuccinic acid (DMSA) renal scintography to evaluate pyelonephritis and differentiate renal scars resulting from reflux (17). Voiding cystourethrograph can then be done to confirm the diagnosis and obtain more detailed information. Scans are particularly attractive because they allow the physician to "see" the pyelonephritic lesion and follow its evolution. DMSA scans are much more definitive than surrogate tests for "upper tract infection" (C-reactive protein, erythrocyte sedimentation rate, antibody-coated bacteria, and various isoenzymes).

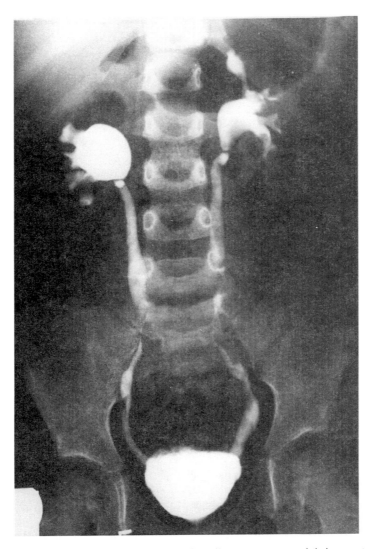

Figure 5.8. Voiding cystourethrogram with radiocontrast material demonstrating vesicoureteral reflux in a young child. (Courtesy of Dr. Stephen A. Koff)

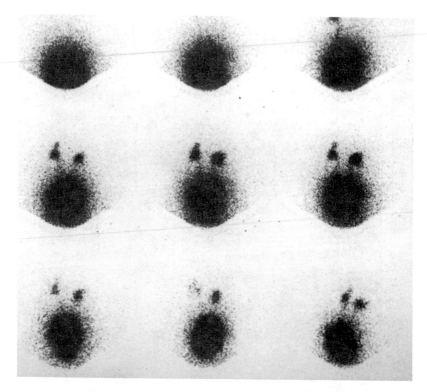

Figure 5.9. Voiding cystourethrogram using radionuclide cystography with
^{99m}technetium pertechnetate in the same child shown in Figure 5.8. The
sequence consist of adding incremental quantities of contrast material
beginning at 50 ml (scan upper left) to 250 ml (last scan row two). A prevoid
film is then obtained (first scan last row), followed by postvoid films (last two
scans). (Courtesy of Dr. Stephen A. Koff)

Key Points About Detection of Vesicoureteral Reflux

- The voiding cystourethrogram is the "gold" standard. It offers the additional advantage of detecting abnormalities of the bladder and dysfunctional voiding.
- ^{99m}technetium pertechnatate cystography uses less radiation and allows physiologic monitoring.
- Renal ultrasonography is noninvasive and is an acceptable method to screen children for reflux and other congenital abnormalities of the urinary tract. Children with abnormal sonograms should be investigated by voiding cystourethrogram.
- Renal scintography with ^{99m}technetium dimercaptosuccinic acid (DMSA) offers excellent visualization of the pyelonephritic lesion and can identify patients who should be investigated by voiding cystourethrogram.
- Intravenous urograms and CT scans should be reserved for special diagnostic problems.
- Because grades I–II reflux disappear spontaneously and rarely produce renal scars, it really does not matter if they are missed.

Associated Bladder Abnormalities

Many children with reflux also have a large and often trabeculated bladder. Some children also have an associated megacolon (Hirschsprung's disease) (18) and constipation (19). The large bladder (megacystis syndrome) was thought to be caused by bladder obstruction. In the past, a Y-V plasty of the bladder neck was performed at the time the ureters were reimplanted to improve emptying of the bladder. These combined procedures are rarely done today because the results have not been entirely satisfactory and other methods have been developed to manage bladder function. Distal urethral stenosis and urethral caliber are not related to reflux, and operations to dilate the urethra are not recommended.

It has been proposed that functional urinary tract obstruction caused by dysfunctional voiding can initiate and perpetuate vesicoureteral reflux (20,21). Koff and Murtagh (22) studied a large group of children with vesicoureteral reflux using urodynamic techniques to identify uninhibited bladder contractions with voluntary sphincteric obstruction (dyssynergia). They divided the patients into two groups. One received anticholinergic drugs and the other served as a control. Both groups received antimicrobial prophylaxis. They reported that anticholinergic drugs reduced the frequency of recurrent urinary infection and significantly reduced the frequency of reflux compared to untreated controls. In another study, Sullivan, Purcell, and Gregory (23) obtained excellent results with intermittent catheterization in children with neurogenic bladders and reflux. Not all patients with vesicoureteral reflux will be cured by management of the bladder alone, particularly when the reflux is severe.

An Illustrative Case

The following case in a 38-year-old woman illustrates the relation between reflux and bladder abnormalities. As a child, she had severe, bilateral reflux and an atonic bladder. The ureters were successfully reimplanted at age 7. She was seen at age 40 because of recurrent episodes of pyelonephritis despite prolonged and intensive therapy. Vesicoureteral reflux was no longer present, but she had a large, poorly emptying, atonic bladder and bilateral hydronephrosis (Fig. 5.10). She has had persistent bacteriuria, which is unresponsive to treatment, for the past eight years. Drugs to improve detrusor function and relax the external sphincter have not been effective. She is not compliant with intermittent self-catheterization. Despite these difficulties, her serum creatinine has remained normal.

Reflux Nephropathy

The term "reflux nephropathy" is used to describe renal damage that results from vesicoureteral reflux. The term "chronic atrophic pyelonephritis" is no

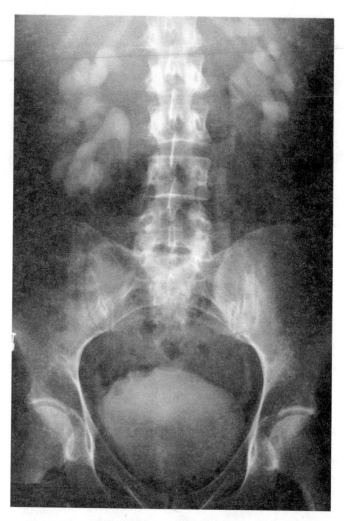

Figure 5.10. Persistent atonic, nonemptying bladder with severe hydronephrosis in a 38-year-old woman who had reimplantation of the ureters for severe vesicoureteral reflux at age 7 years. The reflux is no longer present, but the associated atonic bladder remains. Failure of the bladder to empty spontaneously is associated with "back-up" hydronephrosis.

longer used because the renal damage can occur in the absence of infection. The renal cortical scars and distorted renal calices produced by vesicoureteral reflux are radiographically indistinguishable from those resulting from pyelonephritis. The confusion between pyelonephritis and reflux nephropathy accounts for the high rates of pyelonephritis described in the older literature and the strong association noted between pyelonephritis and hypertension (see Pyelonephritis from a Historical View in Chapter 8). It now appears that so-called *pyelonephritis lenta* and "abacterial" pyelonephritis are actually the result of reflux nephropathy. This conceptual change was brought about by advances in uroradiology and long-term prospective studies of the natural history of reflux (24–26). It is also now possible to differentiate renal scars produced by reflux and acute pyelonephritis in young children by combined use of ^{99m}technesium DMSA scans and cystourethrograms.

The damage from reflux may be limited to cortical renal scars with minimal, if any, reduction in overall renal function. In the more severe cases, the renal lesions may be large enough to produce complete loss of renal function in the affected kidney. Reflux nephropathy is reported to be responsible for about 30% of cases of severe hypertension and 15% of chronic renal failure in children (27). Patients with severe reflux nephropathy may develop massive proteinuria, hypertension, and end-stage renal failure.

The renal lesions consist of linear, discrete sublobar medullary scars that extend from the inner medulla to the cortex (28). Renal biopsies may show mesangial glomerular lesions and focal sclerosing glomerulopathy (29) and interstitial nephritis (30) with deposits of Tamm-Horsfall protein in the renal interstitium (31). It has been postulated by several investigators that the renal damage in reflux nephropathy may be due, in part, to autoantibodies directed against Tamm-Horsfall protein. Some have proposed that measurement of the antibody response to Tamm-Horsfall protein might be helpful to detect obstructive uropathy (32), whereas others have found this to be of no value as a screening procedure for vesicoureteral reflux (33). Measurement of the excretion of N-acetyl-β-D-glucosaminidase (NAG) (34), endothelin-1 (35), and interleukin-8 (36) has been suggested as a means to assess tubular dysfunction associated with reflux, but it should be considered a research tool.

The evidence for the central role of vesicoureteral reflux in producing renal damage, even without infection, is summarized in Table 5.1. Most experts in this field believe that infection superimposed upon vesicoureteral reflux can produce further renal damage and should be detected early and prevented. These issues will be discussed further in the section on Management.

An Illustrative Case

The following case is presented to demonstrate how reflux nephropathy can be confused with acute and chronic pyelonephritis. The case also demonstrates that vesicoureteral reflux in the absence of infection can produce severe renal damage.

The patient was a 23-year-old nulliparous woman who had been in good health all of her life. She denied ever having had urinary tract infections in the past. About 2 years after marriage, she developed the sudden onset of urgency, frequency, dysuria, and severe right flank pain. On admission, she was an acutely ill, lean young woman in obvious pain. Her blood pressure was in the normal range; pulse was 120 per minute and her temperature was 102° F. Physical examination was unremarkable except for exquisite right flank tenderness. The white blood count was 12,000 per cu mm with a shift to the left. The urine was loaded with pus cells and bacteria. Blood cultures were sterile, but the urine culture revealed > 10^5 cfu/ml of *E. coli.* She was treated with 500 mg ampicillin 4 times a day for 10 days and did well. Three months later the same symptoms recurred, but were more mild. Large numbers of *E. coli* were again recovered from the urine. She responded well to a 2-week course of nitrofurantoin. An intravenous urogram revealed a markedly atrophic right kidney with focal thinning of the renal cortex and corresponding clubbed calices. The left kidney was enlarged with normal caliceal architecture. (Fig. 5.11). There were no abnormalities of the ureter or the bladder. A cystourethrogram revealed vesicoureteral reflux on the right, clearly outlining the segmentally dilated calices (Fig. 5.12). Over the next 10 years, she had no further urinary tract infections and both her blood pressure and serum creatinine remained normal. She did not receive prophylactic antimicrobial therapy.

This patient would have been considered to have "chronic atrophic pyelonephritis" in the past. Her current diagnosis is unilateral reflux

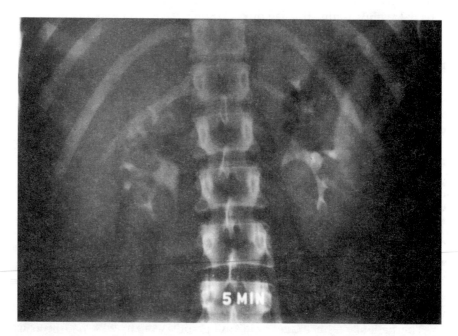

Figure 5.11. Intravenous urogram in a 23-year-old woman with recent onset of acute pyelonephritis. Note the small kidney on right side with blunting of calices and marked thinning of renal cortex. The left kidney is markedly hypertrophic, but the collecting system is otherwise normal.

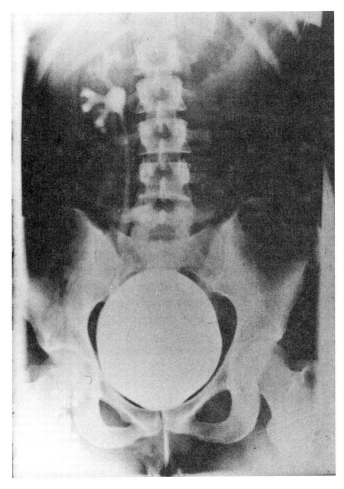

Figure 5.12. Voiding cystourethrogram of the same patient shown in Figure 5.11. Note the presence of marked vesicoureteral reflux on right side.

nephropathy with compensatory hypertrophy of the contralateral kidney. The small right kidney and the hypertrophic left kidney could not have been caused by the episode of acute pyelonephritis a few months earlier. These changes take years to develop. The finding of vesicoureteral reflux on the same side as the damaged kidney strongly argues that the damage was caused by reflux that occurred during fetal life or shortly after birth. It is now well known that reflux can produce severe renal damage in the absence of infection. The underlying vesicoureteral reflux would not have been detected had she not developed acute pyelonephritis. She appears to be relatively insusceptible to urinary tract infections despite the presence of reflux.

Frequency of Vesicoureteral Reflux and Reflux Nephropathy

The frequency of vesicoureteral reflux is closely related to age and sex. It can be detected by antenatal ultrasound as early as 16 to 17 weeks of gestation. The highest rates are found in neonates and during the first 2 to 3 years of life. As the ureterovesical valve mechanism matures, both the magnitude and frequency of reflux gradually fall. Reflux is uncommon among adults, but residual scars may remain.

During Fetal Life

Urinary anomalies are present in about 1 to 2 per 1,000 fetuses, depending on the criteria selected and the stage of pregnancy (37–41). Most of the abnormalities consist of hydronephrosis or hydroureter, multicystic dysplasia of the kidney, vesicoureteral reflux, and bladder obstruction secondary to posterior urethral valves. Hydronephrosis is usually produced by reversible physiologic changes in an elastic system (41). Mild degrees of hydronephrosis tend to disappear by birth. Persistent hydronephrosis, caused by

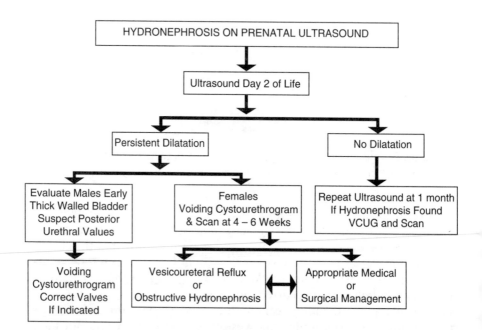

Figure 5.13. An algorithm for neonatal evaluation of hydronephrosis detected by antenatal ultrasound. Adapted and modified from Blyth B, Snider HW, and Duckett JW (41).

obstruction at the ureteropelvic junction, can produce severe renal damage and needs to be repaired. About 10% of prenatal hydronephrosis is caused by primary vesicoureteral reflux. There is a marked predominance in males (more than 4:1); two-thirds will have bilateral reflux (42). An algorithm to evaluate neonates found to have hydronephrosis by antenatal ultrasound is presented in Figure 5.13.

Newborns

The frequency of reflux in newborns with urinary tract infections ranges from about 50% to 70% (43,44). The rates are about the same in boys and girls. Most cases are detected in the first 2 months of life when urinary tract infections are most common.

Older Children and Adults

The frequency of vesicoureteral reflux as determined in a large urologic referral practice is shown in Figures 5.14 and 5.15. Reflux was detected in 70% of children under the age of 1 year and fell to about 10% by age 12. Only 4.4% of adults over the age of 21 years referred because of recurrent urinary tract infection were found to have reflux. The frequency of reflux among school girls with asymptomatic bacteriuria ranges from about 19% to 35% (46). It decreases with age and is not influenced by socioeconomic class. A close correlation exists between the presence of reflux and renal scars (Table 5.2).

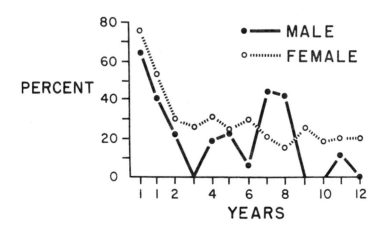

Figure 5.14. Prevalence of reflux by age group for male and female patients relative to the total number of children studied for each age group. Reproduced with permission from Baker R, Maxted W, Maylath J, and Shuman I (45).

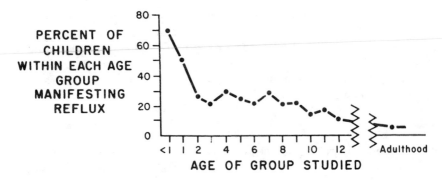

Figure 5.15. Number of patients at a given age manifesting reflux related to the total number of patients of each age group studied that were referred to a urologic practice. Reproduced with permission from Baker R, Maxted W, Maylath J, and Shuman I (45).

Relation To Race

In the large epidemiologic study of urinary tract infections among school children, shown in Table 5.2, the prevalence of vesicoureteral reflux in white girls was twice that in black girls. Similarly, vesicoureteral reflux was found 3.4 times more in white girls than black girls who were evaluated for symptomatic urinary tract infections (47). In a more recent series, the ratio was almost tenfold higher in white girls (48). Reflux also cleared more rapidly among the black girls, without progression of scars.

Table 5.2. Characteristics of School Girls with Asymptomatic Bacteriuria Found to Have Vesicoureteral Reflux on an Initial Cystourethrogram*

Group	Studied No.	Reflux No.	Present %
Race			
White	115	24	20.8
Black	22	2	9.0
Total	137	26*	18.9
Age (White)			
5–9 years	37	13	35.1
10–14 years	52	8	15.3
15 or more years	26	3	11.5
Socio-economic (White)			
High	41	7	17.0
Low	62	13	20.9

*Ten of these girls (35%) also had cortical scars of caliectasis. From Kunin CM (46).

Reflux in Siblings

Numerous reports exist of vesicoureteral reflux among siblings. The rates among siblings and first order relatives range from about 34% to 45%, depending on age and method of study (49–52). Various forms of genetic inheritance have been proposed, including a dominant gene with incomplete expression. Initial reports of an association with histocompatibility antigens B12 and Aw32 have not be substantiated. Because of this high association, some investigators recommend that siblings under 5 years of age undergo cystourethrographic studies.

Frequency of Reflux Nephropathy

Children and adults with uncomplicated urinary infections rarely develop end-stage renal failure unless there are important underlying structural or neurologic lesions (see Chapter 1). It is now well appreciated that reflux nephropathy accounts for much of the renal damage. For example, in various series of adults with end-stage renal disease entering dialysis and transplant programs, about 15% to 25% have reflux nephropathy (53,54). Many of the patients have severe hypertension (29) and significant proteinuria, which at times may be massive (55). Renal calculi, including large staghorn stones, may occur as a consequence of long-standing infection, particularly with urease-producing organisms.

Current Concepts About Vesicoureteral Reflux and Reflux Nephropathy

- Reflux is a congenital defect of the vesicoureteral valve.
- Reflux occurs during intrauterine life at a rate of 4 times greater in boys than in girls.
- Most of the renal damage is produced by high grades of reflux during the first 2 months of life.
- Reflux is frequent among siblings.
- Black children appear to be less prone to reflux than white children.
- Moderate and mild grades of reflux disappear with growth and development and may leave small residual scars.
- Renal scars may be insignificant provided that renal function is not impaired.
- More severe grades of reflux tend to lessen over time.
- Severe renal damage may occur even in the absence of infection.
- Reflux is often associated with bladder and bowel dysfunction.
- The large, trabeculated bladder may mimic obstructive uropathy.

Management

The understanding of the natural history and management of vesicoureteral reflux has markedly improved over the past 30 years. Until recently, it was standard practice to correct reflux by ureteroneocystostomy. The procedure consists of detaching the ureters from the bladder, tailoring them to remove excessive hydroureteric tissue, and reimplanting them into the bladder through a submucosal tunnel of sufficient length to establish a normal closing mechanism. The operations were successful in most cases. Some enthusiastic surgeons did not limit the procedure to children with high grades of reflux, but included cases with mild to moderate grades. YV plasty of the bladder neck was performed in children with the so-called "megacystis syndrome." It was thought that their large, poorly emptying bladders were caused by bladder neck obstruction. It now appears that this syndrome is caused by bladder dysfunction (see the illustrative case in this chapter). Despite the good surgical outcome of ureteroneocystostomy and related procedures, the absence of untreated controls and the use of concomitant antimicrobial therapy made it impossible to determine whether it was truly beneficial in preventing renal damage. In addition, it became increasingly apparent that reflux tended to disappear even when left untreated.

Attitudes toward operative intervention changed dramatically when a group in Christchurch, New Zealand (44) chose to observe infants with vesicoureteral reflux without surgery. The only treatment was for the presenting urinary tract infection and recurrent episodes. They found that gross reflux was accompanied by a high incidence of initial and progressive renal damage. In most instances, mild to moderate reflux disappeared spontaneously and severe grades lessened over time. Similar results were reported by other investigators (8,46). Soon thereafter, Smellie and Normand (25) demonstrated that most children, even with severe grades of reflux, could be managed conservatively if given low doses of prophylactic antimicrobial drugs to prevent urinary tract infections. The results of their 10-year study are shown in Figure 5.16. Reflux disappeared over time in most children, except for those with the most severe grade IV lesions. They also noted normal growth of the effected kidneys over time. They were so convinced that infection superimposed on reflux would result in renal damage that they did not include controls in their series. Their work led to the current practice to use long-term prophylaxis in children with reflux under 3 to 5 years of age until the reflux virtually disappears.

The next development that dramatically changed the management of vesicoureteral reflux, was four large controlled trials with follow-up for 4 to 5 years (56). Medical management with prophylactic antimicrobial drugs was shown to be equally as effective as surgery in preventing progressive renal damage in children with grade III-IV reflux. The current general consensus is that operative intervention should be reserved for children who have persistent or recurrent infection despite prophylaxis.

Does Infection Increase the Risk of Renal Damage?

It seems reasonable that urinary tract infections might produce additional renal damage in patients with reflux. Much of the clinical evidence for this notion is based on uncontrolled observations. These consist of 1) the coincidental

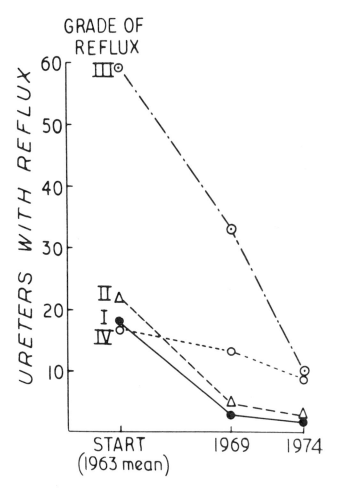

Figure 5.16. Prognosis for vesicoureteral reflux (VUR) of differing severity in 75 children (112 refluxing ureters) managed with low-dose prophylaxis and followed for 9 to 15 years. Grade I VUR is minimal, grades II and III extend up to the kidney, without dilatation, in grade II on voiding only, and grade IV includes all ureters with dilatation of ureter or renal pelvis. Reproduced with permission from Smellie JM (25).

finding of reflux in children with infection, 2) case studies demonstrating additional renal damage associated with acute infection, and 3) fewer attacks of pyelonephritis in children who have undergone reflux surgery.

Evidence in experimental animals that support the notion that infection may produce further damage is based on the following facts: 1) a renal scar always occurs when infection is superimposed on intrarenal reflux in piglets (13); 2) a combination of intrarenal reflux, P-fimbriated *E. coli,* and absence of prior immunization are synergistic in producing reflux nephropathy in piglets (57); and 3) sterile reflux can produce reflux nephropathy in infant monkeys. When bacteria are introduced, maturation of the ureterovesical junction is delayed and reflux persists longer (58).

Arguments that infection may not be as important as once supposed are based on the following observations: 1) most of the renal damage occurs within the first few months of life even in the absence of infection; 2) reflux produces about the same amount of damage in newborn males as females, even though males are less susceptible to infection; 3) adults (as shown in the first illustrative case) may develop severe reflux nephropathy with end-stage renal damage (when both kidneys are involved) despite the absence of infection (59); 4) children with reflux are not at greater risk of developing urinary tract infections than those without (46); and 5) children tend to be infected with less virulent strains of *E. coli* (60).

Indications for Antimicrobial Prophylaxis

It is common practice to continue antimicrobial prophylaxis until reflux disappears. This may take 3 or 4 years. Winberg (61) has argued that this may not be necessary or desirable for all children. He points out the following: 1) most of the infections and damage occur in the first year of life, so why continue prophylaxis longer?; 2) post-infectious scars can be prevented in children by treating symptoms as soon as they occur (62); and 3) recurrent infections are not common among boys. He argues that close follow-up to detect recurrent infection may be preferred over stereotyped programs that do not allow for an individualized approach. Prophylaxis may be most beneficial in children who are socially neglected and not likely to have ready access to medical care.

Current Concepts of Management of Vesicoureteral Reflux

- Prophylactic antimicrobial therapy is as effective as operative repair in preventing renal damage.
- It is customary to continue prophylaxis until reflux disappears.
- Treatment of symptomatic episodes, particularly in boys, may be equally effective.
- Another approach is to use prophylaxis during the first year of life and promptly treat symptomatic infections thereafter.
- Pharmacologic methods and intermittent catheterization are useful in children with bladder dysfunction associated with reflux.
- Operative repair may be indicated in children with severe grades of reflux who have persistent infection despite medical management.

Questions That Need to be Resolved

Despite the major advances in understanding the natural history of vesicoureteral reflux and reflux nephropathy, several questions still need to be resolved: 1) Given the low rate of antenatal hydronephrosis and the fact that it is often physiological, is it worthwhile and cost-effective to perform ultrasound studies on all pregnant women at 20 weeks of gestation? 2) Given the high rate of reflux among siblings, is it worthwhile to perform ultrasound examinations after the first year of life when most of the renal damage has already been done? 3) Should search for reflux and other congenital abnormalities of the urinary tract be reserved for infants with infection? If so, many cases of reflux, obstructive hydronephrosis, and posterior urethral valves would be missed. 4) Is it really necessary to detect reflux early because surgical intervention is usually not warranted and infection can be treated as soon as it occurs? These hot issues can be resolved only by careful assessment of the current information available to us and by clinical trials.

Major Issues About Vesicoureteral Reflux That Still Need To Be Resolved

Screening by Ultrasound
Is antenatal screening worthwhile?
Should all neonates be screened?
Should all siblings of cases be screened?

Management
Should all young children receive long-term prophylaxis?
If so, what is the proper duration of prophylaxis?
Would monitoring for infection and short term treatment be equally effective?
Do circumcised boys need to receive long-term prophylaxis?
What are the indications for operative repair?
Is persistent infection a valid indication for operative repair?

References

1. Sampson J A. Ascending renal infection with special reference to the reflux of urine from bladder into the ureters. Bull Johns Hopkins Hosp 1903;14:334–352.
2. Gruber CM. Ureterovesical valve. J Urol 1929;22:275–292.
3. Hodson J, Edwards D. Chronic pyelonephritis and vesicoureteric reflux. Clin Radiol 1960;11:219–231.
4. Hutch JA, Miller ER, Hinman F Jr. Vesicoureteral reflux. Am J Med 1963;34:338–349.
5. McGovern JH, Marshall VF, Paquin AJ Jr. Vesicoureteral regurgitation in children. J Urol 1960;83:122–149.
6. Stephens FD, Lenaghan D. The anatomical basis and dynamics of vesicoureteral reflux. J Urol 1962;87:669–680.
7. King LR, Surian MA, Wendel R, et al. Vesicoureteral reflux. JAMA 1968;203:169–174.
8. Winberg J, Larson H, Bergstrom T. Comparison of the natural history of urinary infection in children with and without vesico-ureteral reflux. In: Kincaid-Smith P, Fairly KF, eds. Renal inflammation and scarring. Melbourne: Mercedes, 1970:293–302.
9. Smellie J, Norman C. Reflux nephropathy in children. In: Hodson J, Kincaid-Smith P, eds. Reflux nephropathy. New York: Masson et Cie, 1979:14–20.
10. Report of the International Reflux Study Committee. Medical versus surgical treatment of primary vesicoureteral reflux. A prospective international reflux study in children. J Urol 1981;125:277–283.
11. Bailey RR. The relationship of vesico-ureteric reflux to urinary tract infection and chronic pyelonephritis with reflux nephropathy. Clin Nephrol 1973;1:132–141.
12. Rolleston GL, Maling TMJ, Hodson CJ. Intrarenal reflux and the scarred kidney. Arch Dis Child 1974;49:531–539.

13. Hodson CJ, Craven JD, Lewis DG, et al. Experimental obstructive nephropathy in the pig. Br J Urol (suppl) 1969;41:4–51.
14. Ransley PG, Risdon RA. Renal papillary morphology in infants and young children. Urol Res 1975;3:111–113.
15. Lebowitz RL. The detection and characterization of vesicoureteral reflux in the child. J Urol 1992;148:1640–1642.
16. Kangarloo H, Gold RH, Fine RN, et al. Urinary tract infection in infants and children evaluated by ultrasound. Radiology 1985;154:367–373.
17. Rushton HG, Majd M. Dimercaptosuccinic acid renal scintigraphy for the evaluation of pyelonephritis and scarring: a review of experimental and clinical studies. J Urol 1992;148:1726–1732.
18. Swenson O, Fisher JH. The relation of megacolon and megaloureter. N Engl J Med 1955;253:1147–1150.
19. O'Regan S, Schick E, Hamburger B, et al. Constipation associated with vesicoureteral reflux. J Urol 1986;28:394–396.
20. Allen TD. Vesicoureteral reflux and the unstable bladder. J Urol 1985;134:1180.
21. Koff SA. Relationship between dysfunctional voiding and reflux. J Urol 1992;148:1703–1705.
22. Koff SA, Murtagh DS. The uninhibited bladder in children: effect of treatment on recurrence of urinary infection and on vesicoureteral reflux resolution. J Urol 1983;130:1138–1141.
23. Sullivan T, Purcell MM, Gregory JG. The management of vesicoureteral reflux in the pediatric neurogenic bladder. J Urol 1981;125:65–66.
24. Rolleston GL, Shannon FT, Utley WLF. Relationship of infantile vesicoureteric reflux to renal damage. Br Med J 1970;1:460–463.
25. Smellie JM. Reflections on 30 years of treating children with urinary tract infections. J Urol 1991;146:665–668.
26. Winberg J. Commentary: progressive renal damage from infection with or without reflux. J Urol 1992;148:1733–1734.
27. Goldraich NP, Goldraich IH, Anselmi OE, et al. Reflux nephropathy: the clinical picture in South Brazilian children. Contrib Nephrol 1984;39:52–67.
28. Bernstein J, Arant Jr BS. Morphological characteristics of segmental renal scarring in vesicoureteral reflux. J Urol 1992;148:1712–1714.
29. Torres VE, Malek RS, Svensson JP. Vesicoureteral reflux in the adult II. Nephropathy, hypertension and stones. J Urol 1983;130:41–44.
30. Stickler GB, Kelalis PP, Burke EC, et al. Primary interstitial nephritis with reflux. a cause of hypertension. Amer J Dis Child 1971;122:144–148.
31. Cotran RS, Hodson CJ. Extratubular localization of Tamm-Horsfall protein in experimental reflux nephropathy in the pig. In: Hodson J, Kincaid-Smith P, eds. Reflux nephropathy. New York: Masson et Cie, 1979:213–219.
32. Marier R, Fong E, Jansen M, et al. Antibody to Tamm-Horsfall protein in patients with urinary tract obstruction and vesicoureteral reflux. J Infect Dis 1978;138:781–790.
33. Fasth A, Hanson LA, Asscher AW. Autoantibodies to Tamm-Horsfall protein in detection of vesicoureteric reflux and kidney scarring. Arch Dis Child 1977;52:560–562.
34. Carr MC, Peters CA, Retik AB, et al. Urinary levels of renal tubular enzyme N-acetyl-B-D-Glucosaminidase in relation to grade of vesicoureteral reflux. J Urol 1991;146:654–656.
35. Komeyama T, Takeda M, Katayama Y, et al. Value of urinary endothelin-1 in patients with primary vesicoureteral reflux. Nephron 1993;65:537–540.
36. Haraoka M, Senoh K, Ogata N, et al. Elevated interleukin-8 levels in the urine of children with renal scarring and/or vesicoureteral reflux. J Urol 1996;155:678–680.
37. Gloor JM, Ogburn Jr PL, Breckle RJ, et al. Urinary tract anomalies detected by prenatal ultrasound examination at Mayo Clinic Rochester. Mayo Clin Proc 1995;70:526–531.
38. Watson AR, Readett D, Nelson CS, et al. Dilemmas associated with antenatally detected urinary tract abnormalities. Arch Dis Child 1988;63:719–722.
39. Madarikan BA, Hayward C, Roberts GM, et al. Clinical outcome of fetal uropathy. Arch Dis Child 1988;63:961–963.
40. Gunn TR, Mora JD, Pease AP. Outcome after antenatal diagnosis of upper urinary tract dilatation by ultrasonography. Arch Dis Child 1988;63:1240–1243.

41. Blyth B, Snyder HM, Duckett JW. Antenatal diagnosis and subsequent management of hydronephrosis. J Urol 1993;149:693–698.
42. Elder JS. Commentary: importance of antenatal diagnosis of vesicoureteral reflux. J Urol 1992;148:1750–1754.
43. Abbott GD. Neonatal bacteriuria: a prospective study in 1460 infants. Br Med J 1972;1:267–269.
44. Shannon FT. The significance and management of vesico-ureteric reflux in infancy. In: Kincaid-Smith P, Fairly KF, eds. Renal inflammation and scarring. Melbourne: Mercedes, 1970:241–245.
45. Baker R, Maxted W, Maylath J, et al. Relation of age, sex and infection to reflux: data indicating high rate of spontaneous cure rate in pediatric patients. J Urol 1966;95:27–32.
46. Kunin CM. A ten-year study of bacteriuria in school girls: final report of bacteriologic, urologic and epidemiologic findings. J Infect Dis 1970;122:382–393.
47. Askari A, Belman AB. Vesicoureteral reflux in black girls. J Urol 1982;127.747–748.
48. Skoog SJ, Belman AB. Primary vesicoureteral reflux in the black child. Pediatrics 1991;87:538–543.
49. Noe HN. The long-term results of prospective sibling reflux screening. J Urol 1992;148:1739–1742.
50. Bailey RR, Janus E, McLoughlin K, et al. Familial and genetic data in reflux nephropathy. Contrib Nephrol 1984;39:40–51.
51. Aggarwal VK, Jones KV. Vesicoureteric reflux: screening of first degree relatives. Arch Dis Child 1989;64:1538–1541.
52. Van den Abbeele AD, Treves ST, Lebowitz RL, et al. Vesicoureteral reflux in asymptomatic siblings of patients with known reflux: radionuclide cystography. Pediatrics 1987;79:147–153.
53. Bailey RR, Lynn KL, Smith AH. Long-term follow-up of infants with gross vesicoureteral reflux. J Urol 1992;148:1709–1711.
54. Huland H, Bosch R. Chronic pyelonephritis as a cause of end stage renal disease. J Urol 1982;127:642–643.
55. Pillay VG, Battifora H, Schwartz FD, et al. Massive proteinuria associated with vesicoureteral reflux. Lancet 1969;2:1272–1273.
56. Weiss R, Duckett J, Spitzer A. Results of a randomized clinical trial of medical versus surgical management of infants and children with grades III and IV primary vesicoureteral reflux (United States). J Urol 1992;148:1667–1673.
57. Torres VE, Kramer SA, Holley KE, et al. Interaction of multiple risk factors in the pathogenesis of experimental reflux nephropathy in the pig. J Urol 1985;133:131–135.
58. Roberts JA. Pathogenesis of pyelonephritis. J Urol 1983;129:1102–1106.
59. Salvatierra Jr O, Tanagho EA. Reflux as a cause of end stage kidney disease: report of 32 cases. J Urol 1977;117:441–443.
60. Lomberg H, Hellstrom M, Jodal U, et al. Virulence-associated traits in *E. coli* causing first and recurrent episodes of urinary tract infection in children with or without vesicoureteral reflux. J Infect Dis 1984;150:561–569.
61. Winberg J. Commentary: progressive renal damage from infection with or without reflux. J Urol 1992;148:1733–1734.
62. Elo J, Tallgren LG, Alfthan O, et al. Character of urinary tract infections and pyelonephritic scarring after antireflux surgery. J Urol 1983;129:343–346.

Urinary Tract Infections in Adults

*Pregnancy, Diabetes, the Elderly,
Renal Transplantation, Hypertension,
and Other Risk Factors*

Overview

In previous chapters we have delineated the various ways urinary tract infections are expressed and shown how the concept of significant bacteriuria and the quantitative bacterial count are used to diagnose and understand the epidemiology and natural history of urinary tract infections in children. This chapter deals with urinary tract infections in adults. We will begin with a discussion of uncomplicated urinary tract infections in women and consider the key issues that determine their susceptibility to infection. These issues include innate susceptibility, the putative roles of body habits, and sexual activity on acquisition of infection. Urinary tract infections in women are important complications of diabetes and pregnancy and are a contributing factor to premature birth. Urinary tract infections in men exhibit a distinctly different epidemiology and natural history and often are linked to infections of the prostate gland. Urinary infections are common in the elderly, but they are usually benign unless they are associated with urinary catheters, foreign bodies, or neurologic or obstructive uropathy. Other topics include the impact of urinary tract infections on hypertension, polycystic kidney disease, sickle cell disease, renal transplantation, and cancer. The distinction between uncomplicated and complicated infections continues to be emphasized throughout this book as the paramount factor that determines renal damage.

Uncomplicated Urinary Infections in Women

Uncomplicated urinary tract infections in adult women produce considerable morbidity but rarely cause significant renal damage. The diagnosis is readily established from the clinical history and examination of the urine. The invading microorganisms are *E. coli,* other gram negative enteric bacteria, *Staphylococcus saprophyticus,* and enterococci. The infection usually responds within a few days to specific therapy, but recurrence is common. Despite their benign course, uncomplicated urinary infections in women produce considerable discomfort and cause a great deal of concern. Some women never have a urinary tract infection. Others may have an occasional episode of pyuria-dysuria or cystitis or acute pyelonephritis. A relatively small group of women suffer from distressingly frequent symptomatic episodes. This section will consider the epidemiology of urinary tract infections in women, consider the factors that are thought to predispose them to infection, and touch briefly on host-parasite relationships. Special attention is given to the putative role of sexual intercourse and the effect of urinary tract infections on pregnancy and diabetes. A more detailed discussion of the pathogenesis of infection is presented in Chapter 11.

Epidemiology

The epidemiology of urinary tract infections in adult women is presented in Chapter 1 (see Figure 1.1). To recapitulate briefly, urinary tract infections in females occur throughout life and increase with age. About half of adult women report that they had a urinary tract infection at some time during their life. In the United States, there were 5,740,000 office visits to physicians in 1990 for one of the following primary complaints: painful urination, frequency and urgency, or urinary tract infection. Most of the visits (75.8%) were made by females and most of the care is provided by general physicians.

The epidemiologic dynamics are similar to those in school girls (Figure 4.1). The prevalence of significant bacteriuria in Caucasian women aged 16 to 19 years is about 2% to 4% and rises about 1% per decade to about 10% in women over the age of 70 (1) (Fig. 6.1). Higher rates are reported in elderly women in hospitals and nursing homes. The prevalence of bacteriuria is somewhat greater in married women and increases with parity. The lowest rates are found in Roman Catholic nuns, regardless of race (2) (Fig. 6.2).

Figure 6.1. Prevalence of bacteriuria according to age in women in East Boston. Reproduced with permission from Evans DA, Williams DN, Laughlin LW, et al. (1).

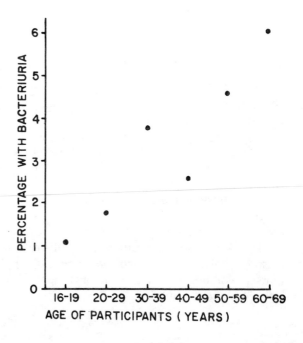

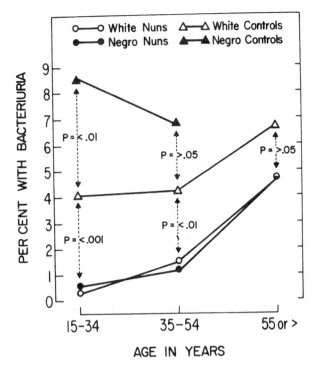

Figure 6.2. Prevalence of significant bacteriuria among black and white nuns and other women. Reproduced with permission from Kunin CM and McCormack RC (2).

Some investigators have reported a higher prevalence of significant bacteriuria among black women, lower socioeconomic classes, and in rural populations. These differences may be related more to the availability of health care services than to susceptibility to infection. Urinary tract infections occur during all months of the year. The highest frequency is reported to occur during the autumn (3). Infections with *Staphylococcus saprophyticus* are more common in late summer and early autumn (4,5).

Confounding by Spontaneous Cure
Some women with asymptomatic bacteriuria or even symptomatic urinary tract infections may undergo spontaneous resolution of their infection even without treatment. This phenomenon appears to be real although difficult to explain. For example, in studies conducted annually in Jamaica and Wales, the prevalence of bacteriuria was constant, but in sequential years about 50% of the population was made up of new individuals (6). It appears as though some previously bacteriuric women develop a sterile urine, even without therapy, and new individuals then enter the pool. In another study, 40% of bacteriuric women became spontaneously free of infection within 1

year, whereas many others had recurrences within a short time after treatment (7). Spontaneous cure might be explained in part by faulty diagnostic methods, wash-out effects of voiding large amounts of fluids, or paraurethral infection without true bladder bacteriuria. It is important to recognize that a single urine culture is not always valid, and not all "cures" reported in clinical trials are caused by the tested drug.

Susceptibility to Infection

It is generally assumed that the short urethra in women accounts for their increased susceptibility to urinary tract infections compared to men. The anatomic differences between women and men fails to explain why urinary tract infections are rare in most women and why some women are prone to recurrent infections. The explanation is much more subtle. There appears to be a special population of females who are more susceptible to recurrent urinary infections throughout life and are at special risk of acquiring urinary tract infections during pregnancy. Considerable evidence now shows that women susceptible to recurrent infections are more likely to be nonsecretors (Lewis blood-group nonsecretor [Le(a+b−)] and recessive [Le(a−b−)] phenotypes) and more frequently belong to B or AB blood groups. In addition, *E. coli* expressing P-fimbriae have the special ability to colonize the gut, attach to the urothelium, and invade the urinary tract of otherwise healthy females. The special pathogenicity of the invading microorganisms and host susceptibility will be considered in greater detail in chapters 10 and 11.

We owe much of our understanding concerning the nature of recurrent infections in women to the work of Stamey and his colleagues (8) and to parallel studies conducted in girls (9–11). In these studies, serotyping of *E. coli* was used to trace the invading microbes as they colonized the gut, established residence in the vaginal vestibule, and predictably caused the next episode of infection. Stamey showed that most healthy females do not harbor uropathogens on the vaginal vestibule, whereas those who develop recurrent urinary tract infection exhibit the following features: 1) infection is preceded by rectal and periurethral colonization with the same organism; 2) the periurethral zone is colonized with enteric bacteria during infection-free periods; and 3) recurrence with the same microbe may occur even after prolonged prophylaxis. He concluded that the ideal drug would eradicate bacteria not only from the urine, but from the periurethral zone as well.

Not all females develop infection even when their periurethral zone is colonized for prolonged periods of time with the same strain of *E. coli* (12,13). In addition, the colonizing strain may change over time depending on the influence of antimicrobial therapy. Thus, recurrence may be caused by persistence with the same microorganism or reinfection with a new strain or species. Most recurrences in girls are caused by reinfection (9,10). In adult women, the proportion of recurrences caused by reinfection with a new microbe or persistence of the same strain depends on the population selected for study. Several recent studies, using sophisticated genotype and pheno-type methods to characterize the strains, provide conflicting results. In a large prospective study in Finland, women with acute cystitis were observed for a year. One-third of the recurrent episodes were caused by the same strain and two-thirds were caused by reinfection with a new microorganism (14). In contrast, in one United States study, the same strain caused half of the recurrent episodes of infection (15), whereas in another the same strain accounted for two-thirds of the recurrences (16). These differences are most likely explained by the case mix. Studies that include a large proportion of women who are known to have recurrent infection are more likely to contain women who are persistently colonized with the same microorganism. A more detailed discussion of the pathogenesis of infection and host susceptibility will be presented in chapter 11.

Key Points Concerning Acquisition of Urinary Tract Infections in Females

- The length and anatomical position of the urethra helps to explain why females are more susceptible to infection than men, but does not explain why some females are more susceptible to infection than others.
- The periurethral zone in most females is colonized by Lactobacilli, alpha hemolytic streptococci, diphtheroids, and coagulase negative staphylococci, and not by uropathogens.
- Uropathogens (*E. coli*, other enteric bacteria, and *Staphylococcus saprophyticus*) must colonize the periurethral zone before they can enter the bladder urine.
- Mechanical factors such as sexual intercourse can only induce urinary tract infections when uropathogens are present in the periurethral zone. They should be considered as permissive rather than causal.
- Some women are much more susceptible to infection than others. Increased susceptibility to infection is determined by interactions between the host and the invading microorganism over time.
- Recurrent infection may be caused by persistence of the same microorganism or reinfection with a new microorganism. Women susceptible to highly recurrent infections are often persistently colonized with the same microorganism.

Mechanical Factors

There is much folklore, often perpetuated by physicians, concerning factors that predispose women to urinary tract infection. Some believe that cold feet, the weather, diet, personal hygiene, bathing, frequency or patterns of urination, failure to void after intercourse, or the direction of wiping after defecation increase susceptibility to infection. These are highly emotional and personal issues that cannot be resolved by "clinical impressions." They require the same level of proof expected of any other important medical finding. Most of the evidence supporting one notion or another is based on case control studies. This is a powerful epidemiologic tool, but it is readily confounded by selection bias, inadequate statistical power, interaction of multiple factors,

Table 6.1. Factors Proposed to Increase Susceptibility to Urinary Tract Infections

Not Associated or the Evidence is Too Weak to Recommend Change in Behavior
    Activities of daily living—diet, clothing, urination habits, bathing (17–20)
    Menstrual protection (tampons versus napkins) (2)
    Direction of wiping after defecation
    Oral contraceptives (21, 22)
    Washing the genitalia before intercourse
    Number of sexual partners
    Position, vaginal lubrication or nature of intercourse (other than for comfort)
    Sexual intercourse in most women, most of the time
Clearly Associated
    Urethral catheterization
    Vaginal diaphragms (23–25)
    Spermicidal jellies containing nonoxynol-9 (25, 26)
    Sexual intercourse in women susceptible to recurrent infection (27–29)
Weakly Associated or Not Clearly Established
    Voiding after intercourse (30)

and other methodological problems. Case control studies also do not take into account the frequency of illness or events in the general population. At best, they provide evidence for an association among risk factors, but do not prove causation. Much more convincing evidence is provided by carefully designed prospective studies, but these require much more effort and expense.

The factors that have been proposed to increase susceptibility to urinary tract infections in women are listed according to the level of certainty in Table 6.1. In this table, clear association is defined as several well conducted case-control studies that demonstrate a consistent pattern. The findings must be statistically significant at a probability of < 0.05 after adjustment for confounding by other factors. Prospective studies are given more weight. It is doubtful that meta-analysis would provide stronger evidence because of differences in methodology and the populations studied. The only factors that meet the criteria for a clear association are the urethral catheter, vaginal diaphragm, spermicide jellies, and sexual intercourse in women who are susceptible to recurrent infection.

Vaginal Diaphragm
The evidence for an association between use of the vaginal diaphragm with spermicidal jelly and urinary tract infections is quite strong in all studies that have examined this relationship. Theories concerning the association between vaginal diaphragms and urinary tract infection are listed in Table 6.2. The most attractive explanation is that spermicides alter the vaginal flora and favor colonization with enteric bacteria. This explanation fits best with the key point that uropathogens must colonize the periurethral zone before they can enter the bladder urine.

Table 6.2. Theories Concerning Vaginal Diaphragms and Urinary Tract Infections

Obstructs the urethra and inhibits voiding after intercourse
Elevates the posterior angle of the bladder causing higher voiding pressure and
    residual volume
Nonoxynol-9 is toxic to *Lactobacillus acidophilus* and may damage normal tissues
Spermicidal jelly with diaphragms or spermicidal foam with condoms favor vaginal
    colonization with *E. coli,* other uropathogens and Candida

Role of Sexual Intercourse

It is commonly held that a close association exists between sexual intercourse and urinary tract infections in females. This notion cannot be taken
for granted. It has strong emotional connotations and is not true for most
women. Generating feelings of guilt or resentment is not a good way to begin a long-term relationship or maintain a happy marriage. The occurrence
of an acute urinary tract infection soon after the first few episodes of sexual

Table 6.3. Evidence that Sexual Intercourse Does Not Have a Role in Causation of Urinary Tract Infections in Most Women

- Association does not prove causation.
    Common events are commonly associated. Let us assume that a woman has inter-
    course on the average of 3 times each week. Any episode of urinary tract infection
    must then occur within 1 to 2 days after intercourse regardless of whether the two
    events are causally related.
- Intercourse is too common in most women to explain occasional episodes of urinary
    infection.
    Women who have sexual intercourse on average of 3 times each week will have 156
    such encounters each year. Most women have fewer than one episode of urinary tract
    infection each year. Therefore, the ratio of intercourse to infection must be quite
    low in most women.
- Uropathogens must colonize the periurethral zone before they can enter the bladder
    urine.
    The periurethral zone in most females is colonized by Lactobacilli, alpha hemolytic
    streptococci, diphtheroids and coagulase negative staphylococci and not by
    uropathogens. Small numbers of commensal microorganisms enter the bladder when
    the urethra is gently milked during gynecologic procedures, but these do not cause
    infection (31). Bacterial counts of vaginal commensual microorganisms transiently
    rise in voided urine after intercourse, but also do not cause infection (32).
- Prior episodes of urinary tract infection set the state for the next infection by
    establishing periurethral colonization with uropathogens.
    The first episode of urinary tract infection predisposes women to further episodes in-
    dependently of sexual activity (20).
- Many women with highly recurrent urinary tract infections do not report an' association
    with sexual intercourse.

intercourse (previously referred to as "honeymoon cystitis") is often cited to support the notion that intercourse predisposes women to urinary tract infection. However, behavioral factors associated with the initial infection (frequency of sexual intercourse, diaphragm use, and voiding after intercourse) do not distinguish between women who do or do not experience a second urinary tract infection (20).

The theory behind the notion that sexual intercourse promotes urinary infections is that vigorous and frequent sexual activity traumatizes the female urethra and forces bacteria into the bladder. This notion is attractive but is somewhat difficult to accept outright or without modification for the reasons noted in Table 6.3. I am not aware of any studies that deal with anal intercourse in women or carefully document the relation of positions of intercourse to urinary tract infection.

Despite these reservations, there are many well documented case control studies that demonstrate a strong relationship between sexual intercourse and urinary tract infection in some women (33–38). The problem with the case control studies is that they do not select women at equal risk of acquiring infection. To accomplish this, they would need to stratify the population according to those with and without periurethral colonization with uropathogens before intercourse. It is likely that those women who develop urinary tract infections associated with sexual intercourse are innately more susceptible to infection than the controls. They may have had asymp-

Table 6.4. Evidence that a Subgroup of Women are at Increased Risk of Urinary Tract Infection After Sexual Intercourse

- Females with asymptomatic bacteriuria in childhood are at increased risk of symptomatic infections as adults.
  About 5% of girls will have significant bacteriuria prior to the onset of sexual activity. Follow-up of these girls reveals that about 50% of those who were bacteriuric during school years develop symptomatic infection with marriage and pregnancy (39).
- Observations in celibate women.
  The frequency of asymptomatic bacteriuria in Roman Catholic nuns is much lower than in women who are not celibate (Fig. 6.2[2]). Sexual intercourse appears to be an additional risk factor.
- Case-control studies.
  Most, but not all studies demonstrate higher rates of urinary tract infections in young women shortly after they become sexually active (33–38,40).
- Temporal relationships.
  Women with recurrent infection exhibited higher rates of infection within 24 hours of sexual intercourse after antimicrobial prophylaxis was discontinued than those without infection (36).
- Efficacy of postcoital prophylaxis.
  Antimicrobial prophylaxis after intercourse is highly effective in preventing infection in women with recurrent urinary tract infection (27–29). This may be equivalent to bedtime prophylaxis in women who frequently engage in intercourse.

tomatic bacteriuria during childhood and adolescence and symptomatic infections in the past. This notion is supported by the work of Stamey discussed previously. The evidence that there is a subgroup of women at increased risk to acquire urinary tract infection with intercourse is presented in Table 6.4.

Key Points About Sexual Activity and Urinary Tract Infections in Females

- Sexual and hygienic practices are highly personal. They have great emotional significance and should not be changed without good reason.
- The motivation for selection of a specific form of contraception, such as use of the diaphragm and spermicidal jellies, can be more important than an increased risk for urinary tract infection.
- Premarital counseling should include a discussion of the potential for "honeymoon cystitis." The patient should be offered a supply of an effective drug to be taken as soon as symptoms occur.
- Most women do not develop urinary tract infections in association with sexual intercourse.
- There is a special group of women with highly recurrent infection in whom sexual intercourse appears to be related to recurrent urinary tract infection. These women benefit from postcoital prophylaxis.

Urological Evaluation

Urologic investigation is not routinely indicated in women with asymptomatic bacteriuria, pyuria-dysuria, or cystitis. The yield of correctable urologic abnormalities is remarkably low even in women with recurrent infections (41–47) (Table 6.5). Less invasive ultrasound examinations of the kidney and bladder might be useful in selected cases. Indications for urologic evaluation include hematuria between infections, pyelonephritis, obstructive symptoms, urea-splitting bacteria, and urinary calculi. Diabetes by itself is not an indication for urologic evaluation (47).

Table 6.5. Findings on Intravenous Urography and Cystoscopy in Women Referred to Urologists for Evaluation of Recurrent Urinary Tract Infection (41–46)

Intravenous Urography

Patients Studied	Normal		Renal Stone		Significant Lesions*	
	No.	%	No.	%	No.	%
876	770	87.9	7	0.8	5	0.6

Cystoscopy

Patients Studied	Significant Lesions**	
	No.	%
276	21	7.6

*Hydronephrosis secondary to uretero-pelvic junction obstruction (1), papillary necrosis (4).
**Rigid or contracted bladders (11), interstitial cystitis (5), urethral diverticulum (2), colorectal fistula (1), transitional cell carcinoma (1), meatotomy (1).

Long-term Follow-up Studies

Uncomplicated Infections

A large number of long-term follow-up studies, including over 1,000 girls and women, have been conducted to ascertain the long-term outcome of uncomplicated urinary tract infections (Table 6.6). These studies include women with asymptomatic bacteriuria, symptomatic infection, and urinary infection of pregnancy. All of the authors agree that these women do not develop progressive renal damage or hypertension. Some exhibit depressed urine concentrating ability during infection, but function returns to normal after therapy. The few exceptions in these series are women who were coincidentally found to have renal scars produced by vesicoureteral reflux in childhood.

Acute Pyelonephritis

We conducted a long-term follow-up of 74 women who had been hospitalized for acute pyelonephritis 10 to 20 years earlier (53). The clinical illness began in most patients in association with marriage, pregnancy, or the postpartum period. Many continued to have repeated episodes of infection (Fig. 6.3). Of these, 17% were bacteriuric at the time of follow-up, 28% had undergone an operative urologic procedure, and 23% had a history of renal stone. Elevated blood pressure was no more common than expected for this age group. One patient had died of the complications of pyelonephritis, one required a renal transplant for end-stage renal disease and two others had azotemia. Seven patients had undergone unilateral nephrectomy for pyelonephritis. These findings strongly support the recommendation that uroradiologic examinations be conducted in all patients with acute pyelonephritis.

Table 6.6. Long-Term Follow-up Studies of Urinary Tract Infections in Women

Author	Year	No. Cases	Years Follow-up	Renal Damage
Pinkerton et al. [†] (48)	1961	50	5	Unilateral nephrectomy in 2
Bullen and Kincaid-Smith (49)	1970	70	4–7	No progression
Zinner and Kass[†] (50)	1971	192	10–14	2 cases of necrotizing papillitis
Freedman (51)	1972	250	12	No progression or hypertension
Asscher et al. (52)	1973	107	4	No progression
Parker and Kunin[‡] (53)	1973	74	10–20	Renal failure in 4
Gower et al.[†] (54)	1976	85	0.5–11	No progression except with analgesic use
Alwall* (55)	1978	94	3–7	No progression

*General population with no underlying risk factors
[†]Urinary tract infections during pregnancy
[‡]Had been admitted to the hospital for acute pyelonephritis

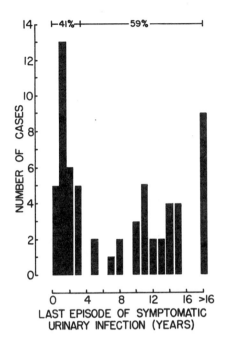

Figure 6.3. Years since the last episode of symptomatic urinary tract infection in a 10 to 20-year follow-up of young women previously hospitalized with acute pyelonephritis. Reproduced with permission from Parker J and Kunin CM (53).

Pregnancy

Urinary tract infections are common during pregnancy. The invading microorganisms are the same uropathogens commonly found in uncomplicated urinary tract infections (*E. coli*, other gram negative enteric bacteria, *Staphylococcus saprophyticus*, and enterococci). Small numbers of group B streptococci, diphtheroids, and Lactobacilli are usually caused by contamination with vaginal secretions (56). Asymptomatic bacteriuria occurs in about 2% to 6% of healthy women early in pregnancy and rises by about 1% during its course (57,58) (Fig. 6.4). The prevalence increases with parity and age (Fig. 6.5) and is higher in diabetics and women with previous urinary tract infections (59). Women in lower socioeconomic strata have a higher prevalence of bacteriuria in countries that do not provide comprehensive health services. The risk for acute pyelonephritis during the later part of pregnancy ranges from 20% to 60%. Treatment of bacteriuria is highly effective in preventing pyelonephritis and reduces the risk of low birth weight infants by about half.

Susceptibility to Infection

Most women acquire bacteriuria before pregnancy. At the first examination, the rates of bacteriuria in pregnant women are similar to nonpregnant women with similar risk factors. About 37% to 57% of bacteriuric school

Figure 6.4. Incidence of bacteriuria in relation to duration of pregnancy at the time of the first prenatal visit. Reproduced with permission from Kass EH (57).

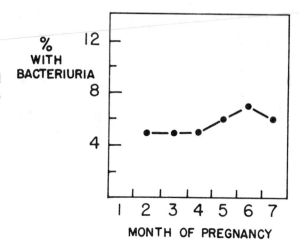

girls develop urinary tract infections during pregnancy (39,60,61). An additional 1% of infections occurs during pregnancy (Fig. 6.4). In a study conducted in Sweden, the risk of acquiring bacteriuria increased with the duration of pregnancy, reaching a maximum between gestational weeks 9 and 17 (58). It is not known whether acquisition of infection is independent of pregnancy because nonpregnant controls were not included.

Pyelonephritis of Pregnancy

Acute pyelonephritis tends to occur during the later stages of pregnancy, usually in the last trimester. Characteristically, the patient is acutely ill with high fever, leukocytosis, and costovertebral angle pain. Bacteremia is com-

Figure 6.5. Incidence of bacteriuria in relation to numbers of previous pregnancies in prenatal patients, Boston City Hospital. Reproduced with permission from Kass EH (57).

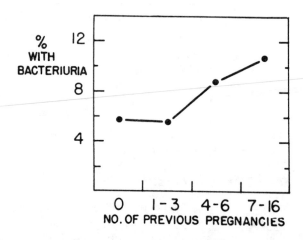

mon, but mortality and complications are low when the patient is treated with effective therapy. The major causes of concern are the presence of underlying urologic abnormalities and associated risks to the mother, such as toxemia, hypertension, prematurity, and perinatal mortality. Before the introduction of the sulfonamides in the 1930s, pyelonephritis of pregnancy was associated with sepsis, premature birth and, in some women, chronic illness, persistent renal pain, and subsequent stone disease (62). The major renal impairment was decreased urinary concentrating ability, but hypertension, renal failure, and death were rare unless there was underlying renal disease. Currently, antimicrobial therapy is so effective that, even with bacteremia, almost all patients with uncomplicated pyelonephritis do well and become afebrile within a few days. Choice of drug and duration of therapy are discussed in Chapter 12.

Early detection and prompt treatment of bacteriuria in pregnancy is highly effective in preventing pyelonephritis (63). For example, the annual incidence of pyelonephritis of pregnancy fell from 1.8% to 0.6% in a large teaching hospital after the introduction of a program to screen and treat asymptomatic bacteriuria (64). Another advance has been the abandonment of the routine practice of catheterizing women just before delivery (65). This practice can no longer be justified (see Chapter 9, Care of the Urinary Catheter).

Predisposing Factors

The factors that predispose bacteriuric women to pyelonephritis of pregnancy appear to be related to the anatomic and physiologic changes in the kidney and urinary tract late in pregnancy. The ureters become dilated above the pelvic brim and the bladder is displaced anteriorly and superiorly by the enlarging uterus. The renal blood flow and glomerular filtration rates increase by about 30% to 40% during pregnancy, and the kidney becomes slightly enlarged and hyperemic. Urine flow may be sluggish, and the bladder may not completely empty. Residual urine is increased from about 3 ml in antenatal patients to a mean of 33 ml 2 days after spontaneous delivery (66). It is important to note that suprapubic discomfort and urinary urgency are common in pregnancy and do not indicate that the patient has a urinary tract infection.

Women who develop high antibody titers to the microorganism in their urine and have defects in urinary concentrating ability are at increased risk of pyelonephritis of pregnancy (67). *E. coli* grows well in urine obtained throughout pregnancy (68). Urine obtained during pregnancy is reported to be more favorable to growth of *E. coli* than urine obtained from nonpregnant women (66). Pregnant rats are more susceptible to ascending infection with *E. coli.* (69) and diethylstilbestrol (70) and estrogen increases susceptibility to infection in rats and mice (71).

Prematurity and Neonatal Mortality

Bacteriuria of pregnancy is associated with a significant increase in low-birth-weight infants (≤ 2500 grams), decreased gestational age (< 37 weeks), and neonatal mortality (72,73). Eradication of bacteriuria reduces these complications (Fig. 6.6) (Table 6.7). Based on data found on birth certificates (74), the risk of prematurity is 2.4 times greater in children born of mothers with urinary tract infection during pregnancy. The Collaborative Perinatal Project of the National Institutes of Health, which included more than 50,000 pregnancies, revealed an association between urinary tract infections of pregnancy, prematurity, and neonatal mortality (75,76). Certain groups of pregnant women are at higher risk of delivering premature infants. These include women with persistent infection despite treatment (77) or evidence of "tissue invasion" as demonstrated by antibody-coated bacteria in their urine (78).

The relationship between toxemia and bacteriuria of pregnancy is less clearly defined. The data are confounded by the strong association of toxemia and socioeconomic status and to the marked decrease in frequency of toxemia encountered in recent years (63).

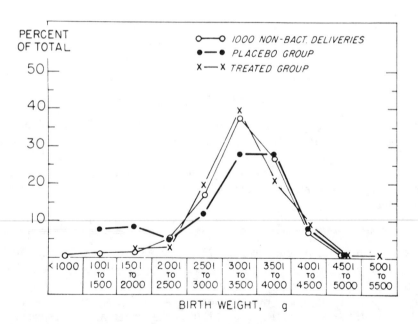

Figure 6.6. Effect of bacteriuria on birth weight of infants. Reproduced with permission from Kass EH (79).

Table 6.7. Meta-Analysis of Studies that Examined the Relationship Between Asymptomatic Bacteriuria of Pregnancy and Preterm Delivery and Low Birth Weight Infants*

Cohort Studies
Relative risk of low birth weight infants born to women without bacteriuria compared to those with untreated bacteriuria (17 studies)
Relative risk of all trials = 0.65; 95% confidence interval 0.56, 0.74
Difference in low birth weight infants = 3.4%; 95% confidence interval 1.8, 5.0%
Relative risk of preterm delivery in women with and without bacteriuria (4 studies)
Relative risk of all trials = 0.51; 95% confidence interval 0.36, 0.69
Difference in preterm delivery = 3.8%; 95% confidence interval 1.1, 6.4%
Randomized Clinical Trials
Low birth rate in patients receiving antibiotics relative to those receiving placebo (8 trials)
Relative risk of all trials = 0.56; 95% confidence interval 0.43, 0.73

*From Romero R, Oyarzun E, Mazorm M, Sirtori M, Hobbins JC and Bracken M. (72)

Confounding by Other Causes of Premature Birth

Low birth rate and preterm delivery are associated with black race, low socioeconomic status, older maternal age, previous preterm delivery, and smoking during pregnancy. Microorganisms associated with prematurity include bacteroides, *Mycoplasma hominis, Gardnerella vaginalis, Ureaplasma urealyticum,* group B streptococci, *Chlamydia trachomatis,* and *Trichomonas vaginalis.* Lactobacilli appear to be protective. Several studies have shown that long-term treatment of pregnant women with tetracycline or erythromycin reduces the rate of prematurity (80), but the antimicrobial spectrum of these drugs is too broad to pin point the causal microorganisms. Bacterial vaginosis is strongly linked to prematurity (81,82). Treatment of bacterial vaginosis during pregnancy with erythromycin base (333 mg three times daily for 14 days) together with metronidazole (250 mg three times daily for 7 days) reduced the rate of preterm delivery from 49% to 31% (p = 0.006) (81). These drugs are not effective for urinary tract infections and appear to work by an independent mechanism.

Treatment of Urinary Tract Infections in Pregnancy

This is discussed in more detail in Chapter 12. Briefly, trimethoprim and quinolones are not approved for use during pregnancy and tetracyclines concentrate in newly forming bone. Beta lactam antibiotics and nitrofurantoin are highly effective, provided that the microorganism is susceptible. A single course of therapy is not always effective. Therefore, follow-up cultures at subsequent visits are recommended. Recurrent infections after delivery frequently occur. Postpartum infections are reported to occur in as many as 25% to 30% of women (49). Important correctable urinary tract abnormalities are not frequent enough to justify routine radiologic or urologic studies during pregnancy except in women with pyelonephritis or those who persistently fail treatment. Ultrasound examinations are useful; radiologic studies are best reserved for after delivery.

Breast Feeding

Several investigators have reported that infants who are breast fed are partially protected from urinary tract infection. In one study, the relative risk of urinary tract infection was 0.38 (95% confidence interval 0.22 to 0.65) in breast fed compared to bottle fed infants (83). Another study found complete breast feeding to be briefer among infants with pyelonephritis than with controls (84). It is possible that the protective effect of breast feeding is related to the anti-adhesive properties of secretory IgA antibodies and receptor analogues against bacteria present in breast milk and that these factors prevent colonization of the gut with uropathogens.

Key Points About Urinary Tract Infections in Pregnancy

- The prevalence of bacteriuria at the beginning of pregnancy is similar to rates in women with similar age and host characteristics.
- The prevalence of asymptomatic bacteriuria increases about 1% during pregnancy.
- Women with a prior history of urinary tract infections and bacteriuric school girls are at high risk of developing bacteriuria with pregnancy.
- Pregnant women with asymptomatic bacteriuria are at high risk of developing pyelonephritis in the later stages of pregnancy.
- Treatment of asymptomatic bacteriuria early in pregnancy prevents pyelonephritis.
- Infants born of bacteriuric mothers are at increased risk of premature birth and fetal mortality.
- Treatment of asymptomatic bacteriuria pregnancy reduces the risk of premature birth.
- Bacterial vaginosis is an important, independent risk factor for premature birth.
- Treatment of bacterial vaginosis during pregnancy reduces the risk of premature birth.

Diabetes

Most diabetics respond to urinary tract infections no differently than nondiabetics and exhibit the same benign course. The invading microorganisms are the same as in patients with uncomplicated infection, and they respond well to antimicrobial therapy. Some diabetics, for reasons that are not entirely clear, are at greater risk of severe forms of pyelonephritis (Table 6.8).

Diabetic women are much more likely to have upper tract infection than controls as shown by localization studies with antibody-coated bacteria (ACB) (85) or bladder wash-out methods (86). Those at greater risk of complicated infection often have a long history of recurrent infections with multiple resistant strains of *E. coli*, *Klebsiella pneumoniae* and other enteric bacteria, enterococci, group B streptococci, Candida, and other yeasts. Dia-

Table 6.8. Severe Forms of Urinary Tract Infections Associated with Diabetes Mellitus*

Emphysematous pyelonephritis
Emphysematous cystitis
Medullary (papillary) necrosis
Xanthogranulomatous pyelonephritis
Metastatic and ascending pyelonephritis
Perinephric abscess
Urinary tract infections with Candida and other yeasts and fungi

*See Chapter 8 for a more detailed discussion of these disorders.

betics are more prone to bacteremia with *Staphylococcus aureus* and to develop metastatic renal abscesses.

Epidemiology

The prevalence of asymptomatic bacteriuria in school age boys and girls with diabetes is the same as nondiabetic controls (87–89). The prevalence of asymptomatic bacteriuria among adult women depends on the clinical setting, duration of diabetes, and age. The rate is not influenced by quality of diabetic control (as measured by hemoglobin A1C) or renal function (90,91). There are conflicting data regarding whether the rate is increased with diabetic retinopathy and renal microangiopathy (90). Several studies report little or no difference in the prevalence of asymptomatic bacteriuria between diabetic and nondiabetic groups, but most investigators report approximately threefold higher rates. It is likely that the higher prevalence of asymptomatic bacteriuria among diabetic women is confounded by factors such as an increased pool of cases due to recurrent infections, more intense medical care, diabetic complications, and urinary catheterization. The prevalence of asymptomatic bacteriuria does not differ between diabetic and nondiabetic men.

Susceptibility to Infection

The reason why diabetics are more susceptible to bacterial and fungal infections is not clearly established, but it is most likely multifactorial. The conditions most often mentioned are delayed mobilization of leukocytes to an area of infection, deficient polymorphonuclear leukocyte (PMN) function, renal microangiopathy, and diabetic uropathy.

Deficient Polymorphonuclear Leukocytes

PMNs obtained from patients with diabetes mellitus show impaired adherence, chemotaxis, phagocytosis, oxidative activity, and antibacterial activity (92). A possible explanation for deficient PMN function in diabetics is elevated levels of cytosolic calcium related to hyperglycemia (93). It has not been shown as yet that improved glycemic control reduces the rate of infections in diabetics.

Bladder Dysfunction

Diabetic cystopathy is an insidious autonomic nerve dysfunction characterized by a loss of sensation of distension, decreased frequency of voiding, and an increased residual volume. It is reported to occur in 26% to 87% of diabetic women, depending on the criteria used, the age, presence of neuropathy, and dependence on insulin (94). The frequency is about 25% in patients with diabetes of 10 years duration and increases to over 50% in patients who had diabetes for more than 45 years. More attention needs to be addressed to voiding disorders in diabetics and their relation to urinary tract infections. Long-term prospective studies are much more feasible now that relatively inexpensive bladder ultrasound and urine flow devices are available.

Experimental Infections

Rats rendered diabetic with alloxan are more susceptible than controls to infection with *E. coli* (95), *Candida albicans,* and *Staphylococcus aureus* and tend to persist longer. Alloxan produces renal tubular lesions as well. These might render the kidney more susceptible independent of glycosuria. Candida infection are often severe in diabetic rats and may produce fungus balls causing ureteral obstruction and gross abscesses.

Glycosuria

Some investigators have found that *Candida albicans and Staphylococcus aureus* grow better in the urine of diabetic rats (96). Others report that addition of glucose to human urine prolongs bacterial multiplication without altering growth rate (97).

Pathogenesis of Kidney Infection in Diabetic Women

It seems reasonable to speculate that diabetic women are more susceptible to severe forms of pyelonephritis because 1) they are more likely to have recurrent urinary tract infections over time, 2) the infections are more difficult to eradicate because of large volumes of residual urine and local tissue invasion, 3) the bladder and kidney are more susceptible to infection because of impaired adherence, chemotaxis, and phagocytosis by polymorphonuclear leukocytes, and 4) renal microangiopathy provides a nidus for ascending or hematogenous infection. The last point is consistent with the classic animal studies of Beeson (98) who demonstrated that local trauma, tubular obstruction, and small burns render the kidney more susceptible to infection.

Key Points About Urinary Tract Infections in Diabetics

- Diabetic school girls are not at increased risk of urinary tract infection.
- Diabetic boys and men are also not at increased risk of urinary tract infection.
- Most diabetic women handle urinary tract infections well and do not develop renal disease.
- The prevalence of bacteriuria in diabetic women is about threefold greater than nondiabetics. This may be caused by the tendency of urinary tract infections to persist in diabetics and increase the size of the pool over time.
- Susceptibility to bacteriuria is not related to control of hyperglycemia.
- The role of bladder dysfunction and residual volumes of urine as a cause of persistent infection needs to be determined by long-term prospective studies.
- Diabetic women as a group are more susceptible to severe forms of cystitis as well as metastatic and ascending pyelonephritis.
- Diabetics have major defects in polymorphonuclear leukocyte chemotaxis and function.
- Microangiopathy may render the kidney more susceptible to infection.

Urinary Tract Infections in Men

Urinary tract infections are much less common in men than in women. They are more likely to be associated with complicated infections and can be more difficult to treat. They rarely cause renal damage or increased mortality in the absence of major structural or functional abnormalities of the urinary tract or catheter-induced sepsis. The diagnosis is readily established from the clinical history and examination of the urine. Contamination of the voided urine is less likely to occur in men than women. Nevertheless, small numbers of gram positive bacteria (*Staphylococcus epidermidis,* streptococci, and diphtheroids) are normally present in the fossa navicularis (99). To minimize potential contamination, it is recommended that the meatus be cleansed and a clean-catch midstream-void urine be obtained. This is particularly important when urine is obtained from a patient with a condom catheter. These procedures may not be necessary when the collection is carefully supervised (100). Colony counts will usually be $\geq 10^5$ cfu/ml, but counts of $\geq 10^3$ cfu/ml with a uropathogen and pyuria are considered significant, particularly if confirmed on repeat cultures (Fig. 6.7). The infection may be asymptomatic or expressed as prostatitis, epididymitis, cystitis, or pyelonephritis.

The invading microorganisms in young men tend to be the same uropathogens commonly associated with uncomplicated urinary tract infections in females (*E. coli,* other gram negative enteric bacteria, *Staphylococcus saprophyticus,* and enterococci). *Hemophilus influenzae* and *Gardnerella vaginalis* are relatively rare causes of infection, but are readily missed if a gram stain is not done. In older men, the microorganisms tend to be those associated with complicated infections (more resistant strains of *E. coli,* enteric gram negative bacteria, Pseudomonas, *Staphylococcus aureus,* and enterococci). Recurrent

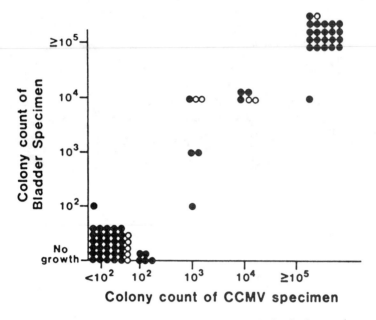

Figure 6.7. Correlation between colony counts (cfu/ml of urine) on culture of clean-catch midstream-void and bladder (suprapubic aspiration or urethral catheterization). The open circles represent patients receiving antibiotics; the closed circles represent patients not receiving antibiotics. Note that almost all the counts were ≥ 10⁴ cfu/ml. Reproduced with permission from Lipsky BA, et al. (100).

urinary tract infections in men are usually caused by microorganisms that persist in the prostate and intermittently colonize the bladder urine. Prostatic infections are exceedingly difficult to eradicate, particularly when prostatic stones are present.

Epidemiology

The overall epidemiology of urinary tract infections in men is presented in Chapter 1 (see Figure 1.1). To recapitulate briefly, bacteriuria and symptomatic infections rarely occur in males under the age of 50 years in the absence of urinary tract instrumentation or prostatitis. The prevalence of asymptomatic bacteriuria in school boys is 0.04% (10). The rate of spontaneous symptomatic infections in healthy young men is about 5 to 8 per 10,000 per year (period prevalence 0.05% to 0.08%) (101,102). The rates are somewhat higher (1.5%) in young men attending clinics for sexually transmitted diseases (103). The prevalence of bacteriuria in men over 70 years of age is about 6% and may exceed 15% in hospitalized elderly men (see Urinary Tract Infections in the Elderly).

Data From the National Ambulatory Medical Care Survey are Instructive (104)
About half (52%) of men with genitourinary problems were seen by urologists. The rate increased steeply with advancing age. Male patients over the age of 65 made eight times as many visits for urinary tract problems as younger men (Table 6.9).

Susceptibility to Infection and AIDS

Circumcision
Uncircumcised men are reported to be more susceptible to urinary tract infections (105), but circumcision is not completely protective. For example, in a series of 38 young men with acute symptomatic urinary tract infections, 87% were circumcised (101).

Masturbation
There are two case reports of urinary tract infection in men associated with masturbation. One, caused by *E. coli,* occurred in a Muslim youth who manually held back the ejaculate (106). The other was caused by *Pseudomonas aeruginosa* in a man who ejaculated into the water jets of a hotel whirlpool. The strains isolated from his urine and the hot tub were the same serologic and pyocin types (107).

Heterosexual Transmission
There are several well documented cases of urinary tract infections in men associated with heterosexual intercourse with women with urinary tract infections (108–110). In each instance, the same strain of *E. coli* was isolated from both partners. There are also well documented cases of urinary tract infections in men caused by *Gardnerella vaginalis.* Microorganisms can be released from a chronic prostatic focus during sexual intercourse and produce acute symptomatic infection (111).

Homosexual Behavior and AIDS
The risk of urinary tract infections among homosexual males is increased in some populations and not others. For example, 12 of 14 men with symptomatic urinary tract infections who attended a clinic for sexually transmitted

Table 6.9. Office Visits by Men and Women to Urologists for Urinary Tract and Associated Infections

	Rate per Year per 1,000 Population	
Disorder	*Male*	*Female*
Cystitis	4	30
Urethritis (nonvenereal)	4	5
Prostatitis	19	–
Orchitis and Epididymitis	4	–

From the National Ambulatory Medical Care Survey: United States (104).

diseases were homosexual or bisexual (112). In another study in a similar setting, the prevalence of significant bacteriuria was 1.5% in both hetero-sexual and homosexual men (103). The presence of AIDS and low CD4+ cell counts < 200 appear to be important risk factors for significant bacteriuria. For example, in a study conducted in Brazil (113), the rate was 1.8% in HIV negative men, 3.2% in HIV positive men without AIDS, and 13.3% in pa-tients with AIDS. In a study conducted in patients with AIDS in the Nether-lands (114), the frequency of significant bacteriuria over a two-year period was 30% in patients with CD4+ cell counts < 200 compared to 17% with CD4+ cell counts of 200–500 and 0% in patients with CD4+ cell counts > 500. The association between urinary tract infection and AIDS was not re-lated to homosexual behavior or anal intercourse. Prophylaxis for *Pneumo-cystis carinii* infection with trimethoprim/sulfamethoxazole and other drugs with antibacterial activity may be a confounding factor in future studies. Pa-tients with AIDS may develop prostatitis with unusual microorganisms, in-cluding Histoplasma, Aspergillus, *Candida tropicalis,* epididymo-orchitis with *Hemophilus influenzae,* cystitis with Toxoplasma, and Mycoplasma infection of the kidneys (115–120). In addition, they may develop urodynamic problems when the central nervous system is involved (121).

Urinary Tract Infections in the Elderly

Elderly men and women are a select population that has survived longer than other members of their cohort. The contribution of urinary tract infec-tions to morbidity and mortality is confounded by the high rates of heart dis-ease, cancer, diabetes, and neurologic, psychiatric, and musculoskeletal disorders. Most elderly men and women live independently. Only about 5% of those 65 years or older reside in long-term care facilities. Nursing home populations tend to be older, more debilitated, and most (about 80%) of the residents are female. Urinary tract infections in the independently-living el-derly are usually uncomplicated and not associated with increased mortal-ity. Urinary tract infections in the more debilitated elderly are complicated more often by incontinence, instrumentation, and indwelling urinary catheters (see discussion of increased mortality in nursing home patients with long-term indwelling catheters later in this chapter).

The important risk factors for urinary tract infections in the elderly are age, gender, ability to perform the functions of every day living, underlying diseases, urinary instrumentation, and voiding disorders (Table 6.10). Es-trogen use in older women with intact uteri is reported to be associated with a twofold increase in the clinical diagnosis of urinary tract infections (122). This report is puzzling because estrogen therapy in postmenopausal women has a protective effect against urinary tract infections. The results may have been confounded by diagnostic problems and selection bias.

Table 6.10. Risk Factors that Account for Increased Urinary Tract Infections in the Elderly

Females
    Accumulation of recurrent infections over time
    Decreased vaginal glycogen and increased vaginal pH
    Increased introital colonization with gram-negative bacteria
    Changes in the anatomy and function of the urethra and bladder
    Incomplete emptying of the bladder
Males
    Benign prostatic hypertrophy
    Prostatic carcinoma
    Prostatic calculi
    Instrumentation
    Urethral strictures
Both Sexes
    Coexisting diseases including diabetes, cerebrovascular accidents, dementia
    Increased hospitalizations and urinary instrumentation
    Management of incontinence with urinary catheters
    Alterations in cellular and immune response to infection

Epidemiology

The prevalence of significant bacteriuria in the independently-living elderly, 70 years or older, is about 6% in men and 16% to 18% in women (123,124). The rates are somewhat higher among elderly male veterans (9.0 % for 65–74 and 15% for 75 years and older) (125). The epidemiologic dynamics are confounded by a high turnover of bacteriuria in both men and women. The prevalence of bacteriuria is considerably higher in nursing home populations. The rates range from 17% to 55% in women and 15% to 31% in men without catheters and 100% with long-term indwelling catheters (125).

Morbidity and Mortality

The relation between urinary tract infections in elderly men and women and morbidity and mortality has been examined in several long-term prospective studies (126–130). The general consensus is that the elderly do not differ significantly from other age groups who have uncomplicated or complicated urinary tract infections. The impact on morbidity and mortality is confounded by concomitant diseases and disability. Symptomatic urinary tract infections should be evaluated and treated in the same manner as younger adults. The studies on which these conclusions are based are briefly outlined as follows.

The Pittsburgh Good Health Study

The incidence of all infections in the noninstitutionalized population 65 years or older was determined over a two-year period (131) (Table 6.11).

Table 6.11. Infections Among Free-Living Persons 65 Years of Age or Older, by Diagnosis and Sex

Diagnosis	Rates of Infection per 100 Person Years		
	Males	Females	Both
Respiratory Disease	34.3	37.0	35.8
Urinary Tract Infection & Prostatitis	12.6	14.0	13.6
Skin Infections	17.7	10.1	12.7
Gastrointestinal Diseases	1.7	2.8	2.5
Other	1.8	1.2	1.4
All Infections	69.4	68.4	68.6

From Ruben et al. (131).

About half the population had one or more infection. Urinary tract infections accounted for about a quarter of all infections. There were 115 infections related to hospitalization. Of these, 34 were urinary tract infections and prostatitis. Urinary tract infections were cited as the secondary cause of death in three cases. The overall mortality associated with urinary tract infections was 3 of 417 in 2 years, or 0.4% per year.

Cohort Study and Controlled Trial of Antimicrobial Therapy in Elderly Ambulatory Women

This long-term study consisted of an observational study of mortality among women with and without bacteriuria conducted over 10 years, and clinical trials of single dose, 3 days, and 14 days versus placebo (130). In the observational study, the death rates were 10.1 versus 18.7 per 100,000 in never-positive versus ever-positive for bacteriuria. Nevertheless, urinary tract infection was not found to be an independent cause of mortality after adjustment for age and other risk factors. In the controlled clinical trials, mortality was not significantly different in the treated versus the untreated groups, 13.8 versus 15.1 per 100,000 respectively.

Elderly Institutionalized Men

In a study of 91 elderly men, there was no difference in survival at 6 years among men who were continuously bacteriuric, intermittently bacteriuric, or nonbacteriuric (128).

Residential Nursing Home

In this study, 408 male and female residents were observed for up to 11 years (126). The mortality ratio was 1.13 in patients with persistent bacteriuria and was not statistically significant (p > 0.20).

Long-term Indwelling Urinary Catheters

A 1-year prospective study of 1,540 nursing home patients revealed that the indwelling urinary catheter was independent of risk factors for death. Patients who were catheterized 76% or more of their days in the nursing homes were three times more likely to die within a year. The number of hospitalizations, duration of hospitalization, and use of antimicrobial drugs were all three times greater among catheterized patients (129) (see "Core of the Urinary Catheter," Chapter 9).

Urinary Tract Infection as a Cause of Bacteremia
Urinary infections account for over 50% of the episodes of bacteremia in the institutionalized elderly and are often associated with long-term urinary catheterization (132–134). Bacteremia is complicated by septic shock in about one-third of patients. The overall case fatality in bacteremic patients is 16% to 23% (125). The typical cases are either a debilitated elderly woman with a urinary catheter who presents with altered mental status, dehydration, fever and hypotension, or an elderly man who recently underwent a traumatic catheterization to relieve obstruction. The most common microorganisms are those associated with complicated urinary tract infection. *E. coli* is most common, followed by *Proteus mirabilis, Klebsiella pneumoniae,* and *Pseudomonas aeruginosa.*

Incontinence in the Elderly

Urinary incontinence affects 5% to 10% of the elderly in the community and about 50% in long-term care facilities (135). Many of these conditions can be managed with careful attention to the cause and do not require catheterization. Patients with central nervous system disease may have detrusor instability, those with bladder neck obstruction will have overflow incontinence, women with stress incontinence often have sphincter insufficiency, and those who have normal urinary tracts, but just wet themselves, may simply not be able to void when convenient or may be receiving drugs that increase the rate of urine flow or alter mental function.

It is estimated that only about 2.5% of elderly patients in a skilled long-term care facility need to be managed with urinary catheters (136). Most can be managed by "prompted voiding" (137). This method has been effective in management of daytime urinary incontinence in one-quarter to one-third of incontinent nursing home residents. It involves 1) focusing the residents' attention on the bladder by asking if they are wet or dry, 2) checking them for wetness and giving feedback, 3) asking if they would like to use the toilet and prompting them up to three times if they refuse, 4) toileting if the residents respond positively to the prompting, 5) verbal positive feedback for dryness and appropriate toileting, 6) offering fluids, and 7) a reminder about the time of the next toileting opportunity. Prompted voiding may take extra effort, but it is well worth trying to reduce the use of catheters. Condom catheters should be used in incontinent men provided that they are not obstructed. Every person for whom a catheter-associated infection can be prevented is one less who will receive antibiotics inappropriately, or be sent to emergency rooms with urosepsis, or die prematurely. Care of the urinary catheter and prevention of nosocomial infections is discussed in Chapter 9.

Key Points About Urinary Tract Infections in the Elderly

- Asymptomatic bacteriuria is benign and often clears spontaneously in both men and women.
- Asymptomatic bacteriuria needs not be treated.
- Symptomatic infections produce considerable morbidity and should be treated.
- Urinary tract infections do not increase mortality in noncatheterized patients.
- A subgroup with diabetes, obstructive uropathy and nephrolithiasis are at increased risk of pyelonephritis and need to be carefully evaluated.
- Urinary incontinence is a major problem in the institutionalized elderly. It usually can be managed by prompted voiding, diapers in women, and condom catheters in men.
- The long-term indwelling urinary catheter is an independent risk factor for premature death and should be avoided whenever possible.
- Debilitated elderly patients with urinary catheters are at increased risk of bacteremia and septic shock.

Renal Transplantation

Patients undergoing renal transplantation are at increased risk of developing urinary tract infection. The frequency ranges from 35% to 79% (138). Women are at about two times greater risk (139–141). The major predisposing factors are prolonged periods of hemodialysis and urinary catheters (142,143). The more severe urinary tract infections tend to appear "early," within the first 3 to 4 months after transplantation. In one large series, most patients with "early" infections had antibody-coated bacteria (ACB) in their urine and there was a 12% incidence of gram-negative bacteremia (138). Urinary tract infections that occur "late," or 6 months after transplantation, tend to be more benign, but there are several reports of bacteremia and acute pyelonephritis even several years later (141,144). Major urologic complications are relatively rare. They include ureteral leakage and obstruction, bladder leakage, urethral stricture, and blood clots in the kidney or the transplant site.

Ascending Infection

Transplant recipients tend to be infected with bacteria commonly associated with nosocomial infections. These infections consist of relatively resistant strains of E. coli, other enteric bacteria, Pseudomonas, staphylococci, enterococci, and yeasts. Because of their immunosuppressed state, transplant recipients are at increased risk of infection with opportunistic organisms, including Cryptococcus, Nocardia, Aspergillus, and Legionella. There are case reports of pyelonephritis caused by *Salmonella enteritidis* and *Gardnerella vaginalis* and ureteropelvic obstruction caused by Candida fungus balls (145).

Infection Acquired from the Donor Kidney
Cytomegalovirus and papovaviruses may be transmitted by an infected transplanted kidney (146,147). The papovaviruses (BK and JC) may be associated with ureteric obstruction (148). Disseminated tuberculosis was acquired in two patients with allografts procured from the same donor (149).

Association of Urinary Tract Infection with Graft Rejection
An association between transplant rejection and *Streptococcus faecalis* urinary infection in men has been reported by some investigators (150) and not confirmed by others (151,152).

Therapy and Prophylaxis
Treatment for 6 weeks is recommended because of the high rate of relapse after 2 weeks (138). Prophylaxis with trimethoprim/sulfamethoxazole (TMP/SMZ) for 4 months after removal of the indwelling catheter reduced the infection rate from 38% in controls to 8% in those receiving once daily prophylaxis. Interstitial nephritis and bone-marrow suppression may occur in transplant recipients receiving TMP/SMZ. Toxicity is presumed to be caused by the additive effects of TMP and azathioprine on folic acid reductase (153,154).

Hypertension

In studies conducted in the 1930s, Longcope and Weiss and Parker (155,156) reported an association between hypertension and end-stage pyelonephritis in some patients. It was thought that chronic pyelonephritis might produce hypertension by damaging the renal arterioles and augmenting the release of renin. This phenomenon is surprisingly rare. Urinary tract infections are not an important cause of hypertension unless the patient has end-stage renal failure as a result of complicated infection (157), or the kidneys are scarred and shrunken as a result of either unilateral or bilateral reflux nephropathy (158).

Elevated blood pressure is distinctly unusual in patients with recurrent urinary tract infections or acute pyelonephritis. For example, in a study among women who had been hospitalized with acute pyelonephritis 10 to 20 years previously, the frequency of elevated blood pressure was no greater in this population than would be expected for their age (53). Autopsy studies among paraplegics reveal that hypertension occurs only at the time the patients develop renal failure (159). In another study, men who had been paraplegic for many years and were chronically bacteriuric did not have elevated blood pressure unless they also had end-stage renal disease (160).

Information from some cross sectional studies suggests that bacteriuric women have higher blood pressure than nonbacteriuric women (6). A study of blood pressure among nuns and age-matched married women revealed higher blood pressure in the married women, but this might be caused by factors other than differences in the frequency of bacteriuria between the two populations (2). In contrast to these reports, hypertension is distinctly unusual among bacteriuric women who have been studied for many years in long-term prospective studies.

Several investigators (161–163) examined the possibility that hypertension may increase the susceptibility to urinary tract infections and pyelonephritis, but the results were inconclusive. In animal studies, the imposition of pyelonephritis on preexisting hypertension exacerbated the disease and its sequelae (164), and hypertensive animals were more susceptible to infection (165).

Key Points About Urinary Tract Infections and Hypertension

- Most hypertensive patients do not have urinary tract infections.
- Most patients with acute pyelonephritis do not have hypertension.
- Long-standing bacteriuria is not associated with hypertension.
- Hypertension may be an important complication of reflux nephropathy.
- Chronic pyelonephritis does not cause hypertension unless it produces end-stage renal failure.

Association of Urinary Tract Infections with Other Diseases

Cancer

The association between urinary tract infection and cancer is largely related to the tendency for neoplasms of the prostate, bladder, or retroperitoneal space to obstruct the flow of urine. Relief of obstruction by catheters may lead to urinary tract infections and sepsis. Hematuria and pyuria caused by renal or bladder cancers may be mistaken for infection. A high index of suspicion needs to exist for urologic neoplastic disease in patients with persistent sterile pyuria.

Most *Enterobacteriaceae* are capable of reducing dietary nitrate in the urine to nitrite. Nitrosamines might be produced by a reaction between secondary amines and nitrite. Small amounts of N-nitrosodimethylamine were detected in the urine of two patients with urinary infections caused by Proteus (166). These observations are intriguing, but I am not aware of a strong association between urinary tract infections and neoplasms of the bladder or kidney.

Granulocytopenia

Granulocytopenic patients with urinary tract infections will usually not exhibit pyuria when the absolute granulocyte counts are 0 to 100/ cu mm;

about two-thirds will have pyuria at counts of 101 to 1,000; and almost all will have pyuria at counts of $> 1,000$ (167).

Chronic Granulomatous Disease

Polymorphonuclear leukocytes in patients with chronic granulomatous disease do not produce the toxic oxygen by-products needed to kill invading pathogens. Genitourinary disorders were present in about half of the patients in one series (168). The lesions consisted of hydroureteronephrosis in association with recurrent episodes of pyelonephritis, retroperitoneal lymphadenitis, and granuloma formation. The bladder may contain large inflammatory masses that mimic bladder carcinoma (169,170).

Glomerulopathies

It has been suggested that the frequency of asymptomatic bacteriuria is increased in patients with glomerulopathies (171), but this has not been confirmed (172).

Chronic Renal Failure and Hemodialysis

A high frequency of asymptomatic bacteriuria, ranging from 27% to 44%, have been reported in patients with chronic renal failure with or without hemodialysis (142,173). It is difficult to determine the specific cause of these infections because of the wide variety of underlying renal diseases involved, lack of information on prior instrumentation of the bladder, the need to correct for age, sex and the presence of diabetes, and poor response to chemotherapy.

Sickle Cell Disease

Urinary tract infections and pyelonephritis are relatively frequent in patients with sickle cell disease and are important complications of pregnancy in this population. Pyelonephritis was reported in 17% of patients with sickle cell anemia in one large series (174). About 10% of patients seen in an emergency room for acute sickle cell crisis had symptomatic urinary tract infections (175). Urinary tract infections accounted for 73% of cases of *E. coli* bacteremia among sicklers (176). The increased susceptibility of patients with sickle cell anemia to pyelonephritis and gram negative bacteremia is thought to be caused by alterations in the blood flow and renal microvascular disease.

References

1. Evans DA, Williams DN, Laughlin LW, et al. Bacteriuria in a population-based cohort of women. J Infect Dis 1978;138:768–773.
2. Kunin CM, McCormack RC. An epidemiological study of bacteriuria and blood pressure among nuns and working women. N Engl J Med 1968;278:635–642.

3. Vorland LH, Carlson K, Aalen O. An epidemiological survey of urinary tract infections among outpatients in northern Norway. Scand J Infect Dis 1985;17:277–283.

4. Hovelius B, Mardh P-A. *Staphylococcus saprophyticus* as a common cause of urinary tract infections. Rev Infect Dis 1984;6:328–337.

5. Pead L, Maskell R, Morris J. *Staphylococcus saprophyticus* as a urinary pathogen: a six year prospective survey. Brit Med J 1985;291:1157–1159.

6. Kass EH, Miall WE, Stuart KL, et al. Epidemiologic aspects of infections of the urinary tract. In: Kass EH, Brumfitt W, eds. Infections of the urinary tract. Chicago: University of Chicago Press, 1975:1–7.

7. Asscher AW, Sussman M, Waters WE, et al. The clinical significance of asymptomatic bacteriuria in the nonpregnant woman. J Infect Dis 1969;120:17–21.

8. Kraft JK, Stamey TA. The natural history of recurrent bacteriuria in women. Medicine 1977;56:55–60.

9. Bergström T, Lincoln K, Ørskov F, et al. Studies of urinary tract infections in infancy and childhood VIII. Reinfection vs. relapse in recurrent urinary tract infections. Evaluation by means of identification of infecting organisms. J Pediatr 1967;71:13–20.

10. Kunin CM, Deutscher R, Paquin AJ. Urinary tract infection in school children: epidemiologic, clinical and laboratory study. Medicine 1964;43:91–130.

11. McGeachie J. Recurrent infection of the urinary tract: reinfection or recrudescence? Br Med J 1966;1:952–954.

12. Kunin CM, Polyak F, Postel E. Periurethral bacterial flora in women. JAMA 1980; 243:134–139.

13. Schlager TA, Hendley JO, Lohr JA, et al. Effect of periurethral colonization on the risk of urinary tract infection in healthy girls after their first urinary tract infection. Pediatr Infect Dis J 1993;12:988–993.

14. Ikäheimo R, Siitonen A, Heiskanen T, et al. Recurrence of urinary tract infection in a primary care setting: analysis of a 1-year follow-up of 179 women. Clin Infect Dis 1996; 22:91–99.

15. Foxman B, Zhang L, Tallman P, et al. Virulence characteristics of *Escherichia coli* causing first urinary tract infection predict risk of second infection. J Infect Dis 1995;172:1536–1541.

16. Russo TA, Stapleton A, Wenderoth S, et al. Chromosomal restriction fragment length polymorphism analysis of *Escherichia coli* strains causing recurrent urinary tract infection in young women. J Infect Dis 1995;172:440–445.

17. Kunin CM, Ames RE. Methods for determining the frequency of sexual intercourse and activities of daily living in young women. Am J Epidemiol 1981;113:55–61.

18. Ervin C, Komaroff AL, Pass TM. Behavioral factors and urinary tract infection. JAMA 1980;243:330–331.

19. Foxman B, Frerichs RR. Epidemiology of urinary tract infection: II. Diet, clothing, and urination habits. Am J Public Health 1985;75:1314–1317.

20. Foxman B, Jen-Wei Chi. Health behavior and urinary tract infection in college-aged women. J Clin Epidemiol 1990;43:329–337.

21. Takahashi M, Loveland DB. Bacteriuria and oral contraceptives. Routine health examination of 12,076 middle-class women. JAMA 1974;227:762–765.

22. Evans DA, Hennekens CH, Miao L, et al. Oral contraceptive use and bacteriuria in a community-based study. N Engl J Med 1978;299:536–537.

23. Gillespie L. The diaphragm: An accomplice in recurrent urinary tract infections. Urology 1984;24:25–30.

24. Remis RS, Gurwith MJH, Gurwith D, et al. Risk factors for urinary tract infection. Am J Epidemiol 1987;126:685–694.

25. Hooton T, Roberts P, Stamm W. Effects of recent sexual activity and use of a diaphragm on the vaginal microflora. Clin Infect Dis 1994;19:274–278.

26. McGroarty JA, Chong S, Reid G, et al. Influence of the spermicidal compound nonoxynol-9 on the growth and adhesion of urogenital bacteria in vitro. Current Microbiol 1990; 21:219–223.

27. Vosti KL. Recurrent urinary tract infections: prevention by prophylactic antibiotics after sexual intercourse. JAMA 1975;231:934–980.

28. Stapleton A, Latham RH, Johnson C, et al. Postcoital antimicrobial prophylaxis for recurrent urinary tract infection. JAMA 1990;264:703–706.

29. Pfau A, Sacks TG. Effective postcoital quinolone prophylaxis of recurrent urinary tract infections in women. J Urol 1994;152:136–138.
30. Lyon RP, Marshall S. Postcoital water flush in the prevention of urinary tract infection. JAMA 1971;218:1828.
31. Bran JL, Levison ME, Kaye D. Entrance of bacteria into the female urinary bladder. N Engl J Med 1972,286:626–629.
32. Buckley RM, McGuckin M, MacGregor RR. Urine bacterial counts after sexual intercourse. N Engl J Med 1978;298:321–324.
33. Kelsey MC, Mead MG, Gruneberg RN, et al. Relationship between sexual intercourse and urinary-tract infection in women attending a clinic for sexually transmitted diseases. J Med Microbiol 1979;12:511–512.
34. Adatto K, Doebele KG, Galland L, et al. Behavioral factors and urinary tract infection. JAMA 1979;241:2525–2526.
35. Elster AB, Lach PA, Roghmann KJ, et al. Relationship between frequency of sexual intercourse and urinary tract infections in young women. South Med J 1981;74:704–708.
36. Nicolle LE, Harding GKM, Preiksaitis J, et al. The association of urinary tract infection with sexual intercourse. J Infect Dis 1982;146:579–583.
37. Leibovici L, Alpert G, Laor A, et al. Urinary tract infections and sexual activity in young women. Arch Intern Med 1987;147:345–347.
38. Strom BL, Collins M, West SL, et al. Sexual activity, contraceptive use, and other risk factors for symptomatic and asymptomatic bacteriuria. Ann Intern Med 1987;107:816–823.
39. Gillenwater JY, Harrison RB, Kunin CM. Natural history of bacteriuria in schoolgirls. N Engl J Med 1979;301:396–399.
40. Kunin CM, White LVA, Tong HH. A reassessment of the importance of "low-count" bacteriuria in young women with acute urinary symptoms. Ann Intern Med 1993;119:454–460.
41. Fair WR, McClennan BL, Jost RG. Are excretory urograms necessary in evaluation of women with urinary tract infection? J Urol 1979;121:313–315.
42. Engel G, Schaeffer AJ, Grayhack JT, et al. The role of excretory urography and cystoscopy in the evaluation and management of women with recurrent urinary tract infection. J Urol 1980; 123:190–191.
43. Fowler JE, Pulaski ET. Excretory urography, cystography and cystoscopy in the evaluation of women with urinary-tract infection. N Engl J Med 1981;304:462–465.
44. Lieberman E, Macchia RJ. Excretory urography in women with urinary tract infection. J Urol 1982;127:263–264.
45. De Lange EE, Jones B. Unnecessary intravenous urography in young women with recurrent urinary tract infections. Clin Radiol 1983;34:551–553.
46. Mogensen P, Hansen LK. Do intravenous urography and cystoscopy provide important information in otherwise healthy women with recurrent urinary tract infection? Brit J Urol 1983;55:261–263.
47. Nickel JC, Wilson J, Morales A, et al. Value of urologic investigation in a targeted group of women with recurrent urinary tract infections. Canadian Journal of Surgery 1991;34:591–594.
48. Pinkerton JHM, Wood C, Williams ER, et al. Sequelae of urinary infection in pregnancy. A five-year follow-up. Br Med J 1961;ii:539–542.
49. Bullen M, Kincaid-Smith P. Asymptomatic pregnancy bacteriuria-a follow-up study 4–7 years after delivery. In: Kincaid-Smith P, Fairley KF, eds. Renal infection and renal scarring. Melbourne: Mercedes Publishing Service, 1971:33–39.
50. Zinner SH, Kass EH. Long-term (10 to 14 years) follow-up of bacteriuria of pregnancy. N Engl J Med 1971;285:820–827.
51. Freedman LR. Natural history of urinary infection in adults. Kidney Int Suppl 1975;4:S96–100.
52. Asscher AW, Chick S, Radford N, et al. Natural history of asymptomatic bacteriuria (ASB) in non-pregnant women. In: Brumfitt W, Asscher AW, eds. Urinary tract infection. Oxford: Oxford University Press, 1973:51–60.
53. Parker J, Kunin C. Pyelonephritis in young women. JAMA 1973;224:585–590.
54. Gower PE, Haswell B, Sidaway MME, et al. Follow-up of 164 patients with bacteriuria of pregnancy. Lancet 1968;1:990–994.

55. Alwall N. On controversial and open questions about the course and complications of non-obstructive urinary tract infection in adult women. Acta Med Scand 1978;203: 369–377.

56. McKenzie H, Donnet ML, Howie PW, et al. Risk of preterm delivery in pregnant women with group b streptococcal urinary infections or urinary antibodies to group b streptococcal and E. coli antigens. Br J Obstet Gynaecol 1994;101:107–113.

57. Kass EH. Bacteriuria and pyelonephritis of pregnancy. Arch Intern Med 1960; 105: 194–198.

58. Stenqvist K, Dahlén-Nilsson I, Lidin-Janson G, et al. Bacteriuria of pregnancy. Frequency and risk of acquisition. Am J Epidemiol 1989;129:372–379.

59. Golan A, Wexler S, Amit A, et al. Asymptomatic bacteriuria in normal and high-risk pregnancy. Eur J Obstet Gynecol Reprod Biol 1989;33:101–108.

60. Selkon JB, Davison JM, Sprott MS. Consequences for subsequent pregnancies of bacteriuria in schoolgirls. Lancet 1984;2:1154.

61. McGladdery SL, Aparicio S, Verrier-Jones K, et al. Outcome of pregnancy in an Oxford-Cardiff cohort of women with previous bacteriuria. Q J Med 1992;84:533–539.

62. Crabtree EF, Prather GC, Prien EL. End-results of urinary tract infections associated with pregnancy. Am J Obstet Gynecol 1937;34:405.

63. Norden CW, Kass EH. Bacteriuria of pregnancy-a critical appraisal. Annu Rev Med 1968;19:431–470.

64. Gratacos E, Torres PJ, Vila J, et al. Screening and treatment of asymptomatic bacteriuria in pregnancy prevent pyelonephritis. J Infect Dis 1994;169:1390–1392.

65. Brumfitt W, Davies BI, Rosser E. Urethral catheter as a cause of urinary-tract infection in pregnancy and puerperium. Lancet 1961;2:1059–1062.

66. Roberts AP, Beard RW. Some factors affecting bacterial invasion of bladder during pregnancy. Lancet 1965;1:1133–1136.

67. Norden CW, Levy PS, Kass EH. Predictive effect of urinary concentrating ability and hemagglutinating antibody titer upon response to antimicrobial therapy in bacteriuria of pregnancy. J Infect Dis 1970;121:588–596.

68. Asscher AW, Sussman M, Weiser R. Bacterial growth in human urine. In: O'Grady F, Brumfitt W, eds. Urinary tract infection. London: Oxford University, 1968:3–13.

69. Prat V, Konickova L, Rizerfeld W, et al. Experimental infection of the kidneys and urinary tract in pregnant rats. Physiologia Bohemoslovenica 1969;18:243–247.

70. Andriole VT, Cohn GL. The effect of diethylstilbestrol on the susceptibility of rats to hematogenous pyelonephritis. J Clin Invest 1964;43:1136–1145.

71. Harle EM, Bullen JJ, Thomson DA. Influence of oestrogen on experimental pyelonephritis caused by *Escherichia coli.* Lancet 1975;2:283–286.

72. Romero R, Oyarzun E, Mazor M, et al. Meta-analysis of the relationship between asymptomatic bacteriuria and preterm delivery/low birth weight. Obstet Gynecol 1989;73: 576–582.

73. Mittendorf R, Williams MA, Kass EH. Prevention of preterm delivery and low birth weight associated with asymptomatic bacteriuria. Clin Infect Dis 1992;14:927–932.

74. McGrady GA, Daling JR, Peterson DR. Maternal urinary tract infection and adverse fetal outcomes. Am J Epidemiol 1985;121:377–381.

75. Naeye RL. Causes of the excessive rates of perinatal mortality and prematurity in pregnancies complicated by maternal urinary-tract infections. N Engl J Med 1979;300:819–823.

76. Sever JL, Ellenbert JH, Edmonds D. Urinary tract infections during pregnancy: maternal and pediatric findings. In: Kass, EH, Brumfitt W, eds. Infections of the urinary tract. Chicago: University of Chicago Press, 1978:19–21.

77. Gruneberg RN, Leigh DA, Brumfitt W. Relationship of bacteriuria in pregnancy to acute pyelonephritis, prematurity and fetal mortality. Lancet 1969;1:1–3.

78. Harris R, Thomas V, Shelokov A. Asymptomatic bacteriuria in pregnancy: Antibody-coated bacteria, renal function, and intrauterine growth retardation. Am J Obstet Gynecol 1976;126:20–25.

79. Kass EH. Prevention of apparently non-infectious disease by detection and treatment of infections of the urinary tract. J Chronic Dis 1962;15:665–673.

80. Elder HA, Santamarina BAG, Smith S, et al. The natural history of asymptomatic bacteriuria during pregnancy: The effect of tetracycline on the clinical course and the outcome of pregnancy. Am J Obstet Gynecol 1971;111:441–462.

81. Hauth JC, Goldenberg RL, Andrews WW, et al. Reduced incidence of preterm delivery with metronidazole and erythromycin in women with bacterial vaginosis. N Engl J Med 1995;333:1732–1736.
82. Hillier SL, Nugent RP, Eschenbach DA, et al. Association between bacterial vaginosis and preterm delivery of a low-birth-weight infant. N Engl J Med 1995;333:1737–1742.
83. Pisacane A, Graziano L, Mazzarella G, et al. Breast-feeding and urinary tract infection. J Pediatr 1992;120:88–89.
84. Marild S, Jodal U, Hanson LA. Breast feeding and urinary tract infection. Lancet 1990; 336:942.
85. Forland M, Thomas V, Shelokov A. Urinary tract infections in patients with diabetes mellitus. JAMA 1977; 238:1924–1926.
86. Ooi BS, Chen BTM, Yu M. Prevalence and site of bacteriuria in diabetes mellitus. Postgrad Med J 1974;50:497–499.
87. Etzwiler DD. Incidence of urinary-tract infections among juvenile diabetics. JAMA 1965;191:81–83.
88. Pometta D, Rees SB, Younger D, et al. Asymptomatic bacteriuria in diabetes mellitus. N Engl J Med 1967;276:1118–1121.
89. Lindberg U, Bergstrom AL, Carlsson E, et al. Urinary tract infection in children with type I diabetes. Acta Paediatr Scand 1985;74:85–88.
90. Zhanel GG, Harding GKM, Nicolle LE. Asymptomatic bacteriuria in patients with diabetes mellitus. Rev Infect Dis 1991;13:150–154.
91. Schmitt JK, Fawcett CJ, Gullickson G. Asymptomatic bacteriuria and hemoglobin A1. Diabetes care 1986;9:518–520.
92. Goetz MB, Proctor RA. Normalization of intracellular calcium: a sweet solution to neutrophil dysfunction in diabetes? Ann Intern Med 1995;123:952–954.
93. Alexiewicz JM, Kumar D, Smogorewski M, et al. Polymorphonuclear leukocytes in non-insulin-dependent diabetes mellitus: abnormalities in metabolism and function. Ann Intern Med 1995;123:919–924.
94. Frimodt-Moller C, Mortensen S. Treatment of cystopathy. Ann Intern Med 1980;92: 327–328.
95. Browder AA, Petersdorf RG. Experimental pyelonephritis in rats with alloxan diabetes. Proc Soc Exp Biol Med 1964;115:332–336.
96. Raffel L, Pitsakis P, Levison SP, et al. Experimental *Candida albicans, Staphylococcus aureus,* and *Streptococcus faecalis pyelonephritis* in diabetic rats. Infect Immun 1981;34:773–779.
97. Weiser R, Asscher AW, Sussman M. Glycosuria and the growth of urinary pathogens. Invest Urol 1969;6:650–656.
98. Beeson PB. Factors in the pathogenesis of pyelonephritis. Yale J Biol Med 1955;28: 81–104.
99. Meares EM, Stamey TA. Bacteriologic localization patterns in bacterial prostatitis and urethritis. Invest Urol 1968;5:492–518.
100. Lipsky BA, Ireton RC, Fihn SD, et al. Diagnosis of bacteriuria in men: specimen collection and culture interpretation. J Infect Dis 1987;155:847–854.
101. Krieger JN, Ross SO, Simonsen JM. Urinary tract infections in healthy university men. J Urol 1993;149:1046–1048.
102. Vorland LH, Carlson K, Aalen O. An epidemiological survey of urinary tract infections among outpatients in northern Norway. Scand J Infect Dis 1985;17:277–283.
103. Wilson APR, Tovey SJ, Adler MW, et al. Prevalence of urinary tract infection in homosexual and heterosexual men. Genitourin Med 1986;62:189–190.
104. National Ambulatory Medical Care Survey: United States, 1977–78. (Advance data. 1980; Number 63, National Center for Health Statistics, U.S. Department of Health and Human Services.)
105. Spach DH, Stapleton AE, Stamm WE. Lack of circumcision increases the risk of urinary tract infection in young men. JAMA 1992;267:679–681.
106. Manzar KJ. Unusual cause of acute urinary tract infection in Muslim youths. Lancet 1990;335:1095.
107. Salmen P, Dwyer DM, Vorse H, et al. Whirlpool-associated Pseudomonas aeruginosa urinary tract infections. JAMA 1983;250:2025–2026.
108. Wong ES, Stamm WE. Sexual acquisition of urinary tract infection in a man. JAMA 1983;250:3087–3088.

109. Bailey RR, Peddie BA, Swainson CP, et al. Sexual acquisition of urinary tract infection in a man. Nephron 1986;44:217–218.

110. Hebelka M, Lincoln K, Sandberg T. Sexual acquisition of acute pyelonephritis in a man. Scand J Infect Dis 1993;25:141–143.

111. De Groen PC, Vukov LF. Sexual intercourse: you, me, and the microbe makes three. JAMA 1987;258:1730.

112. Barnes RC, Roddy RE, Daifuku R, et al. Urinary-tract infection in sexually active homosexual men. Lancet 1986;1:171–173.

113. De Pinho AMF, Lopes GS, Ramos-Filho CF, et al. Urinary tract infection in men with AIDS. Genitourin Med 1994;70:30–34.

114. Hoepelman AIM, Van Buren M, Van den Broek J, et al. Bacteriuria in men infected with HIV-1 is related to their immune status (CD4+cell count). AIDS 1992;6:179–184.

115. Marans HY, Mandell W, Kislak JW, et al. Prostatic abscess due to *Histoplasma capsulatum* in the acquired immunodeficiency syndrome. J Urol 1991;145:1275–1276.

116. Halpern M, Szabo S, Hochberg E, et al. Renal aspergilloma: an unusual cause of infection in a patient with the acquired immunodeficiency syndrome. Am J Med 1992;92:437–440.

117. Yu S, Provet J. Prostatic abscess due to *Candida tropicalis* in a nonacquired immunodeficiency syndrome patient. J Urol 1992;148:1536–1538.

118. Bauer FA, Wear DJ, Angritt P, et al. *Mycoplasma fermentans* (incognitus strain) infection in the kidneys of patients with acquired immunodeficiency syndrome and associated nephropathy. Hum Pathol 1991;22:63–69.

119. Cross J, Davidson K, Bradsher R. *Haemophilus influenzae* epididymo-orchitis and bacteremia in a man infected with the human immunodeficiency virus. Clin Infect Dis 1994;19:768–769.

120. Welker Y, Geissmann F, Benali A, et al. Toxoplasma-induced cystitis in a patient with AIDS. Clin Infect Dis 1994;18:453–454.

121. Kane CJ, Bolton DM, Connolly JA, et al. Voiding dysfunction in human immunodeficiency virus infections. J Urol 1996;155:523–526.

122. Orlander JD, Jick SS, Dean AD, et al. Urinary tract infections and estrogen use in older women. J Am Geriatr Soc 1992;40:817–820.

123. Boscia JA, Kobasa WD, Knight RA, et al. Epidemiology of bacteriuria in an elderly ambulatory population. Am J Med 1986;80:208–214.

124. Nordenstam G, Sundh V, Lincoln K, et al. Bacteriuria in representative population samples of persons ages 72–79 years. Am J Epidemiol 1989;130:1176–1186.

125. Nicolle LE. Urinary tract infection in the elderly. J Antimicrob Chemother 1994;33, Suppl.A:99–109.

126. Dontas AS, Tzonou A, Kasviki-Charvati Popi, et al. Survival in a residential home: An eleven-year longitudinal study. J Am Geriatr Soc 1991;39:641–649.

127. Heinamaki P, Haavisto M, Hakulinen T, et al. Mortality in relation to urinary characteristics in the very aged. Gerontology 1986;32:167–171.

128. Nicolle LE, Henderson E, Bjornson J, et al. The association of bacteriuria with resident characteristics and survival in elderly institutionalized men. Ann Intern Med 1987;106:682–686.

129. Kunin CM, Douthitt S, Dancing J, et al. The association between the use of urinary catheters and morbidity and mortality among elderly patients in nursing homes. Am J Epidemiol 1992;135:291–301.

130. Abrutyn E, Mossey J, Berlin JA, et al. Does asymptomatic bacteriuria predict mortality and does antimicrobial treatment reduce mortality in elderly ambulatory women? Ann Intern Med 1994;120:827–833.

131. Ruben FL, Dearwater SR, Norden CW, et al. Clinical infections in the noninstitutionalized geriatric age group: methods utilized and incidence of infections. Am J Epidemiol 1995;141(2):145–157.

132. Gleckman R, Blagg N, Hibert D, et al. Community-acquired bacteremic urosepsis in the elderly patients: a prospective study of 34 consecutive episodes. J Urol 1982;128:79–81.

133. Setia U, Serventi I, Lorenz P. Bacteremia in a long-term care facility. Arch Intern Med 1984;144:1633–1635.

134. Muder RR, Brennen C, Wagener MM, et al. Bacteremia in a long-term-care facility: a five-year prospective study of 163 consecutive episodes. Clin Infect Dis 1992;14:647–654.

135. Williams ME, Pannill FC III. Urinary incontinence in the elderly. Ann Intern Med 1982;97:895–907.
136. Marron KR, Fillit H, Peskowitz M, et al. The nonuse of urethral catheterization in the management of urinary tract incontinence in the teaching nursing home. J Am Geriatr Soc 1983;31:278–281.
137. Ouslander JG, Schnelle JF, Uman G, et al. Predictors of successful prompted voiding among incontinent nursing home residents. JAMA 1995;273:1366–1370.
138. Tolkoff-Rubin NE, Cosimi AB, Russell PS, et al. A controlled study of trimethoprim-sul-famethoxazole prophylaxis of urinary tract infection in renal transplant recipients. Rev Infect Dis 1982;4:614–618.
139. Pearson JC, Amend WJC, Vincenti FG, et al. Post-transplantation pyelonephritis: Factors producing low patient and transplant morbidity. J Urol 1980;123:153–156.
140. Douglas JF, Clarke S, Kennedy J, et al. Late urinary-tract infection after renal transplantation. Lancet 1974;2:1015.
141. Cuvelier R, Pirson Y, Alexandre GPJ, et al. Late urinary tract infection after transplantation: prevalence, predisposition and morbidity. Nephron 1985;40:76–78.
142. Rault R. Symptomatic urinary tract infections in patients on maintenance hemodialysis. Nephron 1984;37:82–84.
143. Lapchik MS, Filho AC, Pestana JOA, et al. Risk factors for nosocomial urinary tract and postoperative wound infections in renal transplant patients: a matched-pair case-control study. J Urol 1992;147:994–998.
144. Gillum DM, Kelleher SP. Acute pyelonephritis as a cause of late transplant dysfunction. Am J Med 1985;78:156–158.
145. Shelp WD, Wen S-F, Weinstein AB. Ureteropelvic obstruction caused by Candida pyelitis in homotransplanted kidney. Arch Intern Med 1966;117:401–404.
146. Ho M, Suwansirikul S, Dowling JM, et al. The transplanted kidney as a source of cy-tomegalovirus infection. N Engl J Med 1975;293:1109–1112.
147. Muller GA, Braun N, Einsele H, et al. Human cytomegalovirus infection in transplantation. Nephron 1993;64:343–353.
148. Hogan TF, Borden EC, McBain JA, et al. Human polyomavirus infections with JC virus and BK virus in renal transplant patients. Ann Intern Med 1980;92:373–378.
149. Mourad G, Soulillou JP, Chong G, et al. Transmission of *Mycobacterium tuberculosis* with renal allografts. Nephron 1985;41:82–85.
150. Byrd LH, Cheigh JS, Stenzel KH, et al. Association between *Streptococcus faecalis* urinary infections and graft rejection in kidney transplantation. Lancet 1978;2:1167–1168.
151. Whitworth JA, D'Apice AJF, Kincaid-Smith P. *Streptococcus faecalis* urinary-tract infection and renal-allograft rejection. Lancet 1979;1:778–779.
152. Frei D, Guttman RD, Gorman P, et al. Incidence of early urinary tract infections and relationship to subsequent rejection episodes in renal allograft recipients. Am J Nephrol 1981;1:37–40.
153. Smith EJ, Light JA, Filo RS, et al. Interstitial nephritis caused by trimethoprim-sul-famethoxazole in renal transplant recipients. JAMA 1980;244:360–361.
154. Bradley PP, Warden GD, Maxwell JG, et al. Neutropenia and thrombocytopenia in renal allograft recipients treated with trimethoprim-sulfamethoxazole. Ann Intern Med 1980;93:560–562.
155. Longcope WT. Chronic bilateral pyelonephritis: its origin and its association with hypertension. Ann Intern Med 1937;2:149–163.
156. Weiss S, Parker F. Pyelonephritis: its relation to vascular lesions and to arterial hypertension. Medicine 1939;18:221–315.
157. Huland H, Bosch R. Chronic pyelonephritis as a cause of end stage renal disease. J Urol 1982;127:642–643.
158. Jacobson SH, Eklof O, Eriksson CE, et al. Development of hypertension and uraemia after pyelonephritis in childhood: 27-year follow up. Br Med J 1989;299:703–706.
159. Tribe CR, Silver JR. Renal failure in paraplegia. Baltimore: Williams & Wilkins, 1969.
160. Kunin CM. Blood pressure in patients with spinal cord injury. Arch Intern Med 1971;127:285–287.
161. Shapiro AP, Sapira JD, Scheib ET. Development of bacteriuria in a hypertensive population. Ann Intern Med 1971;74:861–868.

162. Grieble HG, Johnston LC, Jackson GG. A search for unsuspected pyelonephritis among patients with hypertension. Clin Res 1958;6:293.
163. Smythe CMcC, Rivers CF, Rosemond RM. A comparison of the incidence of bacteriuria among hypertensives and matched controls. Arch Intern Med 1960;105:899–904.
164. Shapiro AP, Geyskes GG, Scheib E, et al. Mechanisms of blood pressure elevation in pyelonephritic rats after sodium loading. Proc Soc Exp Biol Med 1973;143:959–964.
165. Woods JW, Welt LG, Hollander W, et al. Susceptibility of rats to experimental pyelonephritis following recovery from potassium depletion. J Clin Invest 1960;39:28–33.
166. Brooks JB, Cherry WB, Thacker L, et al. Analysis by gas chromatography of amines and nitrosamines produced in vivo and in vitro by *Proteus mirabilis*. J Infect Dis 1972;126:143–153.
167. Sickles EA, Greene WH, Wiernik PH. Clinical presentation of infection in granulocytopenic patients. Arch Intern Med 1975;135:715–719.
168. Aliabadi H, Gonzalz R, Quie P. Urinary tract disorders in patients with chronic granulomatous disease. N Engl J Med 1989;321:706–708.
169. Southwick FS, Van der Meer JWM. Recurrent cystitis and bladder mass in two adults with chronic granulomatous disease. Ann Intern Med 1988;109:118–121.
170. Walther MM, Malech H, Berman A, et al. The urological manifestations of chronic granulomatous disease. J Urol 1992;147:1314–1318.
171. Phanichphant S, Boonpucknavig V. Asymptomatic bacteriuria in health and glomerulonephropathies. Nephron 1986;44:121–124.
172. Peddie BA, Bailey RR, Lynn KL, et al. Asymptomatic bacteriuria in health and glomerulonephropathies. Nephron 1988;48:336.
173. Saitoh H, Nakamura K, Hida M, et al. Urinary tract infection in oliguric patients with chronic renal failure. J Urol 1985;133:990–993.
174. Karayalcin G, Rossner F, Kim KY, et al. Sickle cell anemia—clinical manifestations in 100 patients and review of the literature. Am J Med Sci 1975;269:51–68.
175. Pollack CV, Jorden RC, Kolb JC. Usefulness of empiric chest radiography and urinalysis testing in adults with acute sickle cell pain crisis. Ann Emerg Med 1991;20:1210–1214.
176. Zarkowski HS, Gallagher D, Gill FM, et al. Bacteremia in sickle cell hemoglobinopathies. J Pediatr 1986;109:579–585.

Dysuria

Syndromes

Infections of the

Urethra, Vagina,

Bladder, and

Prostate

Overview

This chapter considers the wide variety of disorders of the urethra, vagina, bladder, and prostate that cause painful urination. Some are produced by microorganisms, whereas others are the result of immune, neoplastic, chemical, or unknown agents. Careful attention to the history, physical examination, microscopic examination, and culture of the urine will usually lead to the underlying diagnosis. The term "lower" urinary tract infection is often applied to bacterial and fungal infections of the bladder and urethra. This term may be misleading because any part of the urinary tract can be involved regardless of symptoms. Several noninfectious diseases can be confused with urinary tract infections. These include interstitial cystitis, a perplexing disease of unknown origin that can cause severe disability, particularly among women. The urethral syndrome in females is not a single entity, but a mixture of mechanical, chemical, infectious, and other conditions. The pyuria-dysuria syndrome is of particular interest because it appears to be a transitional stage between urethral and bladder infection. Dysuria syndromes in males may be caused by bacterial, fungal, viral, and sexually transmitted diseases, bladder tumors, and disorders of the prostate and epididymis. Chronic bacterial prostatitis is the most common cause of recurrent urinary tract infections in men. The focus of infection is exceedingly difficult to eradicate in the presence of prostatic calculi. It is particularly important to distinguish prostadynia from infectious prostatitis. These are entirely separate entities and are managed differently.

Dysuria Syndromes

Painful urination or dysuria is produced by conditions that irritate the urethra or periurethral structures (Table 7.1). Dysuria is relatively common in women. In one survey, 20% of women, aged 20–54 years, complained of having one or more episode in the previous year (1). The most common cause of dysuria in outpatient practice is vaginitis (2,3). This cause is followed by urinary tract infections and urethritis secondary to gonococcal, chlamydial, and herpes simplex infections. These conditions can usually be distinguished from each other by history, physical examination, and microscopic examination of the urine and other laboratory tests. In about one-third of cases, no etiologic agent can be found even with comprehensive microbiologic studies (2). A diagnostic scheme to differentiate among these conditions is presented in Figure 7.1.

Table 7.1. Causes of Frequent, Painful Urination in Females

Cystitis
   Bacterial
   Viral
   Interstitial
   Eosinophilic
   Other noninfectious causes
Urethral Syndromes
   Mechanical, Physical and Chemical Irritation (nonbacterial)
   Frequency-Dysuria Syndrome (nonbacterial)
   The Pyuria-Dysuria Syndrome (bacterial)
Sexually Transmitted Urethritis
   Neisseria gonorrhea
   Chlamydia trachomatis
   Herpes simplex
Vaginitis/Vaginosis
   Candida albicans
   Trichomonas vaginalis
   Gardnerella vaginalis
Vulvar vestibulitis

Cystitis

Cystitis literally means inflammation of the bladder. The symptoms include the urge to void immediately (urgency), inability to void at once (hesitancy), frequent voiding of small volumes of urine (frequency), and burning and pain on urination (dysuria). A burning or searing pain may be noted at termination of urination. This pain often is accompanied by a sensation of bladder fullness associated with gnawing, suprapubic pressure. The urine contains leukocytes (pyuria) and, frequently, erythrocytes (microscopic or gross hematuria). Cystitis may be produced by a variety of conditions other than urinary tract infection (Table 7.2). Cyclophosphamide and radiation therapy can produce severe hemorrhagic cystitis several weeks after initiation of treatment (4). Dysuria and sterile pyuria are common among males irradiated for cancer of the prostate. Dysuria and hematuria may be the first signs of interstitial nephritis caused by methicillin and other beta lactam antibiotics (5) and toxic chemicals (6). Eosinophiluria may provide an important clue to the diagnosis of immune tubulo-interstitial nephritis.

Bacterial Cystitis

The clinical features of bacterial cystitis are similar to other causes of cystitis and the pyuria-dysuria syndrome. Bacterial cystitis can easily be distinguished by the finding of bacteria and pus cells on microscopic examination of the urine and significant bacteriuria on quantitative culture. The patient

VAGINAL SYMPTOMS	URINARY SYMPTOMS
External Dysuria	Internal Dysuria
Vaginal discharge, itching, swelling, redness, soreness or vulvar burning, fishy odor	Urinary frequency, urgency, small volume of urination, pain on termination of urination, suprapubic pressure, foul odor
Suggests Vaginitis—Perform Pelvic Examination, Microscopic Examination of the Vaginal Secretions	*Suggests Urinary Infection—Perform Microscopic Examination of the Urine, Leukocyte Esterase & Nitrite Tests*

NO PYURIA OR BACTERIURIA	PYURIA WITHOUT BACTERIURIA
Suggests	*Suggests*
Mechanical or Chemical Irritation	Sexually Transmitted Urethritis
If Chronic Consider Cytoscopy for	*Consider Gonorrhea or Chlamydia and*
Bladder Tumors	*Specific Therapy*
Dysuria-Frequency Syndrome	Partially Treated Urinary Tract Infection,
Interstitial Cystitis	Radiation Cystitis
Do Not Treat With Antibiotics	*Do Not Treat for Urinary Infection*

PYURIA WITH LOW-COUNT BACTERIURIA	PYURIA WITH HIGH COUNT BACTERIURIA
Suggests	*Suggests*
Bacterial Urethritis	Bacterial Cystitis
(Pyuria-Dysuria Syndrome)	(Bacteria Are Growing In Urine)
Treat As For Urinary Tract Infection	*Treat Without Waiting For Culture Results*

HEMATURIA WITH BACTERIURIA AND PYURIA	HEMATURIA WITHOUT BACTERIURIA
Suggests Bacterial Cystitis	*Suggests Nonbacterial Cause*
Commonly Seen In Urinary Tract	Stones, Radiation, Cyclophosphamide,
Infections	Virus, Immune (β lactams, NSAIDS)
Should Resolve With Antibiotic Therapy	*Diagnosis Is Suspected From History*

Figure 7.1. Differential diagnosis of painful urination in females (dysuria syndromes).

Table 7.2. Conditions That Cause Inflammation of the Bladder (Cystitis)

Infectious-Intact Immune System
  Bacteria (Uropathogens)
  Viruses (Adenoviruses, *Herpes simplex, Herpes zoster*)
  Fungi (Candida and other yeasts)
  Parasites (Bilharzia-*Schistosoma haematobium*)
Infectious-Immunocompromised (AIDS, bone marrow transplant)
  Viruses (Adenoviruses, Cytomegalovirus, Papovavirus, Polyomavirus)
  Parasites (*Toxoplasma gondii*)
  Fungi (*Cryptococcus neoformans*)
  Others (*Pneumocystis carinii*)
Tumors and Foreign Bodies
  Carcinoma of the bladder, foreign bodies in the bladder
Chemical and Radiation
  Cyclophosphamide, Ether (used to deflate a balloon catheter)
  Radiotherapy in the bladder region (uterine and prostate cancer, lymphoma)
Immune
  Lupus erythematosus, beta lactam antibiotic-induced cystitis, eosinophilic cystitis
Interstitial Cystitis
  Hunner's ulcer

may report a foul odor to the urine. There may be a low grade fever ($\approx 100°$ F). Patients with persistent fever, leukocytosis, and flank pain are more likely to have pyelonephritis. Cystoscopic examination in patients with acute cystitis shows diffuse inflammation and focal areas of hemorrhage in the bladder wall. Chronic cystitis is often associated with lymphocytic infiltration of the submucosa [7]. The cells may aggregate to form germinal follicles (cystitis follicularis). Macroscopic tubercle-like nodules may be visible on cystoscopy as tiny, raised, pearly mucosal lesions (cystitis cystica). The lymphoid follicles produce immunoglobulins in response to long-standing infection. In severe infections, there may be gas in the bladder wall (emphysematous cystitis). This rare condition almost always occurs in diabetics and may be caused by enteric gram negative bacteria or Clostridia [8–10].

Viral Cystitis

Viruria may occur in otherwise healthy people during systemic infection [11]. The condition usually is transient and self-limited. Asymptomatic cytomegaloviruria may persist for prolonged periods of time in immunocompromised patients. Viruses can also produce tubulo-interstitial nephritis and hemorrhagic cystitis. Adenoviruses types 11 and 21 cause hemorrhagic cystitis in healthy children [12,13]. The disease is more common in boys than in girls and is self-limited. Polyomavirus BK virus has been isolated from the urine of a healthy boy with cystitis [14]. Viral particles can be seen in the urothelial cells by electron microscopy or be detected in the urine by the polymerase chain reaction (PCR). Herpes simplex, herpes zoster, and varicella viruses can produce cystitis, urinary retention, and urinary incontinence (15–19). Hemorrhagic cystitis and urinary symptoms have been described during epidemics of influenza A (20).

Immunocompromised patients undergoing bone marrow and renal transplantation and cancer chemotherapy are particularly susceptible to viral cystitis (21–24). The most common viruses in immunocompromised hosts are adenoviruses 7, 11, 21, and 35, cytomegalovirus, JC and BK polyoma viruses, and herpes simplex. It may be difficult at times to distinguish viral cystitis from cyclophosphamide and radiation-induced cystitis in immunocompromised patients. Cytomegalovirus, adeno, and herpes viruses have been implicated in IgA nephropathy (25,26).

Interstitial Cystitis

Interstitial cystitis is a painful disorder of the bladder of unknown origin. The symptoms include urinary frequency, nocturia, urgency, suprapubic pressure, and pain with bladder filling, often relieved by emptying. The typical patient is a 20 to 40-year-old Caucasian woman who has been symptomatic for several years and has seen many physicians before the diagnosis is made (27).

Diagnosis

The disease is diagnosed by the presence of long-standing dysuria, the absence of another etiologic explanation, small bladder capacity, and the characteristic findings on cystoscopy and biopsy (28) (Table 7.3). The mucosa may initially appear normal, but when the bladder is distended, there are multiple patches of reddened mucosa or strawberry-like hemorrhages or glomerulations. The findings on histologic examination depend on the severity of the disease. In the mild to moderate stages, there are submucosal edema, vasodilation, collagen deposition, and fibrosis. In the more severe forms, there are ulcerations, hemorrhage, a marked mononuclear inflammatory infiltrate, increased mast cells in the lamina propria and the detrusor muscles, and perineural infiltrates. The urine often contains red blood cells but is sterile. In 1915, Hunner described a "rare type of bladder ulcer," the so-called Hunner's ulcer (29). Although this lesion is classically associated with the disease, it is rarely found because the entire bladder mucosa usually is involved.

Epidemiology

The disease occurs most often in Caucasian women. It is about 10 times more common in females than males. The age of onset ranges from 15 to 80 years with a median of about 40 years. The prevalence is about 8 to 36 per 100,000 women depending on the methods used and country studied (30).

Table 7.3. National Institutes of Health Definition of Interstitial Cystitis (28)

I. INCLUSION CRITERIA
  A. One of the following cystoscopic findings must be present:
    1. Glomerulations
       a. Diffuse, present in three quadrants with at least 10 glomerulations per quadrant.
       b. Examination for glomerulations is performed with the patients under anesthesia after distention of the bladder to 80–100 cm water pressure for 1–2 minutes.
       c. The bladder may be distended up to two times before evaluation.
    2. The finding of a classic Hunner's ulcer.
  B. One of the following two criteria must be present:
    1. Pain associated with the bladder.
    2. Urinary urgency.
II. EXCLUSION CRITERIA
  1. Bladder capacity greater than 350 ml.
  2. No intense urge to void when the bladder is filled to 100 ml of gas or 150 ml of water with a rate of filling of 30–100 ml per minute.
  3. Involuntary bladder contractions on cystometrogram with a medium rate of filling.
  4. Duration of symptoms less than 9 months.
  5. Absence of nocturia.
  6. Symptoms are relieved following use of antimicrobial, antiseptic, anticholinergic or antispasmodic agents.
  7. The frequency of urination while awake is less than eight times per day.
  8. Bacterial cystitis or prostatitis was present within three months. The patient must have been abacteriuric for 3 months.
The following conditions are not present: bladder or ureteral calculi, active genital herpes, cancer of the female genital organs, urethral diverticulum, cyclophosphamide cystitis, vaginitis, tuberculous cystitis, radiation cystitis, any bladder tumors, age less than 18 years.

Pathogenesis

A variety of theories have been proposed to explain interstitial cystitis (Table 7.4). Evidence for altered permeability of the bladder mucosa is based on findings in patients with interstitial cystitis of increased absorption of urea from the vesical mucosa, decreased excretion of glycosaminoglycans in the urine, and the presence of Tamm-Horsfall protein in the intraurothelial space (31,32). Evidence that does not support this hypothesis is the finding that transvesical absorption of ^{99m}technicium-diethylenetriaminepentaacetic acid does not differ in patients and controls (33).

An immunologic mechanism is suggested by the presence of mast and eosinophil cells in the bladder wall, activation of urinary kallikreins, elevated excretion of methylhistamine, and excretion of eosinophilic cationic proteins into the urine. Evidence against an immunologic explanation includes no

Table 7.4. Proposed Causes of Interstitial Cystitis

Abnormal permeability of the urothelium (epithelial dysfunction)
Deficiency in the bladder glycosaminoglycans (GAG) layer of the mucosal surface
Allergic or autoimmune processes
Altered innervation of the bladder and neuropeptide synthesis
Impaired bladder perfusion
Dormant or fastidious microbes
Psychological factors

difference between cases and controls in urinary excretion of complement, eosinophilic cationic protein, interleukin-1, interleukin-2, interferon-γ, tumor necrosis factor, prostaglandins, or thromboxanes (34), although some patients are reported to have elevated urinary excretion of interleukin-6 (35). The urine obtained from patients with the disease does not act as a mitogen (36). Studies of cellular immunity are equivocal. Although autoantibodies and antinuclear anti-Tamm-Horsfall protein antibodies have been demonstrated in the sera and chemotactic factors have been reported in the urine of patients with interstitial cystitis, it is not clear whether these are produced by an autoimmune mechanism or are the result of chronic inflammation and cell death (37).

Therapy

Treatments for this disorder are mainly palliative and rarely curative. They include intravesical administration of oxychlorosene, dimethyl sulfoxide (DMSO) and silver nitrate, and use of heparin, sodium pentosanpolysulfate, and laser therapy. Patients with incapacitating disease may require cystectomy and total bladder substitution. No other disorder of the urinary tract causes more misery to the patient and a greater sense of inadequacy on the part of the treating physician (38). Antidepressant drugs are often used, but it is unclear whether this calms the patient or the physician. It is not difficult to understand why patients with interstitial cystitis become frustrated by a disease of unknown cause and uncertain cure. This frustration requires considerable effort on the part of the physician to listen and try to be understanding and helpful. The Interstitial Cystitis Association (ICA) has accomplished a great deal in dispelling the belief that it is an emotional disorder. This organization has generated an extensive support network for sufferers of this disease and has stimulated research in the field. For further information, contact the ICA at P.O. Box 1553, Madison Square Station, New York, NY 10159–1553.

Lupus Cystitis

Cystitis may be the early finding in systemic lupus erythematosus. It appears to be caused by local depositions of antigen antibody complexes in bladder mucosa (39–41). It may be confused with bacterial cystitis because both conditions are common in young women. The urine is sterile in lupus cystitis.

Eosinophilic Cystitis

Eosinophilic cystitis is a relatively rare condition characterized by infiltration of eosinophils into the submucosa and muscularis of the bladder. The process may involve the ureters and produce obstruction. The usual presenting signs and symptoms are dysuria, frequency, and hematuria. Peripheral eosinophilia and eosinophiluria may present, but these findings are often absent. The patient may have a history of allergy, asthma, or parasitic infections (42,43). Drugs that are associated with the disease include methicillin, warfarin, and Tranilast (n-3',4'-dimethoxycinnamoyl anthranilic acid), a drug used to treat asthma in Japan. The disease may be self-limited or require treatment with oral or intravesical corticosteroids.

Urethral Syndromes in Females

Only about half of female patients with urinary frequency and dysuria will be found to have significant bacteriuria ($\geq 1 \times 10^5$ cfu/ml) (44–48). The term "urethral syndrome" was coined to describe women with symptoms suggestive of a lower urinary tract infection in the absence of significant bacteriuria with a conventional pathogen (49). Other names for this syndrome include abacterial cystitis, irritable urethral syndrome, cystalgia, and urethrotrigonitis. It is now evident that the urethral syndrome consists of several different clinical entities. These entities need to be distinguished carefully from each other to avoid inappropriate diagnoses and therapy. I prefer the classification shown in Table 7.1, which separates infectious from noninfectious causes.

Mechanical and Chemical Irritation

Urethral irritation may occur in association with bubble baths, tight pants, cold weather, and painful sexual intercourse (dyspareunia). Postmenopausal women not on hormone replacement therapy often will have dry urethral and vaginal mucosae and poor vaginal lubrication. *These women do not have pyuria or bacteriuria and should not be treated for urinary tract infections with antimicrobial drugs.*

Frequency-Dysuria Syndrome

This syndrome is characterized by persistent frequency, urgency, dysuria, suprapubic pressure, and difficulty with voiding. There is often a sensation of incomplete emptying of the bladder. There may be microscopic hematuria, but no pyuria. The condition is poorly understood. It is not caused by infection and does not respond to antimicrobial therapy. The role of fastidious bacteria, particularly Lactobacilli in this syndrome, has been vigorously championed by Maskell and her colleagues (50). This notion has not been confirmed by other investigators (51–53). In several independent studies, fastidious organisms could neither be isolated by suprapubic bladder puncture (SPA) nor be found in higher frequency in the periurethral zone of healthy females compared to those with dysuria. Other proposed causes of the frequency-dysuria syndrome include abnormalities of the detrusor mechanism or external sphincter spasm, allergies, cold weather, and psychosocial factors (54–56). The patient often is miserable and frustrated by her inability to obtain relief. A variety of treatments have been tried but provide only temporary relief. These include urethral dilatation and massage, cryosurgery, topical preparations containing estrogens, nitrofurazone or glucocorticosteroids, and tranquilizers. *These women do not have urinary tract infections and should not be treated with antimicrobial drugs.*

The Pyuria-Dysuria Syndrome

This syndrome is clinically indistinguishable from bacterial cystitis. Pyuria exists without apparent bacteriuria on microscopic examination of the urine. The causative microorganisms include *Escherichia coli, Staphylococcus saprophyticus,* and enteric gram negative bacteria. These are the same uropathogens that are found in bacterial cystitis. The only laboratory difference between bacteria cystitis and the pyuria-dysuria syndrome is the bacterial count. Bacterial counts in the pyuria-dysuria syndrome range from 1×10^2 to $< 10^5$ cfu/ml as opposed to $\geq 10^5$ cfu/ml that are present in most patients with urinary tract infections.

Stamm and his associates have studied the pyuria-dysuria syndrome with low-count bacteriuria in considerable detail and provide strong evidence that it is a valid clinical entity (57–59). They found the following:

- Low counts of the same microorganism are present both in the voided urine and urine obtained by suprapubic or urethral catheterization.
- Low counts persist in the same patient over time.
- Dysuria and pyuria resolve with specific antimicrobial therapy.

Based on these observations, Stamm proposed that the criterion for significant bacteriuria be reduced to $\geq 1 \times 10^2$ cfu/ml. We have been able to partially confirm Stamm's work, but we interpret the results differently (60). The syndrome appears to be an early or transitional stage of urinary tract infection initially localized to the urethra. We found the following:

- "Low-count" bacteriuria could not be explained by dilution of the urine or failure of the bacteria to grow well in the patient's own urine.
- Counts of 1×10^2 cfu/ml are often found in asymptomatic individuals.
- There is a step-wise increase in the association of urinary symptoms and pyuria with the bacterial count (Figs. 2.5 and 2.6).

The adult female urethra is not a simple tube (Fig. 7.2). It is surrounded by an extensive network of paraurethral glands analogous to the male prostate. There are also many small arborized ducts and mucous glands and minute pit-like recesses or lacunae that open into the urethra (61). Some of the tubules are analogous to the glands of Littre present in the penile urethra. Skene's ducts are the two largest structures; they open laterally to the urethra and can be a site for infection. It is not difficult to visualize how bacteria can invade these structures, produce localized infection, and eventually migrate to the bladder.

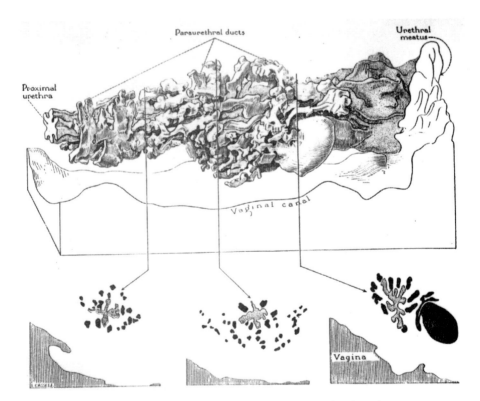

Figure 7.2. Three dimensional anatomy of the female urethra based on wax models. Reproduced with permission from Huffman (61).

Evidence that the Pyuria-Dysuria Syndrome is a Urethral or Paraurethral Infection that May Eventually Develop Into a Urinary Tract Infection

- Low counts cannot be explained by dilution of the urine or failure of the bacteria to grow well in the patient's own urine (60).
- Greater numbers of pus cells are present in the first portion of the voided urine in women with pyuria-dysuria (62).
- The adult female urethra is not a simple tube. It is surrounded by an extensive network of paraurethral glands analogous to the male prostate (Fig. 7.4 [61]).
- The periurethral zone of some women, particularly among those prone to recurrent infections are often colonized with small numbers of uropathogens (63–65).
- About a third to half of women with low-count bacteria will develop counts of $\geq 10^5$ cfu/ml if left untreated (66, 67).

Although low-count bacteriuria clearly is associated with the pyuria-dysuria syndrome, there are good reasons not to lower the standard criterion of $\geq 10^5$ cfu/ml for most urinary tract infections (see Chapter 2 for suggested criteria of significant bacteriuria). The pyuria-dysuria syndrome with "low-count" bacteriuria should be considered a special case.

It also needs to be emphasized that the SPA is not a perfect tool. Bacteria may enter the bladder transiently without producing infection. For example, small numbers of bacteria may be introduced transiently into the bladder when the urethra is massaged or "milked" (68). *Ureaplasma urealyticum* and *Gardnerella vaginalis* may be recovered by SPA from asymptomatic pregnant women (69,70). It is not certain whether this represents infection or contamination. These microorganisms do not grow well in urine and may have refluxed into the bladder without causing infection.

Key Points About the Pyuria-Dysuria Syndrome

- The symptoms are indistinguishable from those of bacterial cystitis.
- Pyuria is defined as ≥ 10–20 leukocytes/mm^3 or a positive leukocyte esterase test.
- A uropathogen is isolated from the urine (*Escherichia coli, Staphylococcus saprophyticus*, or enteric gram negative bacteria).
- The bacterial count may be as low as $\geq 10^2$ cfu/ml, but is preferable $\geq 10^3$ cfu/ml or greater.
- The higher the bacterial count and quantity of pyuria, the more certain is the diagnosis.
- Treatment is the same as for uncomplicated urinary tract infection.
- The syndrome has been studied almost exclusively in young adult women (16–40 years) and may not be applicable to children or older women or men.
- The syndrome appears to be an early or transitional form of urinary tract infection that is best explained by a localized infection in the paraurethral glands.
- If treatment is delayed, many of the patients will develop counts of $\geq 10^5$ cfu/ml.
- It is recommended that for purposes of clinical trials of new anti-infective drugs, the pyuria-dysuria syndrome be regarded as a separate entity.

Sexually Transmitted Urethritis

This condition is divided into gonococcal and nongonococcal urethritis (71). In males, gonorrhea is characterized by a burning sensation on urination, some difficulty with passage of urine, and a penile discharge. The discharge may be clear, milky, or yellowish depending on the severity or chronicity of the process. Gram stain reveals abundant polymorphonuclear leukocytes, and small coffee bean-shaped gram-negative diplococci are usually seen within the cell cytoplasm. Gonorrhea in the female often is more difficult to diagnose and the gram stain is not helpful because the vagina and urethra may contain microorganisms with similar morphology. Culture of the urethra, cervix, and rectum are required.

Nongonococcal urethritis in males tends to be characterized by dysuria and a thin or absent urethral discharge. *Chlamydia trachomatis* accounts for most cases. Culture of the secretions or the newly developed molecular probes are required to make an etiologic diagnosis. Reasonable evidence exists to suggest that *Ureaplasma urealyticum* and *Trichomonas vaginalis* also are causal agents of the syndrome. A full discussion of the diagnosis and management of gonorrhea and nongonococcal urethritis is beyond the scope of this book.

Vaginitis, Vaginosis, and Vulvar Vestibulitis

Vaginitis is the most frequent cause of dysuria in females. It accounts for as much as two-thirds of the cases of dysuria in ambulatory practice (2,3). Dysuria associated with vaginitis is characterized by a sensation of *external* pain as the stream of urine passes over the inflamed vaginal labia. In contrast, dysuria associated with urethritis is more often an *internal* pain (felt inside the body) during urination (72). Some women will describe *both external and internal* dysuria and may have urinary tract infection as well as vaginitis (60) (Fig. 7.1).

The microbial flora of the healthy vagina are unique. The predominant microorganisms are gram positive rods. Gram negative enteric bacteria and other uropathogens are rarely present and, if so, only in small numbers. Vaginal fluid contains about 1×10^8 to 10^9 cfu/g of aerobic and anaerobic microorganisms (73,74). The most abundant species, in order of frequency, are *Lactobacilli spp., Corynebacterium spp., Streptococcus spp., Staphylococcus epidermidis* and other coagulase negative staphylococci, *Bacteroides spp., Eubacterium spp., Mycoplasma hominis,* and *Peptostreptococcus spp.* A wide variety of other microorganisms are present in lower numbers. During the menstrual cycle, the concentration of anaerobes remains constant. The concentration of aerobes decreases during the week preceding menstruation. The vaginal pH in premenopausal women is ≤ 4.5 due to production of lactate by Lactobacilli and streptococcus species.

Alterations in the vaginal microflora may lead to overgrowth with *Candida albicans, Gardnerella vaginalis,* and *Trichomonas vaginalis.* Each of these produces a relatively distinct clinical syndrome, although considerable overlap may exist. Other microorganisms that can produce vaginitis include group A β hemolytic streptococci, which can produce an acute suppurative infection, Shigella in prepubertal girls (75), and pinworms. The toxic shock syndrome, caused by toxin-producing strains of *Staphylococcus aureus*, is not associated with vaginitis, unless a tampon has been left in place too long. The etiologic diagnosis is suggested by the clinical findings.

Vaginosis Caused by Gardnerella vaginalis

This syndrome is referred to as vaginosis rather than vaginitis because inflammatory cells are not present in the vaginal discharge. The symptoms consist of mild itching and irritation of the vulva, a thin, homogenous gray, fishy, odoriferous discharge, and a pH greater than 4.5 (usually in the range of 5.0 to 5.5). The fishy odor is produced by amines and is intensified with addition of 10% KOH. The vaginal epithelial cells often are heavily coated with small gram negative bacilli or coccobacilli (clue cells). Metronidazole (500 mg twice daily for 7 days) is highly effective, but relapses and recurrent infection may be troublesome. There is evidence that bacterial vaginosis doubles the risk of prematurity in some women, particularly those who are also colonized with vaginal bacteroides and *Mycoplasma hominis*.

Vaginitis Caused by Trichomonas vaginalis

This condition may be asymptomatic, or there may be vaginal itching and burning. The discharge may be frothy, white, or yellow and blood-tinged during menses. The vaginal exudate is often filled with polymorphonuclear leukocytes and the inflamed area of the vagina may have a red "strawberry-like" appearance (colpitis macularis). The pH of the vaginal exudate tends to be acid, but is often > 4.5. Trichomonads can be visualized in wet mount preparations by morphology and motility. Treatment is highly successful with a single 2-g dose of metronidazole or with a more standard 7-day regimen of 250 mg given 3 times daily. Vaginal trichomoniasis is considered a sexually transmitted disease and should raise the suspicion of coincident infection with *Neisseria gonorrheae*. Male consorts may become colonized with *Trichomonas vaginalis* and may develop mild symptoms of urethritis. It is also a rare cause prostatitis in the male (76). A single 2-g dose of metronidazole is recommended for treatment of the sex partner to prevent reinfection.

Vaginitis Caused by Candida albicans

This condition is often associated with severe itching and a burning pain on urination. The mucosa is often red and inflamed with a thin exudate and white curds. The vulva is often red, swollen, and painful. Typical yeast cells with pseudohyphi will be seen on gram stain. Excellent clinical response may be obtained with over-the-counter preparations of intravaginal clotrimazole or miconazole creams or oral fluconazole.

Vulvar Vestibulitis

This condition is characterized by tenderness to touch in the ringlike portion of the vulva extending from the hymenal ring to the inner margins of the labia minora. This region includes the posterior fourchette, the clitoris, the urethral meatus, Skene's paraurethral glands, and the openings of the Bartholin's glands. Vulvar vestibulitis should be suspected when a woman complains of vulval irritation and burning that is precipitated by sexual intercourse (77–80). Although *Candida albicans* and *Chlamydia trachomatis* are sometimes isolated from the vaginal vestibule, the cause of this condition is unknown. It does not respond to a variety of topical steroid and antifungal preparations. About half the patients will have spontaneous resolution of the symptoms. Surgical resection of the involved tissue may be needed for patients with persistent dyspareunia.

Prostatitis and Epididymitis

Prostatitis

Prostatitis is an inflammatory condition of the prostate gland (81). It can be infectious or noninfectious (i.e., secondary to trauma or an unknown cause). The process may be limited to the prostate or extend to the contiguous structures of the male genital tract to include the testes (orchitis), the epididymis (epididymitis), and the seminal vesicles. Infections of the prostate gland are classified as acute or chronic prostatitis, prostatic abscess, or nonbacterial prostatitis. A clinical classification based on symptoms, route of infection, and common microorganisms is presented in Table 7.5. Prostadynia is a distinctly different entity and will be discussed separately.

Table 7.5. Infectious Disorders of the Prostate

Clinical Condition	Route of Infection	Common Microorganisms
Acute Bacterial Prostatitis	Ascending and contiguous	Uropathogens*
Prostatic Abscesses	Ascending and contiguous	Uropathogens, anaerobes *Candida* spp., Trichomonas
Prostatic Abscesses	Metastatic	*Staphylococcus aureus, Hemophilus influenzae Mycobacteria tuberculosis*
Prostatic Abscesses (Immunocompromised)	Metastatic	Systemic fungal infections[†] Atypical mycobacteria
Chronic Bacterial Prostatitis	Ascending and contiguous	Uropathogens
Nonbacterial Prostatitis	Unknown	Not established, possibly Chlamydia and Ureaplasma

*These include: *Escherichia coli* and other enteric bacteria, *Pseudomonas aeruginosa* and other water borne bacteria, Enterococci and Staphylococci.
[†]These include: *Cryptococcus neoformans, Blastomyces dermatitidis, Histoplasma capsulatum, Aspergillus fumigatis.*

Clinical Features

Acute bacterial prostatitis is a suppurative process characterized by fever, chills, leukocytosis, and acute perineal and low back pain. In the more severe cases, there may be bacteremia, shock, and disseminated intravascular coagulation (DIC). The prostate is usually enlarged and extremely tender. The epididymis and testes are often tender. Rectal examination should be done gently, if at all. Blood cultures are often positive and will usually reveal the same microorganism found in the urine.

It may be difficult to differentiate acute prostatitis from prostatic abscess. Prostatic abscesses should be suspected when a tender, bulging mass is felt on rectal examination. The urine may be sterile (with metastatic infection) or loaded with bacteria and pus cells (with ascending infection). Blood cultures will usually contain the same microorganism found in the urine. CT scan and rectal ultrasound are extremely helpful in identifying prostatic abscesses (Fig. 7.3).

Chronic bacterial prostatitis may be asymptomatic or characterized by a sensation of perineal fullness, low back pain, dysuria, and pyuria. Fever and constitutional illness are uncommon. The hallmark of chronic, bacterial prostatitis is the presence of the same microorganism with each recurrent episode of urinary tract infection (82). This is undoubtedly the most important cause of recurrent urinary tract infection in the adult male. The focus of infection may be exceedingly difficult to eradicate in the presence of pro-

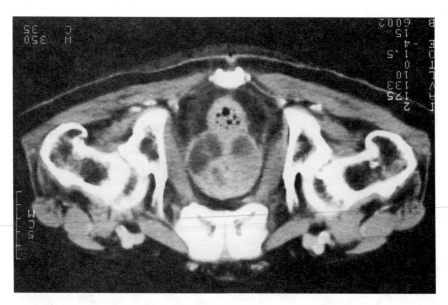

Figure 7.3. Multiple abscesses of the prostate in an elderly man who had been managed with an indwelling urinary catheter. Pseudomonas aeruginosa was isolated from a prostatic biopsy.

static calculi. These small stones consist of deposits of inspissated (dried) salts from urine that has refluxed into the prostatic ducts (83). Surgical removal of all infected calculi may be required for cure.

An example of prostatic calculi in a 56-year-old man with recurrent relapsing infection despite repeated courses of therapy with intravenously administered cephalosporin and aminoglycoside antibiotics is shown in Figure 7.4. He refused surgery and was managed successfully by long-term prophylaxis with trimethoprim.

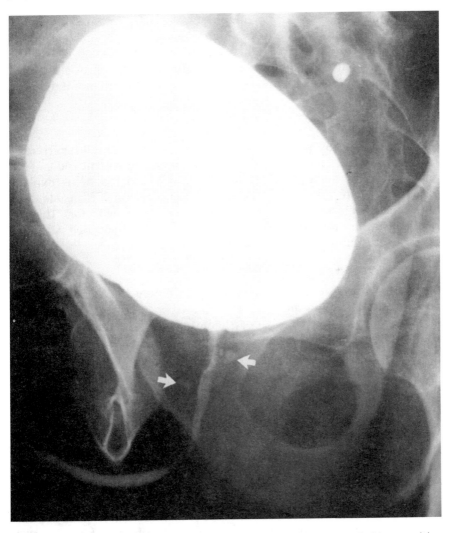

Figure 7.4. Prostatic calculi surrounding the urethra of a 56-year-old man with recurrent urinary tract infection that occurred after use of an indwelling catheter.

Pathogenesis
The prostate gland may become infected by several routes. These include:

Ascending Infection
The infection is often initiated by instrumentation of the urethra and bladder. The microorganisms grow in the bladder urine and reflux into the prostatic ducts. Acute, ascending, bacterial prostatitis is often caused by *E. coli*. Chronic, ascending, prostatitis is caused by more resistant *Enterobacteriaceae*, Pseudomonas, and enterococci. Coagulase negative staphylococci, alpha hemolytic streptococci, and diphtheroids are common commensals of the male urethra and should be interpreted with considerable caution. Coagulase negative staphylococci have been found in prostatic biopsies of some patients with chronic prostatitis and the expressed prostatic secretions of some patients with prostadynia, but more often than not they are contaminants.

Contiguous Infection
The microorganisms presumably enter the prostate from the rectum through lymphatic channels or venules. Although a lymphatic route of infection has not been clearly established, this concept helps explain episodes of acute bacterial prostatitis that emerge "out of the blue" in young and middle-aged men with no known predisposing factors. The microorganisms are the same uropathogens commonly associated with urinary tract infection.

Hematogenous Infection
The microorganisms enter the prostate from a distant site by means of the blood stream. These infections are often caused by *Staphylococcus aureus, Hemophilus influenzae*, tuberculosis, or systemic fungal infections (blastomycosis, histoplasmosis, coccidioidomycosis and cryptococcosis) (84–92). Prostatic infection with unusual microorganisms is often not clinically suspected and is a surprise finding on prostatic biopsy. These microorganisms should be suspected in patients with AIDS and neoplastic disease.

Differential Diagnosis
Acute bacterial prostatitis and prostatic abscesses are readily recognized by their clinical presentation. The prostate specific antigen (PSA) may be extraordinarily high during the acute phase of the illness. It will gradually fall within 2 to 3 weeks in response to antimicrobial therapy. Chronic bacterial prostatitis should be suspected in older males with persistent or recurrent urinary tract infections with the same microorganism. The PSA may be elevated slightly and the condition is easily confused with prostate cancer. PSA levels will usually fall in response to specific therapy.

Nonbacterial Prostatitis

This syndrome is characterized by back pain, discomfort on voiding, and ejaculation and perineal aching. It is differentiated from prostadynia by the presence of leukocytes in the prostatic fluid. The syndrome may be caused by *Chlamydia trachomatis, Ureaplasma urealyticum,* or *Mycoplasma hominis* (93), but the etiology cannot be established in most cases (94). "Nonspecific prostatitis" may be found in transrectal biopsies obtained from men with elevated blood levels of PSA. In some instances, the PSA levels will fall after a short course of antimicrobial therapy, but the long-term outcome is unknown.

Prostadynia

Prostadynia or prostatosis (a term that is now discarded) is a noninflammatory condition of unknown origin (95). It is encountered most often in young men and is characterized by a sense of fullness or pressure in the perineum, testicles, and low back. The expressed prostatic secretions are sterile and do not contain inflammatory cells. The symptoms may be relieved temporarily and sometimes exacerbated by ejaculation or prostatic massage per rectum. Antimicrobial drugs are ineffective. The condition in some men may be caused by sexual problems; others may have detrusor-sphincter dyssynergia, but the cause in most is unknown. Prostadynia can be differentiated from chronic bacterial prostatitis by microscopic examination and culture of the expressed prostatic secretions (EPS) or semen.

Hematospermia

Hematospermia is a benign condition in which blood is present in the ejaculate. It is usually due to rupture of small blood vessels in the prostatic bed. It may be caused by trauma to the prostate, neoplasms, masturbation, and bleeding disorders. It is not a sign of prostatitis.

Epididymitis

Acute epididymitis is characterized by swelling and tenderness of the epididymis. The testicle is swollen and tender. It may be a manifestation of acute or chronic prostatitis or a separate clinical entity. In severe cases, the blood supply to the testes may be compromised and require surgical decompression. There may be a small mucopurulent penile discharge.

Haemophilus influenzae may cause epididymitis in young boys and in men infected with human immunodeficiency virus (96,97). *Chlamydia trachomatis* and *Neisseria gonorrhoeae* are found in sexually active young men (98,99). Epididymitis in older men is usually a complication of indwelling urethral catheters and prostatic surgery. It is believed to be caused by reflux of infected urine into partially obstructed epididymal ducts. The microorganisms consist of the common uropathogens and include *Pseudomonas aeruginosa, Staphylococcus aureus,* and *Staphylococcus epidermidis* (100). Epididymotomy may be needed to drain the infection surgically and to relieve the pressure on the testicles. Other causes of chronic epididymitis include tuberculosis, atypical mycobacteria, and the deep mycoses (blastomycosis, coccidioidomycosis, and cryptococcosis) as seen in chronic prostatitis. Aspiration and biopsy are extremely helpful in making a definitive diagnosis.

Key Points About Prostatitis, Prostatosis, and Epididymitis

- Acute bacterial prostatitis and prostatic abscesses are acute suppurative infections. Ascending and contiguous infections are caused by *E. coli* and other uropathogens as found in urinary tract infections. Hematogenous infections may be caused by *Staphylococcus aureus* and *Hemophilus influenzae.*
- Chronic bacterial prostatitis may be asymptomatic or associated with perineal tenderness. The microorganisms are the same uropathogens as found in urinary tract infections. Coagulase negative staphylococci, alpha hemolytic streptococci, and diphtheroids are part of the normal flora of the male urethra and only rarely cause infection.
- Chronic bacterial prostatitis is the most common cause of recurrent urinary tract infections in men. The focus of infection is exceedingly difficult to eradicate in the presence of prostatic calculi.
- Prostatic abscess should be suspected when a tender, bulging mass is felt on rectal examination, the urine is sterile, the patient fails to respond to antimicrobial therapy, or *Staphylococcus aureus* is isolated from the blood.
- Prostatic abscesses in immunocompromised patients may be caused by systemic fungi, atypical mycobacteria, and tuberculosis.
- Nonbacterial prostatitis is an inflammatory condition that resembles chronic prostatitis. The etiologic agent(s) is not well defined.
- Prostate specific antigen (PSA) often is elevated in patients with acute prostatitis and prostatic abscesses. Levels return to normal after several weeks of specific therapy. Elevated PSA is seen in chronic prostatitis and may be confused with prostate cancer. The levels tend to return to normal with specific therapy.
- Prostatosis is a noninflammatory condition. It is seen most often in young men. Its cause is unknown and it does not respond to treatment with antimicrobial drugs.
- Epididymitis in young men is usually caused by *Neisseria gonorrhea* or *Chlamydia trachomatis.*
- Epididymitis in older men is caused most often by infections induced by urinary catheters and urologic instrumentation. The microorganisms are the same uropathogens as found in complicated urinary tract infections.
- Chronic epididymitis may be caused by bacteria or by systemic fungi, atypical mycobacteria, and tuberculosis in immunocompromised patients.

References

1. Walker M, Heady JA, Shaper AG. The prevalence of dysuria in women in London. J Royal Coll Gen Pract 1983;33:411–415.
2. Berg AO, Heidrich FE, Fihn SD, et al. Establishing the cause of genitourinary symptoms in women in a family practice. JAMA 1984;251:620–625.
3. Komaroff AL. Acute dysuria in women. N Engl J Med 1984;310:368–375.
4. Marshall FF, Klinefelter HF. Late hemorrhagic cystitis following low-dose cyclophosphamide therapy. Urology 1979;14:573–575.
5. Bracis R, Sanders CV, Gilbert DN. Methicillin hemorrhagic cystitis. Antimicrob Agents Chemother 1977;12:438–439.
6. DeVries CR, Freiha FS. Hemorrhagic cystitis review. J Urol 1990;143:1–9.
7. Hansson S, Hanson E, Hjalmas K, et al. Follicular cystitis in girls with untreated asymptomatic or covert bacteriuria. J Urol 1990;143:330–332.
8. West TE, Holley HP, Lauer AD. Emphysematous cystitis due to *Clostridium perfringens*. JAMA 1981;246:363–364.
9. Quint HJ, Drach GW, Rappaport WD, et al. Emphysematous cystitis: a review of the spectrum of disease. J Urol 1992;147:134–137.
10. Devitt AT, Sethia KK. Gangrenous cystitis: case report and review of the literature. J Urol 1993;149:1544–1545.
11. Koss LG. BK Viruria and hemorrhagic cystitis. N Engl J Med 1987;316:108–109.
12. Numazaki Y, Kumasaka T, Yanon N, et al. Further study on acute hemorrhagic cystitis due to adenovirus type 11. N Engl J Med 1973;289:344–347.
13. Mufson MA, Belshe RB. A review of adenoviruses in the etiology of acute hemorrhagic cystitis. J Urol 1976;115:191–194.
14. Padgett BL, Walker DL, Desquitado MM, et al. BK virus and non-hemorrhagic cystitis in a child. Lancet 1983;1:770.
15. Nguyen MLT, Borochovitz D, Thoams G, et al. Hemorrhagic cystitis with *Herpes simplex* virus type 2 in the bladder mucosa. Clin Infect Dis 1992;14:767–768.
16. Amar AD. Hematuria caused by varicella lesions in the bladder. JAMA 1966;196:450.
17. Gibbon N. A case of herpes zoster with involvement of the urinary bladder. Br J Urol 1956;28:417–421.
18. Caplan LR. Mechanisms of genitourinary symptoms in *Herpes simplex* virus infection. N Engl J Med 1983;309:1125–1126.
19. Oates JK, Greenhouse PR. Retention of urine in anogenital herpetic infection. Lancet 1978;1:691–692.
20. Khakpour M, Nik-Akhtar B. Epidemic of hemorrhagic cystitis due to influenza A virus. Postgrad Med J 1977;53:251–253.
21. Koga S, Shindo K, Matsuya F, et al. Acute hemorrhagic cystitis caused by adenovirus following renal transplantation: review of the literature. J Urol 1993;149:838–839.
22. Michaelson RA, Benson GS, Friedman HM. Urinary retention as the presenting symptom of acquired cytomegalovirus infection. Am J Med 1983;74:526–528.
23. Coleman DV, Mackenzie EFD, Gardner SD, et al. Human polyomavirus (BK) infection and ureteric stenosis in renal allograft recipients. J Clin Pathol 1978;31:338–347.
24. Arthur RR, Shah KV, Baust SJ, et al. Association of BK viruria with hemorrhagic cystitis in recipients of bone marrow transplants. N Engl J Med 1986;315:230–234.
25. Tomino Y, Yagame M, Omata F, et al. A case of IgA nephropathy associated with adeno- and *Herpes simplex* viruses. Nephron 1987;47:258–261.
26. Gregory MC, Hammond ME, Brewer ED. Renal deposition of cytomegalovirus antigen in immunoglobulin-A nephropathy. Lancet 1988;1:11–13.
27. Hanno PM, Staskin DR, Krane RJ, et al, eds. Interstitial cystitis. London: Springer-Verlag, 1990.
28. Gillenwater JY, Wein AJ. Summary of the National Institute of Arthritis, Diabetes, Digestive and Kidney diseases workshop on interstitial cystitis. National Institutes of Health, Bethesda, MD. J Urol 1988;140:203–206.

29. Hunner GL. A rare type of bladder ulcer in women: report of cases. Boston Med Surg J 1915;172:660-664.

30. Held PJ, Hanno PM, Wein AJ, et al. Epidemiology of interstitial cystitis. In: Hanno PM, Staskin DR, Krane RJ, et al, eds. Interstitial cystitis. London: Springer-Verlag, 1990:29-48.

31. Fowler JE Jr, Lynes WL, Lau LT, et al. Interstitial cystitis is associated with intraurothelial Tamm-Horsfall protein. J Urol 1988;140:1385-1389.

32. Parsons CL, Lilly JD, Stein P. Epithelial dysfunction in nonbacterial cystitis (interstitial cystitis). J Urol 1991;145:732-735.

33. Chelsky MJ, Rosen SI, Knight LC, et al. Bladder permeability in interstitial cystitis is similar to that of normal volunteers. J Urol 1994;151:346-349.

34. Felsen D, Frye S, Trimble LA, et al. Inflammatory mediator profile in urine and bladder wash fluid of patients with interstitial cystitis. J Urol 1994;152:355-361.

35. Lotz M, Villiger P, Hugli T, et al. Interleukin-6 and interstitial cystitis. J Urol 1994;152:869-873.

36. Miller CH, MacDermott JP, Quattrocchi KB, et al. Lymphocyte function in patients with interstitial cystitis. J Urol 1992;147:592-595.

37. Neal DE Jr, Dilworth JP, Kaack MB. Tamm-Horsfall autoantibodies in interstitial cystitis. J Urol 1991;145:37-39.

38. Ratner V. Rediscovering a 'rare' disease: a patient's perspective on interstitial cystitis. J Urol 1987;S29:44-45.

39. Boyle E, Morse M, Huttner I, et al. Immune complex-mediated interstitial cystitis as a major manifestation of systemic lupus erythematosus. Clin Immunol Immunopathol 1979; 13:67-76.

40. De La Serna AR, Alarcon-Segovia D. Chronic interstitial cystitis as an initial major manifestation of systemic lupus erythematosus. J Rheumatol 1981;8:808-810.

41. Orth RW, Weisman MH, Cohen AJ, et al. Lupus cystitis: primary bladder manifestations of systemic lupus erythematosus. Ann Int Med 1983;98:323-326.

42. Watson HS, Singh EO, Hermans MR, et al. Recurrent eosinophilic cystitis: a case responsive to steroids. J Urol 1992;147:689-691.

43. Okada H, Minayoshi K, Goto A. Two cases of eosinophilic cystitis induced by tranilast. J Urol 1992;147:1366-1368.

44. Mond NC, Percival A, Williams JD, et al. Presentation, diagnosis, and treatment of urinary tract infections in general practice. Lancet 1965;1:514-516.

45. Gallagher D, Montgomerie J, North J. Acute infections of the urinary tract and the urethral syndrome in general practice. Br J Med 1965;1:622-626.

46. Steensberg J, Bartels ED, Bay-Nielsen H, et al. Epidemiology of urinary tract diseases in general practice. Br Med J 1969;4:390-394.

47. Tapsall JW, Taylor PC, Bell SM, et al. Relevance of "significant bacteriuria" to aetiology and diagnosis of urinary-tract infection. Lancet 1975;2:637-639.

48. Brooks D, Mauder A. Pathogenesis of the urethral syndrome in women and its diagnosis in general practice. Lancet 1972;2:893-898.

49. Hamilton-Miller JMT. The urethral syndrome and its management. J Antimicrob Chemother 1994;33(Suppl. A):63-73.

50. Maskell R, Pead L, Allen J. The puzzle of "urethral syndrome": A possible answer? Lancet 1979;1:1058-1059.

51. Brumfitt W, Hamilton-Miller JMT, Gillespie WA. The mysterious "urethral syndrome." Brit Med J 1991;303:1-2.

52. Gillespie WA, Henderson EP, Linton KB, et al. Microbiology of the urethral (frequency and dysuria) syndrome. A controlled study with 5-year review. Br J Urol 1989;64:270-274.

53. Tait J, Peddie BA, Bailey RR, et al. Urethral syndrome (abacterial cystitis)—search for a pathogen. Br J Urol 1985;57:552-556.

54. Abel BJ, Gibbon NOK, Jameson RM, et al. The neuropathic urethra. Lancet 1974; 2:1229-1230.

55. Kaplan WE, Casimir FF, Schoenberg HW. The female urethral syndrome: external sphincter spasm as etiology. J Urol 1980;124:48-49.

56. O'Donnell RP. Acute urethral syndrome in women. N Engl J Med 1980;303:1531.

57. Stamm WE, Wagner KF, Amsel R, et al. Causes of the acute urethral syndrome in women. N Engl J Med 1980;303:409-415.

58. Stamm WE, Running K, McKevitt GW, et al. Treatment of the acute urethral syndrome. N Engl J Med 1981;304:956–958.
59. Stamm WE, Counts GW, Running KR, et al. Diagnosis of coliform infection in acutely dysuric women. N Engl J Med 1982;307:463–468.
60. Kunin CM, White LV, Tong HH. A reassessment of the importance of "low-count" bacteriuria in young women with acute urinary symptoms. Ann Intern Med 1993;119:454–460.
61. Huffman JW. The detailed anatomy of the paraurethral ducts in the adult human female. Am J Obstet Gynecol 1948;55:86–100.
62. Moore T, Hira NR, Stirland RM. Differential urethrovesical urinary cell-count. A method of accurate diagnosis of lower-urinary-tract infections in women. Lancet 1965;1:626–627.
63. Stamey TA, Timothy M, Miller M, et al. Recurrent urinary infections in adult women. Calif Med 1971;115:1–19.
64. Cattell WR, McSherry MA, Northeast A, et al. Periurethral enterobacterial carriage in pathogenesis of recurrent urinary infection. Br Med J 1974;4:136–139.
65. Kunin CM, Polyak F, Postel E. Periurethral bacterial flora in women. JAMA 1980;243:134–139.
66. O'Grady FW, McSherry MA, Richards B, et al. Introital enterobacteria, urinary infection, and the urethral syndrome. Lancet 1970;2:1208–1210.
67. Arav-Boger R, Leibovici L, Danon YL. Urinary tract infections with low and high colony counts in young women. Arch Intern Med 1994;154:300–304.
68. Bran JL, Levison ME, Kaye D. Entrance of bacteria into the female urinary bladder. N Engl J Med 1972;286:626–629.
69. Fairley K, Birch D. Unconventional bacteria in urinary tract disease: *Gardnerella vaginalis*. Kidney Int 1983;23:862–865.
70. McFadyan IR, Eykyn SJ. Suprapubic aspiration of urine in pregnancy. Lancet 1968;1:1211–1214.
71. Wong ES, Stamm WE. Urethral infections in men and women. Annu Rev Med 1983;34:337–358.
72. Komaroff AL, Friedland G. The dysuria-pyuria syndrome. N Engl J Med 1980;303:452–454.
73. Bartlett JG, Onderdonk AB, Drude E, et al. Quantitative bacteriology of the vaginal flora. J Infect Dis 1977;136:271–277.
74. Hooton TM, Stamm WE. The vaginal flora and urinary tract infections. In: Mobley HLT, Warren JW, eds. Urinary tract infections. Molecular pathogenesis and clinical management. Washington: ASM Press, 1996:67–94.
75. Murphy TV, Nelson JD. Shigella vaginitis: report of 38 patients and review of the literature. J Pediatr 1979;63:511–516.
76. Krieger JN, Jenny C, Verdon M, et al. Clinical manifestations of trichomoniasis in men. Annu Intern Med 1993;118:844–849.
77. Woodruff JD, Parmley TH. Infection of the minor vestibular gland. Obstet Gynecol 1983;62:609.
78. Friedrich EG Jr. Vulvar vestibulitis syndrome. J Reprod Med 1987;32:110–114.
79. Dotters DJ, Droegemueller W. Vulvar vestibulitis: common cause of vulvar pain. Clin Adv Infections 1989;3:1–10.
80. Peckham BM, Maki DG, Patterson JJ, et al. Focal vulvitis: a characteristic syndrome and cause of dyspareunia. Am J Obstet Gynecol 1986;154:855–864.
81. Stamey TA. Prostatitis. J Roy Soc Med 1980;74:22–40.
82. Meares EM. Chronic prostatitis and relapsing urinary infections. The Kidney 1975;8:24–28.
83. Meares EM. Infected stones of the prostate gland: laboratory diagnosis and clinical management. J Urol 1974;4:560–566.
84. Inoshita T, Youngberg GA, Boelen LJ, et al. Blastomycosis presenting with prostatic involvement: Report of 2 cases and review of the literature. J Urol 1983;130:160–162.
85. Wise GJ, Silver DA. Fungal infections of the genitourinary system. J Urol 1993;149:1377–1388.
86. Marans HY, Mandell W, Kislak JW, et al. Prostatic abscess due to *Histoplasma capsulatum* in the acquired immunodeficiency syndrome. J Urol 1991;145:1275–1276.
87. Lief M, Sarfarazi F. Prostatic cryptococcosis in acquired immune deficiency syndrome. J Urol 1986;28:318–319.

88. Larsen RA, Bozzette S, McCutchan JA, et al. Persistent *Cryptococcus neoformans* infection of the prostate after successful treatment of meningitis. Annu Intern Med 1989;111: 125–128.
89. Chen KT, Schijj JJ. Coccidioidomycosis of prostate. J Urol 1985;25:82–84.
90. Lentino JR, Zielinski A, Stachowski M, et al. Prostatic abscess due to *Candida albicans*. J Infect Dis 1984;149:282.
91. Meyer RD, Young LS, Armstrong D, et al. Aspergillosis complicating neoplastic disease. Am J Med 1973;54:6–15.
92. Gorse GJ, Belshe RB. Male genital tuberculosis: a review of the literature with instructive case reports. Revs Infect Dis 1985;7:511–523.
93. Poletti F, Medici MC, Alinovi A, et al. Isolation of *Chlamydia trachomatis* from the prostatic cells in patients affected by nonacute abacterial prostatitis. J Urol 1985;134: 691–693.
94. Shortliffe LMD, Sellers RG, Schachter J. The characterization of nonbacterial prostatitis: Search for an etiology. J Urol 1992;148:1461–1466.
95. Meares EM. Bacterial prostatitis vs "prostatosis." JAMA 1973;224:1372–1375.
96. Thomas D, Simpson K, Ostojic H, et al. Bacteremic epididymo-orchitis due to *Hemophilus influenzae* type B. J Urol 1981;126:832–833.
97. Cross J, Davidson K, Bradsher R. *Haemophilus influenzae* epididymo-orchitis and bacteremia in a man infected with the human immunodeficiency virus. Clin Infect Dis 1994;19:768–769.
98. Harnisch JP, Alexander ER, Berger RE, et al. Etiology of acute epididymitis. Lancet 1977;1:819–822.
99. Berger RE, Kessler D, Holmes KK. Etiology and manifestations of epididymitis in young men: correlations with sexual orientation. J Infect Dis 1987;155:1341–1343.
100. Witherington R, Harper WM. The surgical management of acute bacterial epididymitis with emphasis on epididymotomy. J Urol 1982;128:722–725.

Pyelonephritis and Other Infections of the Kidney

Overview

Pyelonephritis is defined as inflammation of the kidney and the renal pelvis. The term is commonly used to describe an infectious process that involves the kidneys and adjacent structures. The infection may be ascending and encompass both the renal pelvis and kidney, or metastatic and limited to the renal parenchyma. The lesion may rupture into the adjacent structures and produce a perinephric abscess. Pyelonephritis includes one or more of the following conditions: 1) an acute or chronic active infection; 2) the residual lesions and scars of past infection; 3) a local immune inflammatory response to infection; or 4) a combination of all of these processes. Pyelonephritis is usually caused by the same gram negative and gram positive bacteria that are commonly associated with all urinary tract infections (bacterial pyelonephritis). It can also be caused by infection of the kidney with mycobacteria, including *Mycobacterium tuberculosis* (renal tuberculosis), yeasts (candida pyelonephritis), fungi, and viruses. Patients with acute, uncomplicated pyelonephritis rarely develop hypertension or permanent renal damage. Patients with complicated infections are more likely to develop sepsis and severe renal damage. The groups at highest risk of severe pyelonephritis are those with urinary obstruction, neurologic abnormalities of the voiding mechanism, diabetes, polycystic kidneys, stones, and urinary catheters. Infections caused by urea-splitting microbes can lead to infection (struvite) stones. Noninvasive methods, such as renal ultrasound with post-voiding studies, help distinguish uncomplicated from complicated infections. Intravenous urograms, CT, and other scanning methods are useful to localize intrarenal and perinephric abscesses and differentiate bacterial pyelonephritis from other forms of renal disease. Diabetics are at special risk of developing destructive forms of the disease, such as emphysematous pyelonephritis and papillary necrosis. Patients with long-standing, complicated infections may develop a rare condition known as xanthogranulomatous pyelonephritis. In the past, pyelonephritis was believed to be one of the most common causes of hypertension and severe renal disease. It is now known that reflux nephropathy accounts for much of the renal damage previously attributed to chronic pyelonephritis. Many other diseases, such as analgesic nephropathy, interstitial nephritis, and renal vascular disease, can mimic bacterial pyelonephritis. This chapter will consider the various causes of infective pyelonephritis and the differential diagnosis. Pathogenesis and management will be presented in greater detail in later chapters.

Pyelonephritis

A scheme for classification of the various forms of pyelonephritis is presented in Table 8.1. Each of these conditions needs to be considered within the clinical framework and underlying diseases outlined in Table 1.6.

Acute, Uncomplicated Pyelonephritis

Acute bacterial pyelonephritis is a term used to describe a well-defined clinical syndrome consisting of the acute onset of fever, flank pain, and cost-vertebral angle (loin) tenderness associated with leukocytosis, leukocyte casts, and bacteria in the urine. These symptoms may be accompanied by cystitis with frequent, painful urination. The accompanying anatomical lesions in the kidneys consist of numerous polymorphonuclear leukocytes in the interstitial spaces of the kidney and tubular lumen, sometimes dense enough to form abscesses. Abscesses may either be multifocal, suggestive of metastatic spread from the bloodstream or, more commonly, appear as focal infection of the renal papillae radiating, within a renal segment, to produce broad, wedge-shaped lesions extending to the cortex. Examples of computed tomography (CT) scans of normal kidneys and with acute pyelonephritis are shown in Figures 8.1 to 8.3.

Table 8.1. Classification of Pyelonephritis

Acute, uncomplicated, bacterial pyelonephritis (focal or diffuse)
   Lobar nephronia
Chronic, complicated bacterial pyelonephritis
   Pyonephrosis
   Emphysematous pyelonephritis
   Renal papillary necrosis
   Xanthogranulomatous pyelonephritis
   Malacoplakia
   Pyelonephritis lenta (infection localized to the "upper" urinary tract)
Renal and perinephric abscesses
Infection superimposed on polycystic kidney disease
Renal infection caused by less common microorganisms
   Renal tuberculosis and other mycobacterial infections
   Fungal infections
   Viral infections

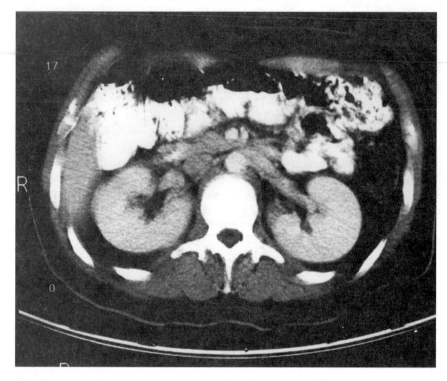

Figure 8.1. Normal kidneys as visualized by CT scanning.

Acute lobar nephronia is a severe localized form of pyelonephritis. It is usually discovered by intravenous urogram, CT scan, or ultrasound examination as a bulging, localized, nonliquified mass involving one or more entire renal lobules. The lesion may be difficult to distinguish from a tumor or abscess (1–6).

Clinical Findings

The classic clinical presentation of acute pyelonephritis in the older child and adult is the abrupt onset of fever (38° to 40° C), shaking chills, and aching pain in one or both costovertebral angles (loin, flank, or costovertebral angle pain) that may radiate to the anterior abdomen and groin. The episode may be preceded or accompanied by symptoms of bladder inflammation, including frequency and dysuria, or be localized only to the kidneys. There may be no prior history of urinary tract infection or the episode may be one of several. Physical examination usually reveals a flushed, acutely ill patient with a rapid pulse with tenderness in the region of one or both kidneys. Patients with acute, uncomplicated pyelonephritis will usually have a normal blood pressure. Patients with acute pyelonephritis, superimposed on a structural or neurologic disease or diabetes, may be hypertensive.

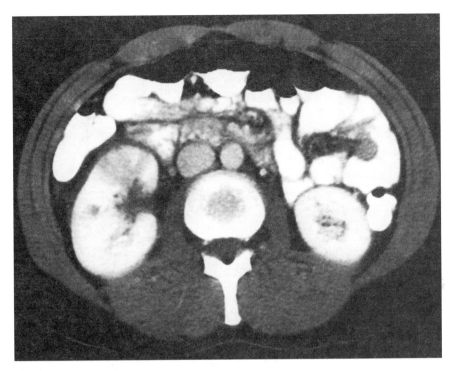

Figure 8.2. A CT scan demonstrating several wedge-shaped lesions of acute pyelonephritis in the right kidney.

This account of the classic presentation of acute pyelonephritis must be modified for infants and young children. They may exhibit only nonspecific signs of irritability and fever. The mother may note an odor to the urine and signs of straining on urination. The diagnosis is strongly suspected when pus cells and bacteria are found in a properly collected specimen of urine. Swedish workers (7) have shown that an elevated serum C-reactive protein level, associated with fever, bacteriuria and pyuria, is a valid indicator of pyelonephritis in young children. Currently, scintillation scans provide more specific information and allow excellent visualization of the evolution of the lesion (8) (Fig. 8.4).

Laboratory Findings
The white blood count is usually elevated with a marked increase in the proportion of neutrophils and band cells. Microscopic examination of the urine reveals numerous bacteria, usually gram negative bacilli, and leukocytes. Leukocyte casts may be present. The blood culture is positive in about 20% of cases. In patients with acute, uncomplicated pyelonephritis, the blood urea nitrogen and serum creatinine are usually normal and there is minimal or insignificant proteinuria. Patients with long-standing, complicated infections

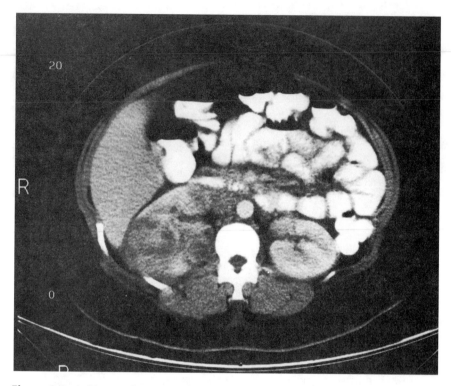

Figure 8.3. A CT scan demonstrating multiple lesions and marked swelling of the right kidney. The patient was initially considered to have a hypernephroma, but the lesions disappeared with long-term antimicrobial therapy.

may be azotemic, and anemic when both kidneys are involved. They may also have proteinuria. The most consistent finding in both uncomplicated and complicated pyelonephritis is a profound defect in urinary concentrating ability (9).

Radiologic Findings
Abdominal films and renal ultrasound studies should be performed early in the course of illness. Intravenous urograms, scintillation, and CT scans are relatively expensive and are reserved for complex or difficult diagnostic problems. They are indicated in patients suspected of having obstructive lesions of the urinary tract and those who are bacteremic, paraplegic, diabetic, or remain febrile for several days after receiving adequate chemotherapy.

ABDOMINAL FILMS. Abdominal films may be entirely normal, or one or both kidneys may appear to be diffusely enlarged. Stones may be obscured by overlying gas-containing bowel. An air-filled segment of small bowel may overlie an infected kidney (sentinel sign).

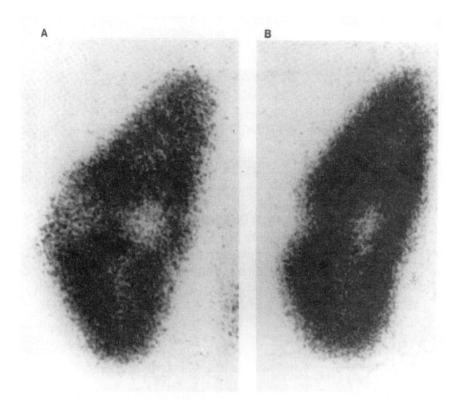

Figure 8.4. Progression of acute pyelonephritis in the left mid kidney (A) to irreversible renal scarring (B) in a 3-year-old girl who presented with acute febrile urinary tract infection. The kidneys were visualized by ^{99m}technetium-DMSA scans. The interval between scans was 2 years. Reproduced with permission from Rushton, Majd, Jantausch, et al. (8).

ULTRASOUND. The renal and bladder ultrasound is the preferred screening procedure for patients with acute pyelonephritis. It is usually adequate to detect obstruction and renal and perinephric abscesses. The most common finding is a diffusely swollen kidney (10). Advantages of the renal ultrasound are listed in Table 8.2.

INTRAVENOUS UROGRAMS. Intravenous urograms are not routinely indicated except to more clearly define lesions found on ultrasound and in patients with complicated infections. Only 8% of patients with acute, uncomplicated pyelonephritis were found to have abnormalities that influenced management—the procedure was performed within 10 days of admission (11). The characteristic findings are listed in Table 8.3 (12,13). Intravenous urograms are not recommended within the first few days after the onset of acute

Table 8.2. Advantages of Ultrasonography as a Screening Procedure in Acute Pyelonephritis

Quick and noninvasive procedure
Less expensive than CT or radionuclide scans
Provides information concerning the extent of renal involvement
Demonstrates large renal and perinephric abscess
Rapidly rules out the presence of obstruction and stones
Provides information on the ability of the patients to empty the bladder

pyelonephritis for the following reasons: 1) the kidney is unable to concentrate contrast material; 2) a dilated segment of the proximal ureter may be confused with ureteral obstruction; and 3) the contrast material may precipitate acute renal failure in a dehydrated patient. Intravenous urograms are not indicated for routine evaluation of women with symptomatic urinary tract infections (14).

COMPUTERIZED TOMOGRAPHY. Renal CT scans will often show a wedge-shaped dense area which will disappear several weeks after successful therapy. It is an excellent method to demonstrate the exact site of the lesion and the presence of perinephric abscesses (Fig. 8.5).

SCINTILLATION SCANS. Radiolabeled technetium (^{99m}technetium-dimercaptosuccinic acid) localizes in the proximal tubular cells in the renal cortex allowing visualization of the functioning renal parenchyma. Renal scans are particularly useful to detect suspected renal involvement in young children and help differentiate reflux nephropathy from focal pyelonephritis (Fig. 8.4). This topic is discussed in the section on vesico-ureteral reflux and urinary infections in childhood.

GALLIUM AND RADIOTAGGED LEUKOCYTES. These studies help localize areas of inflammation. At times they are useful to detect renal and perinephric abscesses, but they may be nonspecific and give false negative results. The CT scan is preferred.

Differential Diagnosis
The clinical presentation of acute bacterial pyelonephritis in older children and adults is rather striking. At times the patient may complain of epigastric

Table 8.3. Characteristic Findings of the Intravenous Urogram During Acute Pyelonephritis

Diminished nephrogram with delayed appearance of contrast material in the
   renal parenchyma
Loss of portions of the renal outline due to renal edema
Enlarged kidney(s), diffuse or localized
Ileus of the proximal segment of ureter due to infection or endotoxin
Striations of the ureter due to mucosal edema

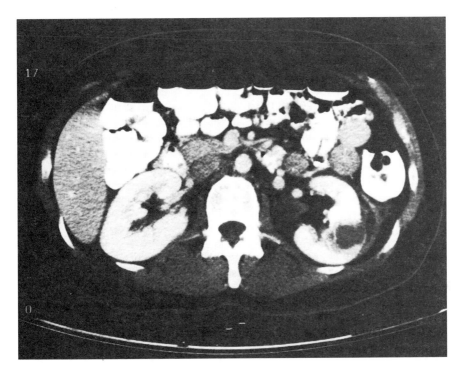

Figure 8.5. A large metastatic abscess caused by *Staphylococcus aureus* in a 45-year-old woman with diabetes mellitus. The abscess is located in the midportion of the left kidney and is beginning to penetrate into the perinephric fascia. The diagnosis was made by renal biopsy and a positive blood culture. She was treated with nafcillin for 6 weeks and did not require surgery.

or lower abdominal pain rather than the characteristic flank or loin pain. The diagnosis may be confused with acute cholecystitis, appendicitis, or diverticulitis and confounded by the coincidental presence of bacteriuria and pyuria (Table 8.4). Appendiceal, tubo-ovarian and diverticular abscesses that adjoin the ureters or bladder may be accompanied by pyuria. The pain from passage of a urinary stone can mimic that of acute pyelonephritis, but

Table 8.4. Clinical Conditions That May Mimic Acute Pyelonephritis

Renal or ureteral stones
Acute cholecystitis
Appendicitis with local abscess or pyelophlebitis
Tubo-ovarian abscesses
Diverticulitis
Acute pancreatitis

the patient usually will not have fever or leukocytosis. The urine will often contain blood without bacteriuria or pyuria unless the patient has a concomitant urinary tract infection.

Course

Acute, uncomplicated pyelonephritis usually responds promptly to antimicrobial therapy with minimal residual renal damage. Recurrent episodes are rare. Hospitalization should be considered when the patient is nauseated, vomiting, noncompliant, or when there is poor supervision at home. If the diagnosis is fairly obvious, radiologic studies should be deferred until the patient has had sufficient time to recover (see previous discussion of radiologic examinations).

Complications

CHILDREN. The acute changes of pyelonephritis are usually reversible and do not lead to new renal scarring or loss of renal function in the majority of cases (8,15). When scars develop, they occur in the areas corresponding to the site of acute pyelonephritis demonstrated on ^{99m}technetium scans (Fig. 8.4). Children with gross vesicoureteral reflux are at high risk of developing focal scars in regions of intrarenal reflux and reflux nephropathy. Children without reflux develop small renal scars at the same or greater frequency as those with reflux (8, 15). Small scars demonstrated on ^{99m}technetium scans do not decrease glomerular filtration rate (GFR) and there is no difference in renal function between children with or without residual scars (15). Children with recurrent episodes of pyelonephritis and scars large enough to be demonstrated on intravenous urograms tend to have a lower GFR than healthy controls (16).

ADULTS. Renal scars and residual renal damage rarely occur following an episode of acute, uncomplicated pyelonephritis. Scars found at the time of diagnosis are usually the residua of reflux nephropathy that originated in childhood (see illustrative case and Figures 5.11 and 5.12 and the long-term follow-up study of women who were hospitalized for acute pyelonephritis, and Figure 6.3). Despite the generally benign course, there are about a dozen case reports of acute renal failure in association with acute, uncomplicated pyelonephritis (17–28). Some of the cases occurred in patients with one kidney or in association with analgesic abuse or pregnancy. The causative microorganism was almost always *E. coli*. Virtually all patients recovered without the need for hemodialysis.

The sepsis syndrome, characterized by hypotension and disseminated intravascular coagulation, is relatively rare in patients with acute uncomplicated pyelonephritis. It is much more likely to occur in patients with diabetes and acute, complicated infections.

Key Points About Acute, Uncomplicated Pyelonephritis in Adults

- The clinical manifestations are acute onset of fever, chills, and flank pain. There is leukocytosis with increased polymorphonuclear leukocytes and band cells. The disease occurs most often in an otherwise healthy female, but may occur in both heterosexual and homosexual males.
- Microscopic examination of the urine usually reveals large numbers of white blood cells and numerous gram negative rods. Gram stain is recommended to visualize gram positive and fastidious bacteria.
- Consider other diseases that have similar clinical presentations if the urine does not reveal bacteria on microscopic examination. These diseases include renal stones, cholecytitis, appendicitis, tubo-ovarian abscess, diverticulitis, and acute pancreatitis.
- *E. coli* is the most common microorganism. *Staphylococcus saprophiticus* presents with an identical clinical picture. Blood cultures should always be performed. About 20% will be positive.
- Hypertension, renal failure, and proteinuria are rare, but concentrating ability is impaired.
- Renal ultrasound is the most useful procedure to immediately rule out urinary obstruction or stones. Intravenous urograms should not be done during the acute phase of the disease because of poor contrast. CT scans characteristically show wedge-shaped lesions.
- Hospitalization and intravenously administered antimicrobial drugs are necessary in patients who are nauseated or cannot be managed safely at home.
- Acute renal failure is rare. Most episodes resolve without residual renal damage.

Chronic, Complicated Pyelonephritis

Chronic bacterial pyelonephritis is a term used to describe the effects on the kidney of long-standing infection. The condition may be either an active process with persistent infection or the residual lesions of past infection. These two entities, *chronic active* and *chronic inactive* (healed) pyelonephritis, are differentiated by the presence or absence of constitutional signs of infection, inflammatory cells, and bacteria in the urine. This distinction is of paramount importance because there is no point in treating an inactive infection. Chronic bacterial pyelonephritis almost invariably occurs in patients with complicated urinary tract infections or conditions, such as diabetes, that decrease host resistance. The process is highly variable depending on the underlying host factors and the presence of structural or functional lesions of the urinary tract. The process may persist for years if the underlying lesions are not corrected. Long-standing infection is associated with general debility and the anemia of chronic disease. In the most severe cases, chronic pyelonephritis may gradually progress to renal amyloidosis, hypertension, and end-stage renal failure.

Few diseases have generated as much controversy and debate as chronic pyelonephritis. The word "chronic" evokes the vision of a persistent, smoldering process, which will inexorably lead to destruction of the kidney if its course is not interrupted. Actually, most patients with urinary tract infections, even those with recurrent attacks, rarely develop end-stage renal failure. For this reason it is exceedingly important to accurately define terminology and the risk factors. Another source of confusion is the tendency to interpret focal renal scars and blunted calices, observed on intravenous urograms, as "chronic pyelonephritis" rather than as old healed pyelonephritic scars or reflux nephropathy. It is now known that scars acquired during acute pyelonephritis and vesico-ureteral reflux in childhood are the major source for those found in adults. The key role of vesico-ureteral reflux in producing renal scars is based on the work of Hodson, Hutch, and Hinman and others (29,30) and new knowledge derived from use of radionuclide scans (8) as discussed in Chapter 5 on vesico-ureteral reflux.

Clinical Findings

The patient may be asymptomatic, have recurrent episodes of acute pyelonephritis, or exhibit nonspecific signs of chronic infection including fever, anemia, and azotemia. Chronic pyelonephritis is one of the causes of fever of unknown origin in some series (31–32).

Laboratory Findings

Laboratory findings are similar to the findings in acute pyelonephritis. Patients with long-standing infection may have the normocytic, normochromic anemia of chronic infection with normal iron binding protein and ferritin. The erythrocyte sedimentation rate (ESR) and C-reactive protein (CRP) are usually elevated in patients with active infection. The serum blood urea nitrogen and creatinine are elevated in patients with severe, bilateral infection. Urinary concentrating ability is greatly diminished, but excessive proteinuria is rare except with end-stage renal disease.

Radiologic Findings

These generally consist of a mixture of the anatomic alterations associated with the underlying structural disease and those due to the infectious process. The renal cortex is often shrunken by multiple, irregular cortical scars with focal clubbing of the renal pelvis. These findings may be indistinguishable from those produced by vesico-ureteral reflux and hypertensive renal disease. Intrarenal abscesses may be visualized on CT scan and may contain gas (emphysematous pyelonephritis) or resemble tumors (xanthogranulomatous pyelonephritis).

Differential Diagnosis

The clinical diagnosis of active, chronic bacterial pyelonephritis is based on the history and clinical, laboratory, and radiologic findings. The diagnosis is usually not difficult in patients with recurrent, complicated infections or diabetes and who have signs and symptoms of infection associated with bac-

Table 8.5. Conditions That May Mimic Chronic Pyelonephritis

Clinical
    Renal stones and ureteral obstruction
    Renal tumors (hypernephroma)
    Psoas and subdiaphragmatic abscesses
    Fever of unknown origin
Radiologic
    Reflux nephropathy
    Hypertensive renal disease
    Renal artery stenosis
    Diabetic nephropathy
    Interstitial nephritis
    Analgesic nephritis
    Gouty nephritis

teriuria and pyuria. The major problem is to distinguish the residual lesions of past infection that are no longer active and with other diseases that have similar radiologic findings (Table 8.5).

Course
The process may be aborted by appropriate urologic surgery combined with antimicrobial therapy. If left untreated, or if treatment is unsatisfactory, the process may persist for many years and be complicated by general debility, anemia of chronic infection, and gradually progress to renal amyloidosis, hypertension, and end-stage renal failure.

Complications
Uncontrolled infections within the kidney may extend to the surrounding renal tissues and produce perinephric abscesses. These may dissect further within the retroperitoneal space. The extent of infection is difficult to determine without radiologic studies. Perinephric abscesses should be suspected when there is persistent flank pain, fever, and leukocytosis unresponsive to otherwise adequate chemotherapy. Surgical drainage is usually required.

The patient may develop the *urosepsis syndrome*. This is a life-threatening complication characterized by a mixed picture of fever, chills, confusion or obtundation, hypotension, and general systems failure, often accompanied by bacteremia and endotoxemia.

Key Points About Chronic, Active Pyelonephritis

- There usually will be a long history of recurrent or persistent infection superimposed on underlying obstruction, stones, neurogenic bladder, and indwelling urinary catheters.
- Diabetes mellitus and renal transplantation are often associated with severe suppurative disease.
- The causative microorganisms are often resistant to commonly used drugs.

- Microscopic examination of the urine will reveal bacteria and pyuria. Urine culture and susceptibility tests are necessary to guide management; blood cultures are required and provide important information about the causative organisms.
- Renal functional abnormalities and hypertension produced by the underlying disease (such as diabetes or obstructive uropathy or reflux nephropathy) may be difficult to differentiate from those due to chronic infection.
- The underlying anatomic lesions must be identified clearly by uro-radiologic studies, including intravenous urograms, voiding cystourethrograms, and CT scans as needed.
- Removal of foreign bodies and correction of anatomic lesions is of paramount importance to preserve renal function.
- Long-standing chronic pyelonephritis may be complicated by renal and perinephric abscesses and unusual conditions, such as emphysematous and xanthogranulomatous pyelonephritis, renal amyloidosis, and renal malacoplakia.

Pyonephrosis

Pyonephrosis is a special form of acute and chronic pyelonephritis associated with obstruction of the ureter by a stone or stricture. The most common site of obstruction is at the uretero-pelvic junction. Characteristically there is a large, dilated renal pelvis filled with purulent urine and severe infection of the renal papillae and medulla.

Emphysematous Pyelonephritis

Emphysematous pyelonephritis is a severe, life-threatening illness characterized by the presence of extensive necrotic renal tissue containing gas. It occurs virtually always in patients with diabetes mellitus (33–44).

Clinical Findings
The patient is usually a middle-aged or elderly diabetic female with a long history of recurrent urinary tract infections, repeated urologic procedures, or chronic pyelonephritis. The onset may be insidious, but it is often abrupt with fever, chills, and flank pain. The patient appears septic and may be obtunded. There may be concomitant diabetic ketoacidosis, hyperglycemia, and disseminated intravascular coagulopathy. A palpable mass may be appreciated in the renal area. Radiographic examination of the abdomen will reveal pockets of air in the kidney that often extends into Gerota's fascia. The perinephric collection of gas may produce a "crescent sign" on radiographic picture. The CT scan is usually diagnostic (Fig. 8.6). Blood cultures are usually positive with the same organism found in the kidney and urine. Several cases associated with *E. coli* meningitis have been described (33,34) and gas may be found in the hepatic veins (44). The mortality is high unless the kidney is removed promptly or the abscess is drained. On pathologic examination the renal tissue is necrotic and liquefied. Renal papillary necrosis and intrarenal vascular thrombi are commonly seen. Clumps of bacteria may be found on microscopic examination in the necrotic tissue.

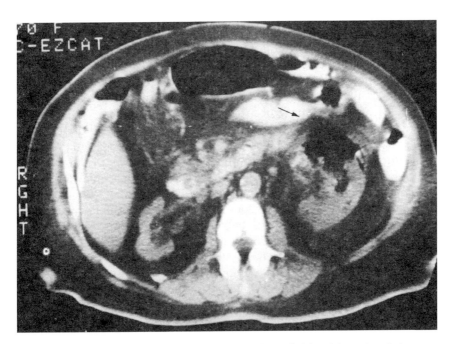

Figure 8.6. An example of emphysematous pyelonephritis with perinephric extension demonstrated by computerized tomography in a 71-year-old woman with long-standing diabetes mellitus. Note the scarred and atrophic right kidney. *E. coli* was grown from her blood and from the fluid aspirated from the abscess cavity.

The disease is fortunately rare, but over 80 cases have been described in the literature and many more cases must have occurred and not have been reported because of the episodic nature of the disease. A remarkable feature is the frequent association with diabetes mellitus. Obstructive disease of the urinary tract is often present. The most common bacteria are *E. coli* followed by Klebsiella, Enterobacter, and Proteus. Anaerobic bacteria are rarely found and Clostridia, which characteristically forms gas, has not been reported in this condition to my knowledge. An unusual case of emphysematous pyelonephritis caused by *Candida tropicalis* was described by Seidenfeld et al. (37). The patient was a 41-year-old male diabetic and a parenteral drug abuser. A complicating feature of this case was the finding of large fungal masses in the renal pelvis and ureter.

The striking association between emphysematous pyelonephritis and diabetes suggests that the gas is derived from glucose fermentation. The key factors appear to be the presence of 1) gas-forming bacteria, 2) high tissue glucose, and 3) impaired tissue perfusion (44). This notion is supported by the finding in the gaseous tissues of a large proportion of hydrogen and carbon dioxide together with an unknown gas, with reduced amounts of nitrogen and oxygen (41).

Renal Papillary Necrosis

Medullary or papillary necrosis may occur as a consequence of severe bacterial pyelonephritis or with excessive use of analgesic drugs. The pyelonephritic form of the disease occurs most frequently in patients with urinary tract infection superimposed on diabetes (with vascular disease or glomerulosclerosis), urinary obstruction, sickle cell disease, and analgesic abuse (45). The process begins with abscesses and obstructed tubules in the renal pyramids and produces infarct-like necrosis extending from the papilla to the inner medulla. Extensive thrombophlebitis of the local venous system may be present in some cases. The clinical findings are similar to those of acute pyelonephritis. There also may be massive hematuria, unilateral renal colic, and oliguria. The diagnosis is usually made by retrograde pyelography or CT scans, but bits of papilla may be found in the urine. The radiologic hallmarks are 1) deformity of the tip of the calyx and excavations extending to the cortex, 2) outlines of necrotic papillae, 3) free masses in the renal pelvis, and 4) replacement of the concave tip suggesting a cavity. Management of this condition, in addition to antimicrobial therapy, will depend on the extent of renal obstruction. It may be necessary to remove the obstructing debris or require nephrectomy in severe cases.

Xanthogranulomatous Pyelonephritis

This is a relatively uncommon, but dramatic, form of chronic pyelonephritis. It is characterized by an extraordinary cellular response by macrophages to long-standing bacterial infection (46–59). Obstructive urologic lesions are present in virtually all cases. Infection stones, particularly staghorn calculi, are common. It may occur at all ages, including infants and children with severe obstructive uropathy (48,53,59). Most series include a few cases with diabetes. It has been described in recipients of renal allografts (58) with bilharziasis (55) and is occasionally accompanied by systemic amyloidosis (56).

Clinical Findings

The typical patient with xanthogranulomatous pyelonephritis is a middle-aged female who has recurrent urinary infections complicated by renal calculi for many years. She will appear chronically ill, reporting prolonged fever, anorexia, weight loss, and persistent unilateral flank pain. On examination there will be flank tenderness and a mass may be felt. Occasionally a sinus track may be noted in the flank. Laboratory findings will demonstrate anemia and leukocytosis and there may be abnormal liver function tests, especially an elevated alkaline phosphatase. The differential diagnosis will include chronic pyelonephritis, intrarenal or perinephric abscess, renal tuberculosis, and renal carcinoma (51). An abdominal radiograph will usually reveal calcification in the kidney or a staghorn calculus. The IVP will show poor or no visualization of the affected side. If the calyces are seen, they will be distorted and clubbed. A renal arteriogram will reveal splayed and attenuated interlobar arteries surrounding multiple nonvascular masses suggestive of tumor or abscesses. A CT scan will demonstrate extensive swelling and lobulation of the kidney, often with extension of the process to the subcapsular space suggestive of an invasive tumor.

The presentation and diagnostic procedures will lead to exploration of the kidney. The surgeon will encounter a large kidney which is either diffusely enlarged or has focal lobular areas with a thick adherent capsule. The kidney usually will be involved so extensively that it will have to be removed, although at times a segmental resection can be done for localized disease. The pathologist will note on slicing the kidney that there are nodular or diffuse, firm, dense, pale, fibrous tissues. Soft yellow nodules are scattered throughout the specimen or they may be confluent. The pathologist's first impression will be carcinoma of the kidney. On microscopic examination there is a dense granulomatous inflammatory infiltrate containing a variety of chronic inflammatory cells associated with sheets of foam cells. These appear to be large histiocytes with small pyknotic nuclei and abundant cytoplasm containing fat and cholesterol esters and PAS-positive material. Xanthoma or foam cells may be found in the urine and provide a helpful preoperative diagnosis.

Enteric gram-negative bacteria, often Proteus, will be isolated, but the infection is often polymicrobic and can contain *E. coli,* Enterobacter, Klebsiella, and Pseudomonas. Gram-positive bacteria, including *Staphylococcus aureus* and *Streptococcus fecalis,* have been isolated alone or in combination with other organisms. The role of anaerobes is obscure, but they may account for reports of the finding of sterile cultures from the kidney (54).

Three stages of the disease have been devised by Malek (49) based upon the extent of involvement of the kidney and adjacent tissue by the process. Stage I is the nephritic with localization only to the kidney. Stage II involves the renal parenchyma with perinephric extension; and Stage III involves the parenchyma, perinephric, and paranephric tissue. The process may also be focal or segmental resembling a round tumor mass.

The nature of the xanthoma cell has generated considerable interest. It has been produced experimentally in animals by inducing chronic infections with *Proteus mirabilis, E. coli,* and staphylococci (60–62). The characteristic lesion is in the macrophages. These macrophages contain periodic acid-Schiff-positive cytosomal granules with myelin figures that bear a strong resemblance to bacterial breakdown products. The foam cells are the macrophages that have taken up lipid from the necrotic tissue.

The clinical findings and presentation of xanthogranulomatous and emphysematous pyelonephritis are usually quite distinct, but there may be considerable overlap (Table 8.6). They may involve both kidneys and occasionally occur together in the same patient.

Renal Malacoplakia

Renal malacoplakia is a chronic form of pyelonephritis characterized by the presence of soft (malakos) yellowish plaques (plakos) or nodules infiltrating

Table 8.6. Clinical Characteristics of Xanthogranulomatous and Emphysematous Pyelonephritis*

	Xanthogranulomatous		Emphysematous	
	No.	%	No.	%
Diabetes	21	10.8	27	100.0
Females	144	74.2	17	63.0
Stones[†]	120	61.9	2	7.4
Mass[‡]	84	43.3	—	—
Gas	—	—	27	100.0
Bacteremia	Rare		19	70.4
Proteus	53	27.3	0	0.0
E. coli	Variable		19	70.4
Klebsiella	Variable		6	22.2
	Often polymicrobial		Usually single microbe	
Total	194	100.0	27	100.0

*These data are compiled from the largest series of cases cited in references 34–59.
†Often staghorn calculi.
‡Often mistaken for tumor.

the renal parenchyma. The disease is relatively rare, but more than 400 cases have been reported (63–66). It resembles xanthogranulomatous pyelonephritis by its insidious presentation and the exuberant proliferation of macrophages containing periodic acid-Schiff-positive cytosomal granules. The unique feature of malacoplakia is the presence of cytoplasmic calcospherules also known as Michaelis-Gutmann or MG bodies. The MG bodies have an owl's eye or target-like appearance. Intact bacteria or bacterial fragments may be seen within the phagolysosomes of malacoplakia cells. The disease is thought to be caused by defective killing of the ingested microorganisms, but the exact mechanism is unknown. E. coli is the most common causative organism.

Clinical Findings
The patient will often be debilitated, have a long history of recurrent urinary tract infections, and present with flank pain, anemia, and fever. The diagnosis is suspected by the finding of a poorly functioning, enlarged kidney, presence of a mass, or hydronephrosis. The diagnosis is made by renal biopsy or at nephrectomy. It may occur from infancy to the very elderly and is about four times more frequent in females. Many of the patients will have an underlying immunodeficiency, or connective tissue disease, a neoplasm, diabetes mellitus, or ethanol abuse (65). Use of immunosuppressive drugs may account for its occurrence in renal transplant recipients.

Malacoplakia of the urinary tract may have protean manifestations because it can involve any portion of the urinary tract. The bladder is the most common site (58%), followed by the kidney (16%), ureter (11%), renal pelvis (10%), ureteropelvic junction (2%), and urethra (2%) (63). The process has also been described in adjacent organs such as the prostate, testis, epididymus, retroperitoneum, stomach, large and small intestine, and female genital tract. It has also been reported to occur in the brain, thyroid, lung, vertebrae, and adrenal gland.

Key Points About Emphysematous and Xanthogranulomatous Pyelonephritis Renal Malacoplakia and Renal Papillary Necrosis

- Emphysematous pyelonephritis is an acute, life-threatening infection characterized by widespread tissue necrosis and production of gas within the kidney. It may be accompanied by septic shock and disseminated intravascular coagulopathy (DIC). The most common causative organisms are *E. coli* and Klebsiella. The disease is almost invariably associated with diabetes mellitus. Prompt surgical intervention or drainage of the abscesses are required.
- Xanthogranulomatous pyelonephritis is an insidious form of chronic pyelonephritis commonly associated with renal stones and staghorn calculi. It often presents as a mass suggestive of a renal neoplasm. The disease is due to a remarkable proliferation of large histiocytes containing fat, cholesterol esters and PAS-positive material in the cytoplasm. Proteus is the most common causative organism, but it may be associated with a variety of gram positive and gram negative bacteria. The infection is often polymicrobial.
- Renal malacoplakia is an insidious form of chronic pyelonephritis that resembles, but is distinctly different from xanthogranulomatous pyelonephritis. The lesions may occur in any part of the urinary tract including the bladder, ureter and renal pelvis and at distant sites throughout the body. The clinical manifestations may be protean depending on the location of plaques that contain macrophages with PAS-positive cytoplasm and Michaelis-Gutmann bodies. Stones are uncommon. The most common causative organism is *E. coli*. The disease commonly occurs in patients with underlying immunologic disorders and with renal transplantation.
- Renal papillary necrosis results from ischemia of the renal medullary vasculature. It can involve either the renal medulla or papilla. It may occur with analgesic abuse and other microvascular disorders in the absence of infection. The infectious form is superimposed on diabetes, obstruction, sickle cell disease and analgesic abuse.

Subclinical Pyelonephritis

Tests used to differentiate "upper" (kidney) from "lower" (bladder) infections may suggest the presence of infection in the kidney or other sites such as the prostate in the absence of the classic symptoms of flank pain or fever (see Localization studies in Chapter 3). Upper tract infection is often equated with pyelonephritis, but this is by no means certain. The finding of decreased concentration ability is the strongest evidence that the kidney is involved, but the diagnosis of pyelonephritis must be presumptive unless confirmed by culture or biopsy of renal tissue.

Infection Superimposed on Renal Cysts and Polycystic Disease

Polycystic kidney disease is the most common of the hereditary renal diseases that result in end-stage renal failure. It occurs in two forms: the adult, which is an autosomal dominant trait; and the child, which is a recessive trait. The adult form accounts for about 10% of patients requiring long-term dialysis or renal transplantation. The course of adult polycystic disease is often complicated by flank pain, hematuria, nephrolithiasis, and urinary tract infection. Infected cysts are a major problem because they are difficult to treat and may progress to intrarenal and perinephric abscesses. Fifty percent to 75% of patients with polycystic disease, mainly females, are said to develop urinary tract infection during the course of their illness (67). Sweet and Keane (68) followed 24 patients with polycystic disease undergoing chronic hemodialysis. Of these, eight (33.3%) developed urinary tract infection and five developed perinephric abscesses. *E. coli* was isolated in the urine in all and in the blood in 2. Three patients died. In view of the hazard of infection in this population, extra precautions need to be taken to avoid instrumentation of the urinary tract and to detect and treat infections early.

The decision to operate to drain or remove the kidney is difficult because the extent of the infection is not easy to assess, and removal of a kidney may severely compromise renal function in patients who could otherwise be maintained off dialysis. Antimicrobial therapy may be ineffective because of poor penetration of drugs into diseased kidneys (69). Most antibiotics, including aminoglycosides, penicillins, and cephalosporins, penetrate polycystic renal cysts poorly. Drugs that penetrate cysts reasonably well include chloramphenicol, trimethoprim/sulfamethoxazole, clindamycin, and ciprofloxacin (70–72).

Simple renal cysts are relatively common and ordinarily of little concern except when they are mistaken for renal tumors or become infected. There are at least 18 case reports of infection in simple renal cysts, mostly occurring in females (73). Infected cysts usually present with the signs and symptoms of acute pyelonephritis. Intravenous urograms are suggestive of intrarenal abscess. The diagnosis of an infected cyst often is not made until the kidney is explored or removed.

The susceptibility to infection of simple renal cysts and polycystic kidneys may be explained by the observations of Beeson, Rocha, and Guze (74). They produced obstruction of nephrons in rabbits by small cautery lesions in the medulla. This resulted in areas described as "intrarenal hydronephrosis." These regions were much more susceptible to ascending or hematogenous infection than cauterized areas of the cortex or the remaining normal or contralateral kidneys.

Renal and Perinephric Abscesses

Renal Abscesses

An abscess is a circumscribed collection of inflammatory cells that may become necrotic and liquefied. As the abscess matures, a rim of fibrous tissue appears and demarcates the abscess from the surrounding tissue. There are two major types of renal abscesses.

1. Severe suppuration of the kidney in patients with urinary obstruction secondary to stones or malformations or in patients with diabetes mellitus. Emphysematous pyelonephritis and renal papillary necrosis are examples

of the most severe forms of infection. The most frequent underlying conditions and causative microorganisms are shown in Table 8.7.
2. Metastatic infection to the kidney from a distant site. They may be single or multiple small abscesses. If left untreated, they may coalesce into large pockets of pus (Fig. 8.5).

Staphylococcus aureus bacteremia accounted for most (about 95%) of renal abscesses or carbuncles during the preantibiotic era. This situation changed with the advent of effective antistaphylococcal drugs. Currently most renal abscesses are caused by enteric gram-negative bacteria, sometimes mixed with obligate anaerobes, in patients with long-standing, complicated, ascending infection. Metastatic renal abscesses with *Staphylococcus aureus* continue to occur in intravenous drug abusers (77), diabetics, vascular line infections, and patients inadequately treated for staphylococcal infections. *Candida albicans* is an important cause of metastatic renal abscesses in leukopenic patients and with vascular line infections. Immunocompromised patients are at risk of metastatic infection with Aspergillus, Blastomyces, Coccidiodomyces, and Histoplasma. Renal abscesses are rare in children (78,79). Unusual cases of perinephric abscesses occur in polycystic kidney disease (68), *Torulopsis glabrata* in a diabetic (80), and Clostridia in a perinephric hematoma (81).

Clinical Findings

Renal and perinephric abscesses simulate those of acute pyelonephritis (leukocytosis, fever, and flank pain). Blood cultures are often positive. The diagnosis is suspected when the patient fails to respond promptly to antimicrobial therapy or when a mass lesion is seen on abdominal radiograph, renal ultrasound, CT, and scintillation scans (Fig. 8.7). Arteriograms are helpful in localizing the abscess. Percutaneous injection of contrast material into the renal pelvis or perinephric space can delineate extension within the fascial planes. Percutaneous drainage has been shown to be as effective as open

Table 8.7. Major Predisposing Factors and Microorganisms in Renal and Perinephric Abscesses*

Major Predisposing Factors	%	Organisms Causing the Abscesses	%
Diabetes mellitus	37.7	*Escherichia coli*	37.4
Renal calculi	18.4	*Proteus mirabilis*	16.5
Ureteral obstruction	4.4	*Klebsiella pneumoniae*	10.4
Immunosuppression	3.5	Other *Enterobacteriaceae*	8.7
Intravenous drug abuse	1.8	*Pseudomonas aeruginosa*	8.7
Chronic urinary retention	8.8	*Staphylococcus aureus*	10.4
Pregnancy	1.8	*Enterococcus* spp.	2.6
Blunt flank trauma	2.6	*Candida albicans*	0.9
Renal biopsy	1.8	Anaerobe	0.9
None**	19.3	Other	3.5

*Combined data of 115 cases reported by Thorley JD, Jones SR, Sanford JP (75) and Fowler JE, and Perkins T (76).
**No identifiable systemic or urologic disorder.

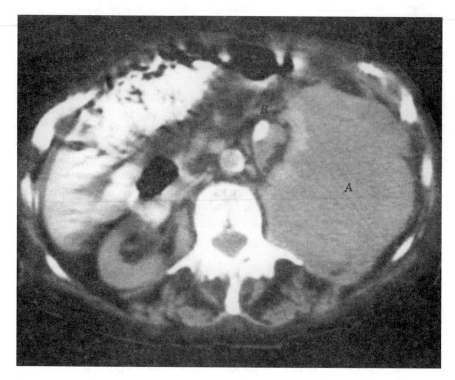

Figure 8.7. A large peri-renal abscess in an 82-year-old nondiabetic woman who had recurrent urinary tract infections. She was afebrile and had no urinary symptoms or flank tenderness. An ultrasound of the kidney was performed because of azotemia and leukocytosis. On computerized tomography, there is a large left renal mass extending to the psoas muscle and peri-renal space (A). A stone is present at the ureteropelvic junction (B). There is a huge liquefied renal abscess with extension to the perinephric space. Over 300 ml of purulent fluid containing *Proteus mirabilis* was aspirated percutaneously.

surgery for large and medium sized renal abscesses, and small abscesses may be effectively treated with antimicrobial drugs (82). Nephrectomy may be required to control infection or to remove a destroyed kidney.

Perinephric Abscesses

Renal abscesses may perforate into the retroperitoneal space between the kidney and Gerota's fascia to form perinephric abscesses. These may extend in several directions, inferiorly towards Petit's triangle or superiorly toward the diaphragm (Fig. 8.8). They may produce subphrenic abscesses with pleural effusions. They rarely perforate intraperitoneally or into the colon, but may evoke localized distention of the large and small bowel. They may occasionally bleed into the retroperitoneal space.

Key Points About Renal and Perinephric Abscesses

- The diagnosis should be suspected when the patient fails to promptly respond to antimicrobial therapy, when there is persistent bacteremia or fungemia despite appropriate antimicrobial therapy or when a mass lesion is seen on radiologic studies.
- Metastatic abscesses should be suspected in patients with bacteremia or fungemia when the same organism is found in the urine.
- Patients with urinary obstruction secondary to stones or congenital abnormalities are at increased risk of renal abscesses.
- Patients with diabetes mellitus may develop the most severe forms of renal abscess including emphysematous pyelonephritis and papillary necrosis.
- Percutaneous drainage is preferred over surgery. Nephrectomy may be life-saving when the kidney is severely damaged.

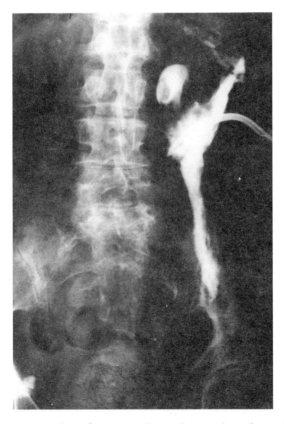

Figure 8.8. Demonstration of a retroperitoneal extension of a perinephric abscess to the region of the iliac crest by injection of contrast material through a percutaneous nephrostomy tube. Over 500 ml of purulent fluid was drained from this site. The patient refused surgery, but remarkably improved with continuous nephrostomy drainage and antimicrobial therapy.

Metastatic Infections Arising from the Urinary Tract

Microorganisms may spread from the urinary tract to other sites during the course of bacteremia, or by means of Batson's vertebral plexus (83). This plexus consists of a network of vertebral veins that extend from the sacrum to the base of the brain. Microorganisms that enter the blood from the penis and pelvic organs may go directly to bone and soft tissues via Batson's plexus and thus escape clearance by the hepatic and pulmonary reticuloendothelial systems. This concept appears to explain the occurrence of metastatic vertebral osteomyelitis after installation of BCG into the bladder (84) and urologic manipulation in men.

Table 8.8. Metastatic Infections Originating in the Urinary Tract Reported in 188 Cases*

Type of Infection	Cases		Major Microorganisms
	No.	%	
Osteomyelitis	92	48.9	(*Staphylococcus aureus, E. coli, Pseudomonas*
Septic arthritis	14	7.4	*aeruginosa, Klebsiella pneumoniae,*
			Enterobacter spp., *Proteus*
Chest infections	8	4.3	*mirabilis, Serratia marcescens,* Bacteroides,
Miscellaneous	5	2.7	Providencia, Salmonella)
Endocarditis	51	27.1	(*Enterococcus faecalis* (54.9%), gram-negative
			bacteria (34.7%), Group B streptococci,
			Staphylococcus aureus)
Meningitis & CNS	9	4.8	*E. coli, Pseudomonas aeruginosa, Klebsiella*
			pneumoniae, Enterobacter spp.
Endophthalmitis	13	6.9	*E. coli, Klebsiella pneumoniae*

*These data were compiled from references 33, 34, and 85–87.

Meningitis and ophthalmitis are rare complications of septic pyelonephritis. They are usually caused by *E. coli* and occur most commonly in women with diabetes. Endocarditis may occur in men with prior heart disease following lower genitourinary manipulation. The most striking feature is the high frequency of *Enterococcus faecalis,* but other bacteria may also be responsible (Table 8.8). Prevention of endocarditis is the major reason for avoiding

Table 8.9 Sites of Skeletal Metastases in Patients with Metastatic Infections*

Metastatic Site	No.	%
Spine	88	83.0
Lumbar	39	—
Thoracic	35	—
Cervical	13	—
Unspecified	1	—
Joints	14	13.2
Long bones	4	3.8

*From Siroky MB, et al. (86).

urologic procedures in infected patients and for the use of prophylaxis if the infection cannot be eradicated before the procedure. Any part of the spine may be involved by metastatic infection (Table 8.9).

Key Points About Metastatic Infections Arising from the Urinary Tract

- Meningitis and endophthalmitis are rare, but important complications of acute pyelonephritis in patients with diabetes mellitus. *E. coli* and *Klebisiella pneumoniae* are the most common causative organisms.
- Spinal and long bone osteomyelitis are late (months) complications of urologic manipulation. A wide variety of gram positive and gram negative bacteria may cause these infections.
- Osteomyelitis must be strongly considered in patients with a remote history of a urologic procedure who complain of back pain or unexplained fever. Bone scans may be extremely helpful to make the diagnosis.
- Endocarditis is a major complication of urologic manipulation, particularly in men with a previous history of heart disease. *Enterococcus faecalis* is the most common causative organism. Urinary infection should be eradicated prior to urologic procedures.

Pyelonephritis as an Autoimmune Disease

There is evidence that renal damage from pyelonephritis may be caused, in part, by an autoimmune response against bacterial and host proteins (88,89). This is based on several lines of evidence. First, healthy rats develop sterile interstitial nephritis when linked parabiotically to infected animals (90). Second, tubulointerstitial nephritis can be produced by injecting animals with Tamm-Horsfall protein (THP) (91,92). This protein lines the renal tubular lumen, coats casts, and binds to mannose receptors on bacterial fimbriae (93). THP is thought to be excluded from the mechanism of immune self-recognition. Andriole and his collaborators (91) demonstrated that an autoimmune response to THP occurs after intravenous challenge of rabbits with THP, in vesicoureteral reflux in pigs, and in recurrent infection and urinary obstruction in man. THP is also known as uromodulin and has been shown to be a renal ligand for lymphokines (94). Third, THP and bacterial antigens have been shown by immunofluorescent methods to persist for long periods of time in kidney tissue obtained from humans at autopsy and experimental animals (95–97).

Immune Complex Nephritis Secondary to Distant Microbial Infection

During the course of infectious diseases, microbial antigens enter the blood stream and induce an antibody response. Antibody-antigen immune complexes, formed under conditions of antigen excess, are rapidly cleared by the reticuloendothelial system under most conditions. When relatively large amounts of antigens are released, some may escape clearance and may be deposited on the glomerular basement membrane. The complexes may elicit a local inflammatory response characterized by deposition of complement and fibrinogen, proliferation mesangial cells within the glomerular tufts, and thickening and damage to the glomerular membrane. The lesions resemble those of membranous or membrano-proliferative glomerulonephritis. Damaged glomeruli may leak serum proteins into the urine, at times resulting in massive proteinuria and the nephrotic syndrome. There may be hematuria, low serum complement, rheumatoid factor and cryoglobulins in patients with severe glomerular damage. Immunohistologic and elution studies reveal the presence of microbial antigens in the glomeruli. Immune complex nephropathy can be distinguished readily from pyelonephritis by the presence of proteinuria, absence of bacteriuria, and the lack of associated symptoms of inflammation of the urinary tract.

The infectious diseases associated with immune complex nephritis include subacute bacterial endocarditis, Q fever endocarditis, syphilis, malaria, and infected ventriculo-atrial shunts ("shunt nephritis"). These infections have the following common features: 1) a microorganism with low virulence, 2) slowly progressive infection, 3) an intravascular location, and 4) continuous production of antigens. The bacteria commonly associated with this lesion include viridens streptococci, enterococci, *Staphylococcus epidermidis*, Corynebacterium species, and occasionally *Staphylococcus aureus*. The indolent infection allows antigens released from the site to stimulate the immune system over a prolonged period of time. Several months or even years may elapse before the nephrotic syndrome is produced. The disease is reversible when the site of infection is eradicated, as with cure of endocarditis, or removal of a shunt. "Shunt" nephritis caused by *Staphylococcus epidermidis* used to occur in children with hydrocephalus treated with ventriculo-atrial shunts. The disease virtually disappeared when the distal end of the shunt was placed into the peritoneal cavity.

Pyelonephritis as Seen by the Pathologist

On gross inspection, the pathologist may have considerable difficulty distinguishing bacterial pyelonephritis from other inflammatory conditions. This is because both acute bacterial pyelonephritis and interstitial nephritis can produce diffusely swollen kidneys and because chronic pyelonephritis, vascular diseases, and severe grades of vesico-ureteral reflux can produce scarred and shrunken kidneys. The distinction between pyelonephritis and other causes of renal damage is much less difficult in the presence of obstruction, stones, or gross abscesses. The hallmarks of acute ascending bacterial pyelonephritis are a dilated and inflamed renal pelvis with focal, wedge-shaped, segmental areas of inflammation extending from the papilla towards the cortex. In long-standing infection, these areas become fibrosed, leaving a shrunken cortical scar. Large areas of the kidney may remain entirely normal. This explains why infection may be missed with percutaneous renal biopsy.

Hematogenous (metastatic) pyelonephritis presents a much different picture. The pathologist usually has little difficulty in recognizing multiple small spherical abscesses distributed fairly evenly throughout an otherwise normal kidney or a kidney that has undergone long-standing infection. The abscesses may be uniform in size if produced by a single bacteremic shower, or be of different ages with multiple infections. An overview of the renal lesions of pyelonephritis is presented in Table 8.10.

Autopsy Studies in Children

Pyelonephritic lesions in children may be divided into acute lesions associated with sepsis and chronic lesions secondary to obstruction. In the study of Neumann and Pryles, 21 of 31 cases were in infants (98). There were twice as many males than females in this group. "Sepsis" in the absence of obstructive lesions accounted for 17 of the 31 cases. Pyelonephritis in these

Table 8.10. Pyelonephritis as Seen at Autopsy or Nephrectomy

Acute Ascending Infection
Gross
 The kidney is irregularly or diffusely enlarged with scattered blanched areas over the cortex.
 The pelvis is inflamed and dilated.
 Most of the inflammation is localized to the calices and fornices.
Microscopic
 Segmental areas of acute interstitial inflammation with polymorphonuclear cells extend from the papillae to the cortex in a wedge-shaped manner.
 There are areas of interstitial inflammation with pus-cell casts.
Chronic Ascending Infection
Gross
 The kidney is small and shrunken with asymmetric distortion of the kidney and cortical scars.
 Segmental areas of atrophy infiltrated with mononuclear cells and wedge-shaped areas of fibrosis.
Microscopic
 Long-term chronic infection or vascular disease may result in localized obstruction of tubules producing dilatation and proteinaceous intraluminar inclusions or casts.
 These blind, obstructed tubules superficially resemble the normal histologic features of the thyroid acini and are called "thyroid-like areas."
 Initially the glomeruli are spared, but in later stages the glomerular tufts may undergo shrinkage and hyalinization as in most other forms of end-stage renal disease.
 Periglomerular fibrosis is a nonspecific lesion. There are concentric rings of collagen fibers within Bowman's capsule.
Metastatic Abscesses
 These often are small, multiple cortical abscesses. They may coalesce to form large abscesses.
Perinephric Abscesses
 The infection has spread beyond the renal cortex and through the capsule into the perinephric fat and fascial planes.

cases was caused largely by hematogenous infection producing renal abscesses. These abscesses were due to mainly gram-positive bacteria arising from another infected site such as endocarditis, pneumonia, or infected burns producing renal abscesses. The obstructive lesions were more often seen in older children, were mostly caused by gram-negative enteric bacteria, and were more chronic in nature. The underlying lesions included severe reflux, urethral valves, and other congenital abnormalities.

Renal Biopsy

Renal biopsy is rarely necessary for diagnostic purposes because acute pyelonephritis can be recognized readily by noninvasive procedures and because chronic pyelonephritis is associated in most cases with obstructive disease of the urinary tract. It is also somewhat hazardous to biopsy an area of active infection. Pyelonephritis is often focal in the acute and subacute phases so that the needle may miss the active lesion. The process may, however, involve the entire kidney in the late chronic atrophic stage.

An extensive experience with renal biopsy reported by Jackson, Poirier, and Grieble (99) is instructive. They performed renal biopsies in 50 patients who had various forms of urinary tract infection. Biopsy and culture were negative in 4 patients with asymptomatic bacteriuria. In the total group, 75% had evidence of pyelonephritis on biopsy and 36% had positive cultures from the kidney. Gram-negative bacteria were isolated from 8 patients, generally those with acute symptoms, whereas gram-positives were isolated from 10 patients, generally with chronic infection. Biopsy was associated with a potentially serious complication in 5%, including bacteremia in 3 patients.

"Abacterial Pyelonephritis"

Angell, Relman, and Robbins (100) examined renal tissue in a series of 12 patients with "active pyelonephritis" who did not exhibit evidence of bacterial infection. Seven were male and 5 were female. All of these patients had the classic histologic lesions consisting of chronic interstitial inflammatory reaction, tubular atrophy and dilation, and periglomerular sclerosis. Some degree of calyceal distortion was observed radiologically in those studied. Cultures of renal biopsy or autopsy specimens were sterile. Several had progressive renal failure in the absence of infection, indicating that the process did not require infection to continue to be active. In retrospect, these cases were probably caused by reflux nephropathy that was not appreciated at the time.

Renal Diseases Resembling Pyelonephritis

The major problem that faces the pathologist in diagnosing pyelonephritis is that many other inflammatory or ischemic processes will produce segmental local areas of disease indistinguishable from those produced by bacterial infection. Some of the entities readily confused with pyelonephritis at postmortem examination are discussed below.

Ischemic Changes

Vascular lesions of the renal arterial system, usually caused by arteriolar nephrosclerosis, frequently result in wedge-shaped scars with intervening areas showing lesser degrees of involvement. The major feature that distinguishes vascular lesions from bacterial pyelonephritis is relative lack of involvement of the pelvi-caliceal region. Wedge-shaped scars in the kidneys of elderly patients who have extensive proliferative vascular lesions and absence of inflammation in the pelvis and papillae are now generally ascribed to ischemic changes rather than to pyelonephritis.

Obstruction and Vesico-Ureteral Reflux

These conditions may occur in the absence of infection. When severe, they may lead to extensive dilatation of the renal pelvis and marked renal atrophy. Small atrophic kidneys in infants have been attributed to bacterial infection, but it is more likely that infection is a late and secondary complication. The role of severe vesicoureteral reflux as a primary cause of renal failure in the absence of urinary infection has been well documented (see Chapter 5 on Reflux and Reflux Nephropathy).

Sickle Cell Disease

Sickle cell disease produces profound alterations in the renal microvasculature, presumably by multiple microinfarction of blood vessels in the renal medulla where oxygen content is diminished. There are associated urinary concentration defects and occasionally papillary necrosis.

Papillary Necrosis

Necrotizing papillitis may be produced by excessive use of analgesic drugs, sickle cell disease, and other disorders of the microcirculation. It may be difficult to differentiate the various causes of papillary necrosis from severe bacterial pyelonephritis on radiologic studies.

Analgesic Nephropathy

Analgesic nephropathy is perhaps the most preventable form of renal disease. The disease was first thought to be caused by phenacetin, a common pain reliever, and the disorder was initially called phenacetin nephritis. The implication that phenacetin or its active metabolite acetaminophen is the sole causal agent in the disease is now less certain, and the term analgesic nephropathy has been substituted. The kidney lesion in analgesic nephropathy is characterized by interstitial nephritis and necrosis of the renal papilla.

Continued long-term use of analgesic compounds containing phenacetin, aspirin, and related agents may lead to progressive renal disease.

Interstitial Nephritis

Interstitial nephritis is a noninfectious acute or chronic inflammatory condition usually caused by hypersensitivity to drugs or drug toxicity. The patient may present with renal failure accompanied by microscopic hematuria and pyuria, but the urine culture will usually be sterile. The kidneys are often diffusely enlarged with normal calices and without focal lesions. In the early stages, there may be extensive infiltration of the interstitium and tubules with polymorphonuclear leukocytes.

The important offenders include sulfonamides, methicillin, and other beta lactam antibiotics, nonsteroidal anti-inflammatory drugs (NSAIDs), amphotericin B, phenytoin, and phenindione. NSAIDs are particularly important because they are among the most commonly used drugs and are now available in the United States without prescription. There have been numerous reports of reversible renal failure, papillary necrosis, and nephrotic syndrome associated with zomepirac, ibuprofen, fenoprofen, and naproxen (to name a few of the many currently available). They appear to elicit an immunologic reaction distinct from their effect on renal prostaglandin synthesis. The finding of eosinophiles in the urine may be an important clue that one is dealing with an immune reaction rather than infection. Other causes of interstitial nephritis include Alport's syndrome, an autosomal dominant hereditary interstitial nephritis associated with deafness.

Pyelonephritis from a Historical Perspective

Pyelonephritis was a major cause of uncontrollable sepsis and renal failure in the pre-antibiotic era. Staphylococcal bacteremia was the most important cause of renal abscesses. The early investigators clearly understood the consequences of ascending infection complicated by congenital abnormalities, stones, obstruction, and diabetes. In retrospect, they placed undue emphasis on the role of urinary tract infections as a cause of hypertension and end-stage renal failure (101–103) (Table 8.11).

Early Studies

In 1933 Longcope and Winkenwerder (104) focused attention on the clinical features of patients found to have contracted kidneys at autopsy. They believed that this was the end-stage of the long and insidious course of progressive pyelonephritis. Much of the evidence for pyelonephritis was based on intravenous urograms. These findings would now be considered the result of reflux nephropathy. Most of the cases occurred in women under the

Table 8.11. Change in Concepts Concerning the Role of Urinary Tract Infection as a Cause of Hypertension and End-Stage Renal Disease

Former Concept*	Current Concept
Pyelonephritis occurs most commonly during infancy and childhood, during childbearing and with the aging process associated with lower urinary tract obstruction.	Unchanged.
Pyelonephritis more frequently causes Bright's disease than chronic glomerulonephritis at all ages and is the most common renal lesion in uremia.	Chronic glomerulonephritis is the most common cause of end-stage renal failure.
Pyelonephritis is frequently associated with hypertension. It is associated with malignant hypertension in 15%–20% of all cases. Pyelonephritis is present in about 20% of cases of hypertension.	Hypertension is rare in acute pyelonephritis. It occurs mainly in patients with long-standing bilateral chronic pyelonephritis who have renal failure.
Pyelonephritis is the commonest renal lesion found at necropsy and is present in 15%–20% of all autopsies.	1.4% (Freedman[†]), 2.8% (Kimmelstiel[‡]) of autopsies.
Diabetic patients have pyelonephritis about four times as often as nondiabetics.	Diabetics are among those at greatest risk for the most severe forms of pyelonephritis.
Renal infections are present in 20% of cases of toxemia of pregnancy.	The renal lesion in toxemia is glomerular capillary endotheliosis, not pyelonephritis.

*Keefer CS (101).
[†]Freedman LR (102).
[‡]Kimmelstiel P, Kim OJ, Beres JA, et al. (103).

age of 40 years who had gradual loss of weight, anemia, and died with uremia and hypertension. In 1940 Weiss and Parker (105) described young women with severe renal disease caused by bilateral renal infection. Hypertension and end-stage renal failure were observed commonly. They were particularly struck by sclerosis of the renal arterioles in the absence of generalized arteriosclerotic disease and believed that this may have had a role in producing hypertension. Both Weiss and Parker and Longcope emphasized that hypertension was not seen in acute pyelonephritis, but only after renal insufficiency had developed as long as 10 to 15 years later.

Weiss and Parker (105) appreciated the importance of pyelographic changes, the focal nature of the renal lesions, and the histologic findings of acute interstitial inflammation and abscesses. Their cases were real, and similar isolated cases of renal failure secondary to bilateral pyelonephritis were described in the postantibiotic era (28). The major problem arose with the interpretation of what Weiss and Parker termed chronic or healed pyelonephritis. They stated: " . . . in the healed stage it is often difficult to determine whether one is dealing with a healed pyelonephritis . . . or with a primary vascular kidney disease." They developed a series of arbitrary criteria for chronic pyelonephritis from which they concluded that pyelonephritis was more frequent than glomerulonephritis as a cause of Bright's disease. The lesions consisted of 1) inflammatory reaction of the interstitial tissues; 2) colloid casts in the tubules, which are lined with atrophic epithelium; 3) periglomerular fibrosis; and 4) evidence of infection or inflammation within the tubules.

In 1952, Saphir and Taylor (106) coined the term *pyelonephritis lenta* or silent pyelonephritis to describe the insidious appearance of endstage renal disease, often accompanied by hypertension occurring mostly in young adult women. The situation was compounded further by Gall (107) who believed that the severely shrunken kidney was the "stigma" of pyelonephritis and that pyelonephritis accounted for a third of all renal disorders found at autopsy and for half the patients who developed chronic uremia. In another study, MacDonald et al. (108) reported that 18% of their autopsy series had healed pyelonephritis.

Modern Studies

The situation changed dramatically in 1961 when Kimmelsteil and his associates (103) reexamined the criteria for chronic, healed pyelonephritis. They found no correlation between urine and kidney cultures and the morphology of the renal lesions. They emphasized the difficulty of establishing an etiology based on morphologic grounds alone. Using rigid criteria to define pyelonephritis, Kimmelstiel could identify pyelonephritis in only 2.8% of autopsies. Only 18 of 97 cases thought to have pyelonephritis also had azotemia. In most of these, the disease could be explained by obstruction or dysplasia or calcinosis. The male to female sex distribution was 1 to 1.3.

Freedman (102) has provided what I consider to be the most convincing of the modern autopsy studies. He combined anatomic and clinical data and excluded patients with genitourinary abnormalities, serious infections, or bacteremia during a terminal illness. Pyelonephritis was found in only 1.4% of autopsies. There was a slight preponderance of males (57%). Renal insufficiency was found in one-fourth of the cases of pyelonephritis. The anatomic findings in these patients were distributed equally in both kidneys and lacked the broad scars expected in pyelonephritis. These lesions could be explained by severe vascular disease, papillary necrosis, or medullary cysts. Most importantly, his analysis of the cases revealed that the role of urinary infection appeared to be negligible based on the clinical course.

An excellent analysis of conditions that produce chronic interstitial nephritis in relation to etiologic factors was undertaken by Murray and Goldberg (109) (Table 8.12). They studied 101 patients with interstitial

Table 8.12. Etiologic Factors in End-Stage Nephritis Identified in 101 Patients with Chronic Renal Failure*

Factor	Frequency (No.)	Characteristics
Anatomic abnormalities	34	Obstruction (32), vesicoureteral reflux (2)
Bacterial infection	27	All had structural causes for infection
Analgesic abuse	20	80% females, 80% with headaches
Nephrosclerosis	20	Most had preceding hypertension
Hyperuricemia	17	Felt to be the primary cause in 11 patients
Stones	12	Most were located in the renal pelvis or calices
Idiopathic or indeterminate	11	No primary cause could be identified
Multiple causes	7	Not further identified
Sickle cell disease	2	One had papillary necrosis
Renal tuberculosis	1	Only identified cause

*These data are retabulated from Murray T and Goldberg M (109). The total number of conditions exceeds the number of patients because many had more than one problem.

nephritis among 320 patients with newly diagnosed chronic renal disease. Histologic data were available in 37 of 101 patients studied. They point out that infection, other than tuberculosis, was not observed as a primary cause of renal failure in these patients, but was often a secondary complication of another process. In the 27 patients with bacterial infection, primary causes were anatomical abnormalities in 14, stones in 7, gout in 2, nephrosclerosis in 1, and analgesic abuse nephropathy in 3. These observations further substantiate the critical roles of obstructive and neurologic disorders of the voiding mechanism in the pathogenesis of chronic bacterial pyelonephritis.

References

1. Rosenfield AT, Glickman MG, Taylor KJW, et al. Acute focal bacterial nephritis (acute lobar nephronia). Diag Radiol 1979;132:553–561.
2. McDonough WD, Sandler CM, Benson GS. Acute focal bacterial nephritis: focal pyelonephritis that may simulate renal abscess. J Urol 1981;126:670–673.
3. Lawson GR, White FE, Alexander FW. Acute focal bacterial nephritis. Arch Dis Child 1985;60:475–477.
4. Zaontz MR, Pahira JJ, Wolfman M, et al. Acute focal bacterial nephritis: a systematic approach to diagnosis and treatment. J Urol 1985;133:752–757.
5. Wegenke JD, Malek GH, Alter AJ, et al. Acute lobular nephronia. J Urol 1986;135: 343–345.
6. Nosher JL, Tamminen JL, Amorosa JK, et al. Acute focal bacterial nephritis. Am J Kidney Dis 1988;11:36–42.
7. Jodal U, Hanson LA. Sequential determination of C-reactive protein in acute childhood pyelonephritis. Acta Paediatr Scand 1976;65:319–322.
8. Rushton HG, Majd M, Jantausch B, et al. Renal scarring following reflux and nonreflux pyelonephritis in children: Evaluation with [99m]technitium-dimercaptosuccinic acid scintography. J Urol 1992;147:1327–1332.
9. Kaitz AL, London AM. Osmolar urinary concentrating ability and pyelonephritis in hospitalized patients. Am J Med Sci 1964;248:41–49.

10. Johnson JR, Vincent LM, Wang K, et al. Renal ultrasonographic correlates of acute pyelonephritis. Clin Infect Dis 1992;14:15–22.
11. Kanel KT, Kroboth FJ, Schwentker FN, et al. The intravenous pyelogram in acute pyelonephritis. Arch Intern Med 1988;148:2144–2148.
12. Little PJ, McPherson HE, de Wardener HE. The appearance of the intravenous pyelogram during and after acute pyelonephritis. Lancet 1965;1:1186–1191.
13. Harrison RB, Shaffer HA Jr. The roentgenographic findings in acute pyelonephritis. JAMA 1979;241:1718.
14. Mushlin AI, Thornbury JR. Intravenous pyelography: the case against its routine use. Ann Intern Med 1989;111:58–70.
15. Jakobsson B, Berg U, Svensson L. Renal scarring after acute pyelonephritis. Arch Dis Child 1994;70:111–115.
16. Berg U. Long-term follow up of renal morphology and function in children with recurrent pyelonephritis. J Urol 1992;148:1515–1720.
17. Bailey RR, Little PJ, Rolleston GL. Renal damage after acute pyelonephritis. Br Med J 1969;1:550–551.
18. Whalley P, Cunningham F, Martin F. Transient renal dysfunction associated with acute pyelonephritis of pregnancy. Obstet Gynecol 1975;46:174.
19. Greenhill AH, Norman ME, Cornfeld D, et al. Acute renal failure secondary to pyelonephritis. Clin Nephrol 1977;8:400–403.
20. Baker L, Cattell W, Fry I, et al. Acute renal failure due to bacterial pyelonephritis. Q J Med 1979;48:603–612.
21. Olsson P, Black J, Gaffney E, et al. Reversible acute renal failure secondary to acute pyelonephritis. South Med J 1980;73:374–376.
22. Woolley P, Wyman A, Nicholls A, et al. Acute renal failure due to bacterial pyelonephritis. Br J Urol 1986;58:733.
23. Thompson C, Verani R, Evanoff G, et al. Suppurative bacterial pyelonephritis as a cause of acute renal failure. Am J Kidney Dis 1986;8:271–273.
24. Atkinson L, Goodship T. Acute renal failure associated with acute pyelonephritis and consumption of non-steroidal anti-inflammatory drugs. Br Med J 1986;292:97–98.
25. Weinstein T, Zevin D, Gafter U, et al. Acute renal failure in a solitary kidney due to bacterial pyelonephritis. J Urol 1986;136:1290–1291.
26. Lorentz WB, Iskandar S, Browning MC, et al. Acute renal failure due to pyelonephritis. Nephron 1990;54:256–258.
27. Nunez JE, Perez E, Gunasekaran S, et al. Acute renal failure secondary to acute bacterial pyelonephritis. Nephron 1992;62:240–241.
28. Jones SR. Acute renal failure in adults with uncomplicated acute pyelonephritis: case reports and review. Clin Infect Dis 1992;14:243–246.
29. Hodson J, Edwards D. Chronic pyelonephritis and vesicoureteric reflux. Clin Radiol 1960; 11:219–231.
30. Hutch JA, Miller ER, Hinman F Jr. Vesicoureteral reflux. Am J Med 1963;34:338–349.
31. Petersdorf RG, Beeson PB. Fever of unexplained origin: Report on 100 cases. Medicine 1961;40:1–30.
32. Jacoby GA, Swartz MN. Fever of undetermined origin. N Engl J Med 1973;289:1407–1410.
33. Goergen TG. Unusual abdominal gas collection. JAMA 1976;239:347.
34. Carris CK, Schmidt JD. Emphysematous pyelonephritis. J Urol 1977;118:457–459.
35. Dunn DR, Dewolf WC, Gonzalez R. Emphysematous pyelonephritis: report of 3 cases treated by nephrectomy. J Urol 1975;114:348–350.
36. Eun Lee S, Ki Yoon D, Kyoon Kim Y. Emphysematous pyelonephritis. J Urol 1977;118: 916–918.
37. Seidenfeld SM, Lemaistre CF, Setiawan H, et al. Emphysematous pyelonephritis caused by Candida tropicalis. J Infect Dis 1982;146:569.
38. Michaeli J, Mogle P, Perlberg S, et al. Emphysematous pyelonephritis. J Urol 1984;131: 203–208.
39. Ahlering TE, Boyd SD, Hamilton CL, et al. Emphysematous pyelonephritis: a 5-year experience with 13 patients. J Urol 1985;134:1086–1088.
40. Michaeli J, Mogle P, Perlberg S, et al. Emphysematous pyelonephritis. J Urol 1984;131: 203–208.
41. Yang WH, Shen NC. Gas-forming infection of the urinary tract: An investigation of fermentation as a mechanism. J Urol 1990;143:960–964.

42. Lowe BA, Poage MD. Bilateral emphysematous pyelonephritis. J Urol 1991;37:229–232.
43. Jeng-Jong H, Kuan-Wen C, Mirng-Kuhn R. Mixed acid fermentation of glucose as a mechanism of emphysematous urinary tract infection. J Urol 1991;146:148–151.
44. Chen KW, Huang JJ, Wu MH, et al. Gas in hepatic veins: a rare and critical presentation of emphysematous pyelonephritis. J Urol 1994;151:125–126.
45. Eknoyan G, Qunibi WY, Grissom RT, et al. Renal papillary necrosis: An update. Medicine 1982;55–73.
46. McCullough DL, Tignor MR. Xanthogranulomatous pyelonephritis. Am J Med 1972; 52:395–398.
47. Carson CC, Weinerth JL. Xanthogranulomatous pyelonephritis in a renal transplant recipient. Urology 1984;23:58–61.
48. Bagley FH, Stewart AM, Jones P. Diffuse xanthogranulomatous pyelonephritis in children: an unrecognized variant. J Urol 1977;118:434–435.
49. Malek RS, Elder JS. Xanthogranulomatous pyelonephritis: a critical analysis of 26 cases and of the literature. J Urol 1978;119:589–593.
50. Goodman M, Curry T, Russell T. Xanthogranulomatous pyelonephritis (XPG): a local disease with systemic manifestations. Report of 23 patients and review of the literature. Medicine 1979;58:171–181.
51. Schoborg TW, Saffos RO, Urdaneta L, et al. Xanthogranulomatous pyelonephritis associated with renal carcinoma. J Urol 1980;124:125–127.
52. Tolia BM, Iloreta A, Freed SZ, et al. Xanthogranulomatous pyelonephritis: Detailed analysis of 29 cases and a brief discussion of atypical presentations. J Urol 1981;126:437–442.
53. Danielli L, Zaidel L, Raviv U, et al. Xanthogranulomatous pyelonephritis in an infant. J Urol 1982;127:304–305.
54. Winn RE, Hartstein AI. Anaerobic bacterial infection and xanthogranulomatous pyelonephritis. J Urol 1982;128:567–569.
55. Bazeed MA, Nabeeh A, Atwan N. Xanthogranulomatous pyelonephritis in bilharzial patients: A report of 25 cases. J Urol 1989;141:261–264.
56. Lauzurica R, Felip A, Serra A, et al. Xanthogranulomatous pyelonephritis and systemic amyloidosis: report of 2 new cases and the natural history of this association. J Urol 1991; 146:1603–1606.
57. Cheng-Keng C, Ming-Kuen L, Phei-Lane C, et al. Xanthogranulomatous pyelonephritis:experience in 36 cases. J Urol 1992;147:333–336.
58. Elkhammas EA, Mutabagani KH, Sedmak DD, et al. Xanthogranulomatous pyelonephritis in renal allografts: report of 2 cases. J Urol 1994;151:127–128.
59. Matthews GJ, McLorie GA, Churchill BA, et al. Xanthogranulomatous pyelonephritis in pediatric patients. J Urol 1995;153:1958–1959.
60. Cotran RS. The renal lesion in chronic pyelonephritis. Immunofluorescent and ultrastructural studies. J Infect Dis 1969; 120:109 -117.
61. Tan HK, Heptinstall RH. Experimental pyelonephritis: a light and electron microscopy study of the periodic acid-Schiff positive interstitial cell. Lab Invest 1969;20:62–69.
62. Povysil C, Konickova L. Experimental xanthogranulomatous pyelonephritis. Invest Urol 191972;9:313–318.
63. Stanton MJ, Maxted W. Malacoplakia: a study of the literature and current concepts of pathogenesis, diagnosis and treatment. J Urol 1981;125:139–146.
64. Sexton CC, Lowman RM, Nyongo AO, et al. Malacoplakia presenting as complete unilateral ureteral obstruction. J Urol 1982;128:139–141.
65. Mitchell MA, Barkovitz DM, Killen PD, et al. Bilateral renal parenchymal malacoplakia presenting as fever of unknown origin: case report and review. Clin Infect Dis 1994;18:704–718.
66. Chen CS, Lai MK, Hsueh S, et al. Renal malacoplakia with secondary hepato-duodenal involvement. J Urol 1994;151:982–985.
67. Danovitch GM. Clinical features and pathophysiology of polycystic kidney disease in man. In Gardner KD, ed. Cystic diseases of the kidney. New York: John Wiley and Sons, 1976: 125–150.
68. Sweet R, Keane WF. Perinephric abscess in patients with polycystic kidney disease undergoing chronic hemodialysis. Nephron 1979;23:237–240.
69. Whelton A, Walker WG. An approach to the interpretation of drug concentrations in the kidney. Johns Hopkins Med J 1978;142:8–14.
70. Elzinga LW, Golper TA, Rashad AL, et al. Ciprofloxacin activity in cyst fluid from polycystic kidneys. Antimicrob Agents Chemother 1988;32:844–847.

71. Elzinga LW, Tolper TA, Rashad AL, et al. TMP/SMZ in cyst fluid from autosomal dominant polycystic kidneys. Kidney Int 1987;32:884–888.
72. Schwab SJ, Hinthorn D, Diederich D, et al. pH-dependent accumulation of clindamycin in a polycystic kidney. Am J Kidney Dis 1983;3:63–66.
73. Kinder PW, Rous SN. Infected renal cyst from hematogenous seeding: a case report and review of the literature. J Urol 1978;120:239–240.
74. Beeson PB, Rocha H, Guze LB. Experimental pyelonephritis: influence of localized injury in different parts of the kidney on susceptibility to hematogenous infection. Trans Assoc Am Physicians 1957;70:120–126.
75. Thorley JD, Jones SR, Sanford JP. Perinephric abscesses. Medicine 1974;53:441–451.
76. Fowler JE, Perkins T. Presentation, diagnosis and treatment of renal abscesses: 1972–1988. J Urol 1994;151:847–851.
77. Hoverman IV, Gentry LO, Jones DW, et al. Intrarenal abscess. Arch Intern Med 1980;140:914–916.
78. Rote AR, Baurer SB, Retik AB. Renal abscess in children. J Urol 1978;119:254–258.
79. Timmons JW, Perlmutter AD. Renal abscess: a changing concept. J Urol 1976;115:299–301.
80. Khauli RB, Kalash S, Young JD. Torulopsis glabrata perinephric abscess. J Urol 1983;130:968–970.
81. Sago AL, Novicki DE, McDonald RE. Clostridial infection of a perinephric hematoma. J Urol 1983;129:126–127.
82. Siegel JF, Smith A, Moldwin R. Minimally invasive treatment of renal abscess. J Urol 1996;155:52–55.
83. Batson OV. The function of the vertebral veins and their role in the spread of metastases. Ann Surg 1940;112:138–149.
84. Civen R, Berlin G, Panosian C. Vertebral osteomyelitis after intravesical administration of Bacille Calmette-Guerin. Clin Infect Dis 1994;18:1013–1014.
85. Rahav G, Levinger S, Frucht-Pery J. *Escherichia coli* endophthalmitis secondary to pyelonephritis: another complication of diabetes? Clin Infect Dis 1994;18:117–118.
86. Siroky MB, Moylan RA, Austen Jr G, et al. Metastatic infection secondary to genitourinary tract sepsis. Am J Med 1976;61:351–360.
87. Kunin CM, Bender AS, Russell CM. Meningitis in adults caused *by Escherichia coli* 04 and 075. Arch Intern Med 1965;115:652–658.
88. Miller TE, Smith JW, Lehmann JW, et al. Autoimmunity in chronic experimental pyelonephritis. J Infect Dis 1970;122:191–195.
89. Feye GL, Hemstreet GP III, Klingensmith C, et al. Auto-antibody to kidney tubular cells during retrograde chronic pyelonephritis in rats. Nephron 1985;39:371–376.
90. Kalmanson GM, Glassock RH, Montgomerie JZ, et al. Pyelonephritis transferred by parabiosis. Proc Soc Exp Biol Med 1974;146:1097–1100.
91. Andriole VT. The role of Tamm-Horsfall protein in the pathogenesis of reflux nephropathy and chronic pyelonephritis. Yale J Biol Med 1985;58:91–100.
92. Nagai T, Nagai T. Tubulointerstitial nephritis by Tamm-Horsfall glycoprotein or egg white component. Nephron 1987;47:134–140.
93. Kuriyama SM, Silverblatt FJ. Effect of Tamm-Horsfall urinary glycoprotein on phagocytosis and killing of type I-Fimbriated *Escherichia coli*. Infect Immun 1986;51:193–198.
94. Kawahima E, Schmeissner U, Heletky S, et al. Uromodulin (Tamm-Horsfall glycoprotein): a renal ligand for lymphokines. Science 1987;237:1479–1484.
95. Aoki S, Imamura S, Aoki M, et al. "Abacterial" and bacterial pyelonephritis. Immunofluorescent localization of bacterial antigen. N Engl J Med 1969;281:1375–1382.
96. Cotran R. Retrograde Proteus pyelonephritis in rats. Localization of antigen and antibody in treated sterile pyelonephritis kidneys. J Exp Med 1963;117:813–82.
97. Zager RA, Cotran RS, Hoyer JR. Pathologic localization of Tamm-Horsfall protein in interstitial deposits in renal disease. Lab Invest 1978;38:52–57.
98. Neumann CG, Pryles CV. Pyelonephritis in infants and children: autopsy experience at the Boston City Hospital 1933–1960. Am J Dis Child 1962;104:215–299.
99. Jackson GG, Poirier KP, Grieble HG. Concepts of chronic pyelonephritis. Experience with renal biopsies and long term clinical observations. Ann Intern Med 1957;47:1165–1183.
100. Angell ME, Relman AS, Robbins SL. "Active" chronic pyelonephritis without evidence of bacterial infection. N Engl J Med 1968;278:1303–1308.

101. Keefer CS. Pyelonephritis: its natural history and course. Bull Johns Hopkins Hosp 1957;100:107.
102. Freedman LR. Chronic pyelonephritis at autopsy. Ann Intern Med 1967;66:697–710.
103. Kimmelstiel P, Kim OJ, Beres JA, et al. Chronic pyelonephritis. Am J Med 1961; 30:589–607.
104. Longcope WT. Chronic bilateral pyelonephritis: its origin and its association with hypertension. Ann Intern Med 1937;2:149–163.
105. Weiss S, Parker F. Pyelonephritis: its relation to vascular lesions and to arterial hypertension. Medicine 1939;18:221–315.
106. Saphir O, Taylor B. Pyelonephritis lenta. Ann Intern Med 1952;36:1017–1041.
107. Gall EA. Pyelonephritis. Bull NY Acad Med 1961;37:367–382.
108. MacDonald RA, Levitin H, Mallory GK, et al. Relation between pyelonephritis and bacterial counts in the urine. N Engl J Med 1957;256:915–922.
109. Murray T, Goldberg M. Chronic interstitial nephritis. Etiologic factors. Ann Intern Med 1975;82:453–459.

9

Care of the Urinary Catheter

Overview

The urinary catheter is an essential part of modern medical care. It is widely used to relieve anatomic or physiologic obstruction, facilitate surgical repair of the urethra and surrounding structures, provide a dry environment for comatose or incontinent patients, and permit accurate measurement of urinary output in severely ill patients. Unfortunately, when used inappropriately or left in place too long, the catheter is a hazard to the very patients it is designed to protect. The indwelling urinary catheter is the leading cause of nosocomial urinary tract infection and gram-negative bacteremia. Systemic antimicrobial therapy may temporarily reduce the bacterial count in the bladder urine but cannot eradicate infections in patients with indwelling urinary catheters. Inappropriate and excessive use of antimicrobial drugs in catheterized patients leads to the selection of antibiotic-resistant microorganisms and accounts for nosocomial outbreaks of infection with multi-resistant strains. Catheters drain the bladder but obstruct the urethra. Indwelling urethral catheters can produce urethral strictures, epididymitis, orchitis, and prostatitis in males.

Urinary tract infections and other complications can be prevented by using catheters only when necessary and by removing them when no longer needed. Indwelling catheters should always be attached to closed drainage. Alternatives to the indwelling catheter include intermittent catheterization for patients with spinal cord injury and neurogenic bladders, condom drainage for the non-obstructed male, and absorbent pads for incontinent females. These measures are particularly important in long-term-care institutions. It is surprising that in the current era of biomedical technology, few improvements have been made in the "low-tech" catheter. This chapter will consider the indications, complications, and management of the urinary catheter. It is hoped that the concepts presented here will stimulate the development of improved urinary collection and drainage systems.

Indications and Risks of Catheterization

The decision to use a urinary catheter depends on the clinical indication and the relative risk of the procedure. A single (in and out) catheterization may be all that is needed to obtain a urine specimen or relieve obstruction. The risk of infection is relatively low. Intermittent (single) catheterizations may be used for several days in acutely ill patients or for months to years in patients with neurogenic bladders. The risks are trauma to the urethra and infection. The indwelling catheter is more convenient and requires less nursing time, but is the major cause of nosocomial urinary tract infections. The risk of infection is low when the catheter is attached to aseptic closed drainage during the first few days after insertion. But when the catheter is left in place for several weeks or longer, the infection is inevitable and the risk of trauma to the urethra and bladder is markedly increased. Suprapubic catheters bypass the urethra but traumatize the bladder; infection is inevitable.

Single Catheterization

Indications
A single urinary catheterization provides ready access to the bladder urine.

Indications for Single Catheterization
- temporarily relieve obstruction or inability to void
- obtain urine from patients who cannot provide a clean-voided specimen because of weakness, obesity, or major medical problems
- determine the volume of residual urine (when ultrasound or post-void studies are not feasible)
- permit examination of the anatomy of the urethra and perform cystourethrograms
- allow intermittent catheterization

Contraindications
Catheters should not be used *routinely* in the following instances:
- to collect urine for culture
- prior to delivery or immediately postpartum
- postoperatively

Risks
The rate of acquisition of urinary tract infections in healthy individuals after a single catheterization is relatively low, on the order of 1% to 2 % (1). The rate of infection is much higher in those who cannot empty their bladders and who retain a significant volume of urine. Patients at increased risk include women catheterized just before delivery or postpartum, men with prostatic obstruction, the elderly, the debilitated, and the diabetic. The rate of infection may exceed 20% in women who are catheterized peripartum (2,3).

Prophylaxis of Infection
It is not necessary to use prophylaxis for single catheterizations in otherwise healthy individuals. The reasons are that uropathogens are not ordinarily present in the periurethral area, the small number of microorganisms introduced at the time of catheterization are washed-out by the urine, and a foreign body is not left in place. High-risk patients may be given a single dose of an effective drug, such as trimethoprim, trimethoprim/sulfamethoxazole (TMP/SMZ), nitrofurantoin, or a quinolone. An alternate method is to irrigate the bladder with an antimicrobial solution containing neomycin/polymyxin or chlorhexidine just before removal of the catheter.

The Indwelling Urethral Catheter

The indwelling urethral catheter is one of the most commonly used instruments in hospitals. It is inserted in about 10% of patients admitted to general hospitals and about 7.5% to 10% of patients in nursing homes (4–6). In hospitalized patients, indwelling catheters are used for relatively short-term periods ranging from several days to few weeks. The greatest use occurs in intensive care units, neurosurgical and urologic services, postoperatively, and in elderly incontinent patients. Most patients leave hospitals without catheters. Hospital-acquired urinary tract infections are usually caused by a single microorganism and can be treated successfully with antimicrobial drugs after the catheter is removed. In contrast, patients in nursing homes and rehabilitation units are catheterized for months to years. They tend to be colonized with multiple microorganisms. Treatment is unsuccessful as long as the catheter remains in place.

Indications
The indwelling catheter is used to drain the bladder for prolonged periods of time.

Indications for the Indwelling Catheter
- Measure urine output in acutely ill patients and after major surgical procedures
- Relieve obstruction before prostatectomy or other urologic procedures
- Bypass an obstructed lower tract
- Serve as a landmark for urologic and gynecologic procedures
- Prevent skin breakdown in incontinent females when other measures fail
- Protect the kidney from damage in patients with neurogenic bladders when condom drainage or intermittent catheterization cannot be used
- Irrigate the bladder with amphotericin B or antineoplastic drugs

Contraindications

The indwelling catheter is contraindicated when used:

- to collect timed urine specimens of urine if the patient can void spontaneously
- to save nursing time for the care of incontinent patients
- as routine postoperative care
- when alternate methods such as condom drainage or intermittent catheterization are available
- when it is no longer needed

Risks

The risks depend on the duration of catheterization, age, sex, and underlying disease (such as diabetes). The rates are highest among females, the elderly, and the critically ill (4,7). Virtually all patients on open drainage will develop significant bacteriuria within 2 to 3 days (8). With aseptic closed drainage, only half the patients will be colonized within 10 days to 2 weeks (4) (Fig. 9.1).

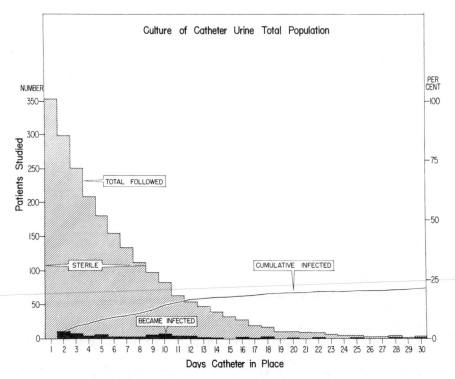

Figure 9.1. Daily cultures of urine obtained directly from the urinary catheter attached to closed urinary drainage bags in consecutive patients who initially had sterile urine. Reproduced with permission from Kunin and McCormack (4).

When a urinary catheter is left in place for longer periods, all the patients will develop urinary tract infections. Most patients with catheter-associated urinary tract infections are asymptomatic. Accordingly, the definition of nosocomial urinary tract infections should be acquisition of bacteriuria after catheterization regardless of the presence of fever, pyuria, bacteremia, or symptoms.

Complications of Indwelling Catheters
- Urinary tract infection
- Acute pyelonephritis
- Bacteremia and sepsis
- Late sequellae, including metastatic osteomyelitis and meningitis
- Prolonged hospital stay
- Increased mortality among bacteriuric patients in general hospitals
- Increased mortality among patients with long-term catheters in nursing homes
- Increased costs of antimicrobial drugs and hospital admissions for sepsis
- Formation of encrustations and obstruction to flow
- Urethral strictures, prostatitis, and orchitis
- Acquisition and spread of yeasts and multi-resistant bacteria

Prophylaxis or Treatment While the Catheter is in Place
Antimicrobial prophylaxis may temporarily delay the onset of bacteriuria in patients with indwelling catheters, but it predisposes to superinfection with resistant microorganisms (9). For example, prophylactic use of a fluoroquinolone has reduced the rate of gram negative, but not gram positive, bacteriuria in patients catheterized for several weeks (10,11). However, excessive use of fluoroquinolones in catheterized patients is associated with the emergence of ciprofloxacin-resistant *E. coli* (12). The rate of nosocomial urinary tract infection at a university medical center doubled between 1982 and 1991 as a result of the selective pressure of antibiotic use (12). There was an increase in infections caused by yeasts, *Klebsiella pneumoniae,* and group B streptococci. The current problem with gentamicin and vancomycin-resistant enterococci may be traced in part to excessive use of cephalosporins in catheterized patients (13).

Attempts to use antimicrobial drugs to eradicate microorganisms adherent to the internal surface of the catheter or in the zone between the external surface of the catheter and the urethral mucosa may be initially successful (14,15), but are doomed to failure because of the problem of emergence of resistant microorganisms. Superinfection with urease-producing microorganisms, such as Proteus and Providencia, produces further complications. Alkaline urine formed by the breakdown of urea to ammonia leads to precipitation and aggregation of struvite crystals on the catheter surfaces. Encrustations block the channel and render it useless. The challenge is to develop better methods to drain the bladder without altering its defense. These issues will be discussed later on in the section on Methods to Improve the Indwelling Catheter.

Treatment After the Catheter is Removed

Bacteriuria will resolve spontaneously in about one-third of women after an indwelling catheter is removed (16). Those who remain bacteriuric often develop symptomatic infection. A single dose of trimethoprim/sulfamethoxazole (TMP/SMZ) given to those who are still bacteriuric at 48 hours after removal of the catheter is as effective as a 10-day course for women older than 65 years (16). Longer treatment with a drug to which the microorganism is susceptible should be used in men and older women. Treatment is usually ineffective in men who develop infection in the presence of prostatic calculi. Prophylactic antibiotics should not be used while the patient is catheterized. Treatment should be reserved for documented infection after the catheter is removed.

Percutaneous Suprapubic Catheters

Suprapubic drainage is a useful alternative to urethral catheters. Urethral catheters drain the bladder but obstruct the urethral glands and the prostatic and ejaculatory ducts. They may also produce epididymitis or prostatitis and provide a passage around the catheter for entry of bacteria into the bladder. Suprapubic catheters (Malecot and de Pezzer types) are placed in the bladder surgically. This placement limits their widespread use. Several types of plastic catheters may be inserted through a trocar directly into the bladder (Fig. 9.2). These devices are often used in patients undergoing gynecologic surgery, but they should also be extended to general medical and surgical patients. The coiled end of the Bonanno catheter permits its retention in the bladder; the narrow lumen does not seem to impair flow.

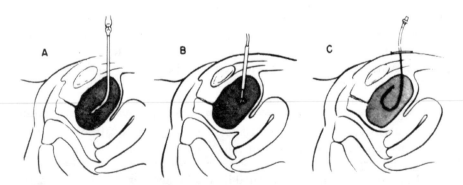

Figure 9.2. Several types of suprapubic catheters. A, device of Taylor and Nickel (17); **B,** trocar cystostomy of Hodgkinson and Hodar (18); **C,** Bonanno suprapubic drainage catheter with coiled tip.

Condom (External) Drainage

Condom drainage offers the opportunity to collect urine from males without instrumenting the urethra (Fig. 9.3). The risk of infection is reduced markedly, but care is needed to avoid strangulation and maceration of the penis. Even the best condom catheters tend to fall off in paraplegic males with intermittent erections and are often pulled off by demented patients. New condom catheter designs include "sticky" internal surfaces and Velcro bands to hold

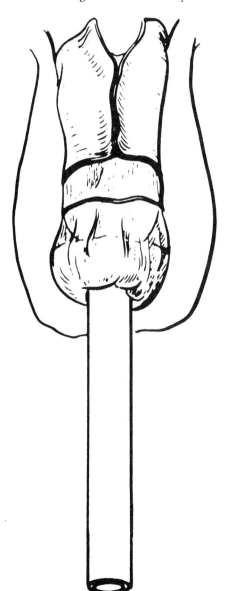

Figure 9.3. Condom drain in place in an adult mate. A band of elastic adhesive tape or Velcro is rolled around the base of the penis to secure the condom in position.

them in place, but a need exists for better fitting devices. Condom catheters should be changed daily after thorough cleansing of the perineal area.

The risk of infection is low in most patients. It is highest in patients who pull it off repeatedly (19). Urine pools around condom catheters and can become colonized with large numbers of bacteria. This poses a risk of cross infection with multi-resistant bacteria (20,21).

Urine cultures should not be obtained from the drainage tube. The condom should be removed, the penis washed, and a clean voided urine obtained (22). The positive predictive value of infection is 86% when the bacterial count is 10^5 cfu/ml. The negative predictive value for counts $< 10^5$ cfu/ml is 90% (23).

Indications
Condom drainage is reserved for comatose or incontinent males who cannot completely empty their bladder.

Contraindications
Urethral or bladder neck obstruction

Risks and Problems
- Maceration of the penis
- Strangulation and gangrene of the penis
- Urinary infection when repeatedly pulled off by the patient

Treatment of Infections
Condom catheter-induced urinary infections may occur in men who use the device for prolonged periods of time. The incidence is reported to be 0.08 episodes per patient month at risk (24). Short courses of therapy may be used, but treatment needs to be individualized depending on the susceptibility of the microorganism and whether the prostate is involved.

Intermittent Catheterization

The concept of intermittent catheterization for the early treatment of patients with traumatic paraplegia was introduced about 40 years ago by Sir Ludwig Guttmann at the Stoke Mandeville rehabilitation hospital in the United Kingdom (25). Tribe and Silver (26) working at the same institution, noted that urinary sepsis and pyelonephritis, complicated by hypertension and renal failure, were the chief causes of febrile illness and death among paraplegics. Guttmann reasoned that aseptic, intermittent catheterization would eliminate the presence of the foreign body and mimic the normal cycle of bladder emptying. This technique has markedly reduced the incidence of urinary tract infections and morbidity among paraplegic patients. Intermittent catheterization was adopted by Lapides for use in children with neurogenic bladders (27). The care of the neurogenic bladder and the methods of Guttmann and Lapides are described in greater detail later in the chapter.

Intermittent catheterization is now widely used for the short-term management of incontinent or acutely ill patients and after renal transplantation. I am not aware of any studies that demonstrate that diabetics with large atonic bladders are better off when managed with intermittent catheterization. There is a need for controlled trials to determine whether the benefits outweigh the risks. Intermittent catheterization is not currently recommended for diabetics with neurogenic bladders as long as their renal function remains stable.

Indications
The general indications for intermittent catheterization include the following:

- Short-term treatment of acute urinary retention
- Monitoring of urine output in intensive care units
- Postoperative care
- Management of the patients with strokes or spinal cord injury
- Management of children and adults with neurogenic bladders

Contraindications
Difficulty in inserting the catheter

Risks
The frequency of urinary tract infections is decreased but not eliminated by intermittent catheterization. Complications may occur in paraplegic males who require long-term management of neurogenic bladders.

Complications
- Bleeding
- Development of urethral strictures and false urethral passages (28)
- Epididymitis

Treatment and Prophylaxis of Infections
A major advantage of intermittent catheterization is that infection can be detected early and treated successfully in most patients. This advantage is possible because a specimen of urine is obtained with each catheterization, the bladder is fully drained, and no foreign body is left in place to cause irritation or serve as a nidus of infection.

There is no standard protocol for treatment. In general, each episode of infection may be treated with a brief three-day course of specific antimicrobial therapy. Short-term treatment is as effective as suppressive or long-term therapy (29). Some patients who develop persistent, symptomatic infection may require long-term prophylaxis (30). One must recognize failure and not treat persistent asymptomatic bacteriuria in patients with resistant microorganisms.

Periodic decompression of the bladder, even in the presence of persistent bacteriuria, is often sufficient as long as the patient has stable renal function.

A variety of methods have been claimed to be effective in the paraplegic patient. These methods include routine irrigation of the bladder with a solution of neomycin-polymyxin after each catheterization (31), oral prophylaxis with nitrofurantoin (30), trimethoprim/sulfamethoxazole, and methenamine mandelate combined with ammonium chloride to acidify the urine (32). Bladder irrigations with polymyxin/neomycin may be complicated by superinfection with yeasts and enterococci. In one controlled trial, neomycin irrigation was found to be ineffective (33).

Catheter Care

Sterile rubber or plastic catheters lubricated with surgical jelly should be used for intermittent catheterization in hospitalized patients. More slippery disposable, hydrophilic, prelubricated catheters are available. They are reported to have good patient acceptance, but it is not clear whether they reduce the frequency of urethral strictures or other complications (34,35). Most patients on long-term home intermittent catheterization can use the same rubber catheter repeatedly, provided that it is kept clean, but not necessarily sterile, by washing between uses. Catheters can be sterilized by a short exposure in a microwave oven (36).

Management of the Neurogenic Bladder

The pioneer in this field is Sir Ludwig Guttmann (25). He adapted intermittent catheterization after finding that urethral or suprapubic drainage of patients with spinal cord injury carried unacceptable risks of urinary tract infection and sepsis. He noted three stages after transection of the spinal cord in man. These are the stage of muscular flaccidity, the stage of reflex activity, and the stage of toxemia or the septic stage. It is now possible to virtually eliminate the third stage by careful aseptic intermittent catheterization. Guttmann demonstrated that intermittent catheterization performed by the "nontouch" technique using meticulous control, including routine culture and treatment of any positive culture, markedly reduced the risk of urinary tract infections in patients with spinal cord injuries.

Lapides (27) introduced clean, but not necessarily aseptic, "self-catheterization" to manage children with neurogenic disorders of bladder function. His contribution lead to a marked decrease in the need for urinary diversion procedures. Remarkable success has been reported in children with neurogenic bladders treated by intermittent catheterization. Most are able to function well, have only rare episodes of urinary sepsis, and have stable upper urinary tracts on pyelography. The procedure is particularly effective for children with vesicoureteral reflux when associated with an atonic bladder (37).

Not all patients with a neurogenic bladder require intermittent catheterization for long-term care. Paraplegic males can often be managed without catheters by use of rectal stimulation and manual pressure over the bladder (the Crede maneuver) and condom drainage. Cholinergic agents enhance detrusor function and alpha adrenergic agents relax the external sphincter. They may be used as adjuncts but are not always effective. Males who are managed successively with intermittent catheterization may eventually develop urethral hemorrhage strictures and false passages. They can be converted to condom drainage by sphincterotomy and, if necessary, by insertion of an endoluminal urethral stent (38). The key points are that drainage is designed to protect the kidney, each patient is different, and there are numerous trade-offs among the different procedures (39). The key role of patient cooperation is illustrated by the following case.

An Illustrative Case

A 28-year-old quadriplegic man was brought to the emergency room because of fever, chills, and hypotension. He had fractured C6 four years earlier in an accident while driving a motor bike. On examination, his temperature was 38°C, pulse 120, blood pressure 80/60, and respirations 22 per minute. He was lean, malodorous, and dehydrated, a cigarette was dangling from his mouth, and he reluctantly provided his history. The physical examination was unremarkable except for a suprapubic catheter surrounded by purulent material at the stoma. The catheter was removed and found to be encrusted heavily and blocked by a mucous plug. The urine had an ammonia-like odor and was loaded with white blood cells and gram negative bacteria. The pH was 8.0. Urine and blood cultures revealed *Proteus mirabilis.* Laboratory examination revealed a white blood count of 18,000 with 80% segmented forms and 10 bands. He had normochromic normocytic anemia, BUN 40, creatinine 1.4, and electrolytes revealed hyponatremia and hypokalemia. A radiograph of his pelvis revealed multiple bladder calculi (Fig. 9.4). He was repleted with fluids and electrolytes and treated with gentamicin and cefazolin to which the microorganisms were susceptible. He improved over several days and the BUN and creatinine returned to normal. He demanded to be discharged home. He was offered removal of the bladder calculi, a sphincterotomy, and a condom catheter, but refused.

This case presents the dark side of paraplegia in an uncooperative patient. Many young male paraplegics are dare-devils who take risks by driving too fast, being shot, falling from trees, or jumping into shallow water. They often reject medical care until they become desperately ill. They will not or cannot self-catheterize and often end up with suprapubic catheters complicated by life-threatening episodes of sepsis. One wonders whether they might do just as well without artificial urinary drainage. It may be preferable not to use an indwelling catheter in paraplegic patients who refuse catheterization or cannot self-catheterize.

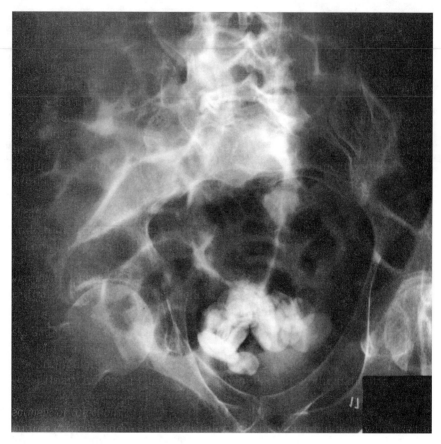

Figure 9.4. Multiple bladder calculi in a paraplegic male with a long-term suprapubic catheter. Large numbers *Proteus mirabilis* were grown from his urine.

Methods of Guttmann and Lapides

Intermittent Catheterization of the Spinal Cord Injury Patient (Method of Guttmann)

"Instrumentation is not attempted for the first 12 to 24 hours after the injury. The bladder is usually not distended during this period, since at this stage, there is a tendency for a low urinary output. If, after this period, there is no spontaneous urination, and gentle manual pressure upon the bladder region or digital massage per rectum has proved unsuccessful and the bladder has become distended, intermittent catheterization is instituted. This is done 2 to 3 times each 24 hours and is performed by the "non-touch" technique by the medical officer in charge for males or well-trained nurses for females. The patient is encouraged to void as best as he can or by manual or abdominal pressure. Diuresis usually occurs by the 4th to 6th day and is controlled by some fluid restriction and more frequent catheterizations. Fluid output is maintained at about 2 liters per day. The urine is cultured several times weekly and, if infected, is immediately treated."

Self-Catheterization by Children (Method of Lapides)
"The basic principles and goals of frequent emptying of the bladder by catheterization are discussed with the patient and parent. Emphasis is placed upon frequency of catheterization rather than sterility. The patients report for their catheterization lesson with a full bladder, if possible. The female subject sits on the examining table with feet on the table, lower limbs flexed and knees held apart to help expose the introitus and urethral meatus. In the sitting position the patient is able to visualize the perineum in a mirror at the foot of the table. The labia are separated and the clitoris, urethral meatus and vaginal outlet are pointed out. The subject is then given a 14F plastic or rubber Robinson catheter and is instructed to insert the catheter through the urethral meatus into the bladder. She is directed to hold the catheter about 0.5 inch from the tip with the hand used for skilled performance and with the fingers of the other hand to hold the labia apart with the index and fourth fingers while pressing on the meatus with the third finger. The third finger is then raised from the meatus and the catheter is passed into the urethral lumen. The patient is advised to partially empty the bladder, withdraw the catheter completely and re-catheterize herself. Thereafter, she catheterizes herself several times again until she feels confident about the procedure. The catheter can be carried in a dry state. No sterilizing solution is used and no lubricant is needed for the female subject. For the sake of cleanliness and prevention of odor the patient washes her hands with soap and water and the outer surface of the catheter with the same soapy lather and rinses the inside and outside of the catheter with clear water. Males are instructed to apply water-soluble surgical lubricant to the outer terminal portion of the catheter to avoid traumatic urethritis. The patients are warned to never forego catheterization at the prescribed time regardless of the circumstances."

Key Points about Intermittent Catheterization

Advantages
- Mimics the normal emptying of the bladder
- Eliminates a persistent foreign body
- Prevents overflow incontinence
- Improves patient self-esteem
- Allows antimicrobial therapy to be more effective
- Decreases complications of catheter care
- Fewer episodes of sepsis
- Less stone formation
- Protects the upper tract
- Decreases the need for urinary diversion procedures

Disadvantages
• Requires more nursing time in hospitals
• Requires patient cooperation or assistance at home
• May ultimately require bladder neck surgery in males

Unresolved Issues
• Do antimicrobial irrigation solutions decrease infections?
• Should asymptomatic bacteriuria be treated?
• Is prophylaxis effective?
• Is it superior to short-term indwelling catheters for postoperative patients?

Clinical Problems

Postoperative Urinary Retention

Catheters should not be used routinely in the postoperative patient who has difficulty voiding. It is common for a male patient to trace the onset of recurrent prostatitis or a female patient to relate recurrent urinary infections to postoperative or postpartum catheterization. The patient should be given adequate time, placed in a comfortable position to void, and, most important, have the privacy to relieve inhibitions. A single or several intermittent catheterizations may suffice for the patient who cannot void after several hours. The surgeon may elect to use an indwelling catheter for 1 to 2 days instead of intermittent catheterization. In one study (40), short-term use of the indwelling catheter reduced the occurrence of urine retention and bladder distention without increasing the rate of urinary tract infection. It is even possible to remove the urinary catheter within 1 to 2 days after prostate surgery (41). *Regardless of the method used to relieve postoperative urinary retention, it is recommended that microscopic examination of the urine or culture be done after the catheter is removed and that infection be eradicated.*

Management of Sepsis in the Catheterized Patient

Acute episodes of fever and chills sometimes accompanied by septic shock may occur in patients with indwelling catheters. Detection of sepsis may be difficult in elderly patients. They may have only low grade fever, appear to be dehydrated, and develop mental confusion. The first step is to remove the catheter. It may be kinked or blocked by encrustations. The urine should be examined by gram stain to obtain a preliminary assessment of the possible causative organisms. Ordinarily, one suspects gram negative bacteria, but gram positive bacteria (staphylococci and enterococci) or yeasts may be seen. Blood cultures and standard laboratory tests should be obtained and attention be directed at managing hypotension and repletion of fluids and electrolytes. Antibiotics therapy is directed initially at resistant gram negative bacteria, enterococci, and staphylococci (when seen in the urine).There is no standard therapy. Some experts recommend the use of an aminoglycoside combined with a cephalosporin or extended spectrum penicillin. Others use a cephalosporin or extended spectrum penicillin or quinolone alone. Ampicillin and ampicillin/sulbactam should not be used for initial therapy because of the high frequency of ampicillin-resistant *E. coli*. There is no standard duration of therapy. Bacteremia is often transient and rarely metastatic. The patients may succumb to endotoxin shock regardless of the choice of antimicrobial drug. Those who survive the first day or two of hospitalization often do remarkably well once good drainage is established and fluids and electrolytes are repleted.

Key Points about Management of Sepsis in Catheterized Patients

- Clues in the elderly are altered mental status, anorexia, low grade fever, and hypotension.
- Remove the catheter and inspect for encrustations and blockage.
- Do not insert a new catheter unless there is obstruction.
- Obtain blood cultures and find out what antimicrobial drugs were used recently.
- Patients with blocked catheters and alkaline urine will be infected with urease-producing bacteria, including Proteus, Providencia, and Morganella.
- Gram stain the urine to determine the presence of gram positive and negative bacteria and yeasts.
- Replete fluids and electrolytes and pressure drugs as necessary.
- Obtain an ultrasound of the kidneys and bladder to look for obstruction and stones.
- Assume that the patient is infected with several multi-resistant uropathogens. *E. coli* has special epidemic virulence.
- Initiate presumptive therapy with an extended spectrum penicillin, cephalosporin, or fluoroquinolone with optional use of an aminoglycoside. Add drugs effective against enterococci and yeasts if gram positive cocci in chains or yeasts are seen in the urine.
- Simplify therapy to a single drug as soon as susceptibility data are available.
- The optimum duration of therapy is not established, but it need not exceed 1 week.
- Reevaluate the need to use an indwelling catheter for the patient.

Nosocomial Urinary Tract Infections

It is estimated that there are two million nosocomial infections among the 35,000,000 admissions annually to hospitals in the United States (42). The annual rate of nosocomial infections is 5.7%. Urinary tract infections account for about 40% of nosocomial infections (43) or about 800,000 nosocomial infections annually. About 80% of nosocomial urinary tract infections are associated with urinary catheters. The rates appear to be rising. In one university hospital over a course of a decade, the rate rose from 2.63% to 4.35% of patients—presumably due to increased intensity of care (44). These estimates are conservative because about 5% of United States citizens over the age of 65 reside in nursing homes. There are more than 1.5 million nursing home beds in the United States (45) and nosocomial infections are common. Virtually all of the 5%-10% of nursing home patients managed with a long-term urinary catheter will have urinary tract infections.

Bacteremia

There are about 250,000 cases of nosocomial bacteremia each year in the United States. The rates vary from 1.3 to 14.5 per 1000 hospital admissions depending on the type of population studied (46). About 18% to 25% of nosocomial bacteremias are caused by urinary tract infection (47,48). The overall case fatality may exceed 50% in patients with septic shock.

Mortality

It is estimated that nosocomial urinary tract infections directly caused 947 deaths and contributed to 6,503 deaths for a total of 7,450 deaths in 1992 (42). This number is conservative because it does not take into account patients who were admitted to the hospital from home or an extended care facility with catheter-associated infections and sepsis. A threefold increase in mortality was noted in catheterized patients in an acute general hospital (49).

Costs

The estimated cost of nosocomial infections was over 4.5 billion dollars in 1992 and is increasing each year (42). Part of the costs stem from prolonged hospital stay. The excess days for urinary tract infection range from an average of 1 to 2.4 (42,50) and are longer in patients with bacteremia, shock, and other complications. Additional costs are generated by diagnostic tests and antimicrobial therapy. Control of nosocomial urinary tract infection should have a profound effect on hospital costs.

Outbreaks

There are numerous reports of outbreaks of nosocomial urinary infections associated with indwelling catheters. The epidemics often are caused by an endemic multi-resistant microorganism, such as Serratia, Proteus, Pseudomonas, Klebsiella, and Enterococcus (51–55). These causes are only the "tip of the iceberg." The source of infection is the reservoir of contaminated urine in the drainage system. The selective force for multi-resistance is the high concentration of antibiotics in the urine. The spread from patient to patient is caused by contaminated urine on hands of attendants (52). This spread leads to contamination of open wounds, tracheotomy sites, and ventilators. Good aseptic technique is often violated by failure of physicians and nurses to wash their hands between patients and failure to wear disposable gloves when emptying drainage systems or caring for the catheter. The most egregious break in technique is the use of the same irrigation system for several patients. These are ideal conditions for microepidemics. They usually go unnoticed until the patients develop fever, sepsis, and bacteremia.

Surveillance needs to be focused on the urine as the site of contamination, on detection of breaks in aseptic techniques, and on excessive use of antimicrobial drugs. Cross contamination can be prevented by geographic dispersal of patients with catheters (56). This may be accomplished in hospital rooms, but it is difficult in crowded intensive care units that have become cesspools of infection.

Overuse of Catheters

Catheters are often overused in hospitals and nursing homes. In a study of catheter use in a tertiary care hospital, the investigators judged use to be unjustified in 21% of patients, and continued catheterization was unjustified in 47% (57). Much of the excessive use in intensive care units was for monitoring urine output when no longer needed. The excessive use in noncritical areas is for management of incontinence.

Catheter-associated Infections in Long-term Care Facilities

Most nursing home residents are elderly and infirm. About 80% are female and about half are incontinent of urine. The major causes of death are cerebrovascular, hypertensive, infectious, and neoplastic diseases. A strong association exists between decreased ability to perform activities of daily living and mortality (58). The overall prevalence of infections in nursing home patients is about 16% (59) with incidence of rates of 3.6 to 7.1 per thousand patient days (60,61). In a three-year surveillance study of residents with infections in nursing homes, 18% had symptomatic urinary tract infections (62). Genitourinary infections accounted for 12% of hospital admissions of nursing home residents (63).

Use of Antibiotics and Antibiotic Resistance

Antibiotics are often prescribed for nursing homes in the absence of fever, culture information, or examination of the patient (64). Over half the courses are deemed inappropriate or unjustified (65). It is therefore not surprising that virtually all patients with indwelling catheters are infected with several species of multiply-resistant microorganisms.

Fever and Bacteremia

Fever is an important sign in bacteriuric elderly nursing home patients. It is relatively uncommon (1.1 episodes per 100 patient days), often transient, and generally about 100° F, but important (66). The authors found that low grade fever was often associated with bacteremia and that mortality was 60 times greater during febrile periods. Unfortunately, fever in the institutionalized elderly may be due to a variety of causes and less than 10% is attributable to urinary tract infections (67). Asymptomatic bacteremia among catheterized patients is relatively common. For example, in one study, bacteremia was detected about 10% of the time when the urethral catheter was changed (68).

Pyelonephritis

Silent pyelonephritis is common among elderly, catheterized patients. An autopsy study revealed acute inflammation of the renal parenchyma in 35% of nursing home patients who had a catheter in place at the time of death, compared with 5% in noncatheterized patients (69).

Increased Mortality

Death caused by the use of indwelling catheters is difficult to assess in nursing home patients because of confounding by other fatal conditions (70). In one study, catheter and noncatheter care was compared in two different wards of the same facility (71). There were no differences in mortality at 4 years. Nevertheless, it was shown that catheters could be removed with relative ease from most patients, bacteriuria disappeared spontaneously, it was easier to eradicate infection, there was improved contact with the staff, decrease in odors, absence of pressure sores, reduction in the number of gram negative nosocomial strains of bacteria, and marked reduction in the use of antibiotics.

The author found catheter-associated mortality to be an independent risk factor for death in elderly in nursing homes patients after adjustment for all other risk factors for death (6). There was a stepwise increase in mortality with duration of catheterization. Patients who were catheterized for 76% or more nursing homes days were three times more likely to die within a year. The number of hospitalizations, duration of hospitalization, and use of antimicrobial drugs were three times greater among catheterized patients.

The rates of infection, death, and excessive antibiotic use can be reduced markedly by strict attention to the indications for use of catheters in nursing home patients and removal of catheters when not essential. Alternative methods of care of incontinence are available and should be used (72,73).

Key Points about Use of Indwelling Catheters in Nursing Homes

- Indwelling catheters are used in about 7.5% to 10% of patients in many U.S. facilities.
- Lower rates can be achieved by use of prompted voiding and incontinence pads.
- All patients catheterized for more than a month will have urinary tract infections.
- Antibiotics are overused in nursing home patients and are inappropriate 50% of the time.
- Multi-resistant, polymicrobial bacteriuria is common in catheterized patients.
- Bacteremia is often silent and occurs in 10% of patients when catheters are changed.
- Fever is relatively uncommon, transient, and low grade, but is an important finding.
- Urinary infections are common causes of hospital admission of catheterized patients.
- Silent pyelonephritis is present at autopsy in about one-third of catheterized patients.
- Catheter-associated infections are an independent risk factor for death.

Prevention of Catheter-associated Infections

Prevention of catheter-associated urinary tract infections remains the major unsolved problem in hospital infection control. The first step is to avoid unnecessary catheterization and to remove the catheter when it is no longer needed (Table 9.1).

The Ascending Route of Infection and Closed Drainage

Patients on open drainage develop bacteriuria and infection within 2 to 3 days. The source of infection is contaminated tubing and drainage bottles. The microorganisms readily ascend the urinary stream and enter the bladder where they continue to grow. Aseptic closed drainage prevents contamination of the system. The efficacy of closed drainage was first demonstrated by Dukes in 1928 (74), but did not become a standard practice in the United States until the introduction of plastic, disposable closed drainage systems about 30 years ago. The first disposable system extensively evaluated is shown in Figure 9.5. Note that most catheters were removed within a week (Fig. 9.1). The system was tested on all services of a general hospital. The time required to produce bacteriuria in 50% of males was 13.5 days and 11.0 days for 50% of females (4).

Table 9.1. Methods to Avoid the Use of the Indwelling Catheter

Population	Methods
Postsurgical patients	Do not overhydrate
	Avoid anticholinergic drugs
	Provide urine containers at bedside
	Allow privacy and time to void
	Apply warm suprapubic pressure
	Consider drugs that stimulate the detrusor muscle and relax the sphincter
	Consider single catheterization if the patient does not void in 4–6 hours
Intensive care	Remove the indwelling catheter when stable
	Use intermittent catheterization as needed
	Condom catheters in males
Oliguric renal failure	Avoid catheterization; consider bed-side ultrasound
Elderly, incontinent patients	Prompted voiding
	Absorbent perineal pads
	Condom catheters with penile prostheses, if needed
Neurogenic bladder	Intermittent catheterization
	Sphincterotomy and condom catheters if needed
	Suprapubic catheters to avoid epididymitis

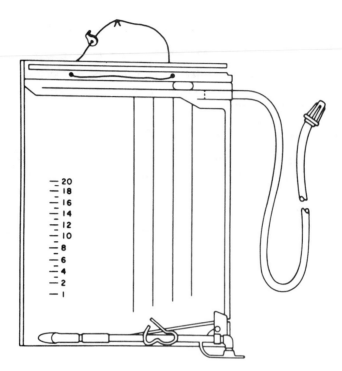

Figure 9.5. The original disposable, closed drainage bag used to demonstrate the efficacy of closed drainage. Reproduced from Kunin CM and McCormack RC. (4). The bag was manufactured by Bard-Parker Division, Becton-Dickinson, Inc., Rutherford, New Jersey, but is no longer commercially available.

Entry of Bacteria into the Drainage System

Both careful attention to aseptic technique and avoiding contamination of the system is essential when inserting the catheter. Bacteria may gain entrance to the bladder by the following mechanisms.

Mechanisms by Which Bacteria Gain Entry into the Bladder During Catheterization

- Poor aseptic technique at the time the catheter is inserted
- Disconnection of the catheter and drainage tube
- Contamination during irrigation
- Colonization of the drainage bag with retrograde flow to the bladder
- Colonization of the distal urethra and ascent around the catheter

The four major sites of introduction of bacteria into the system are illustrated in Figure 9.6.

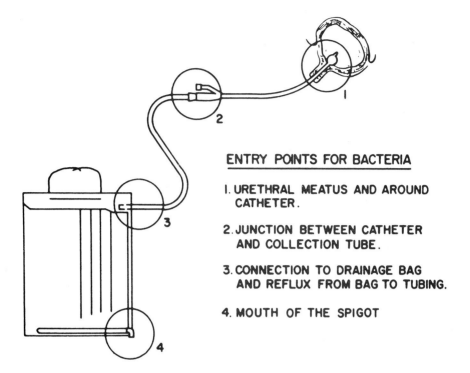

ENTRY POINTS FOR BACTERIA

1. URETHRAL MEATUS AND AROUND CATHETER.

2. JUNCTION BETWEEN CATHETER AND COLLECTION TUBE.

3. CONNECTION TO DRAINAGE BAG AND REFLUX FROM BAG TO TUBING.

4. MOUTH OF THE SPIGOT

Figure 9.6. Entry points for bacteria into the closed drainage system.

Care of the System

The following procedures are necessary to prevent contamination of the closed system and avoid injury to the urethra.

Key Points to Maintain Aseptic Closed Drainage*

- The junction of the catheter with the drainage tube must not be broken once it is attached to the catheter.
- The only indication to disconnect the system is obstruction.
- The column of urine in the drainage tube is usually interspersed with segments of air. A full column of urine in the drainage tube indicates the presence of an air-lock. The air-lock can be broken by brief insertion of a needle into the catheter drainage port allowing urine to flow freely.
- Urine for culture should be obtained by needle aspiration of the catheter or tubing port after cleaning with an alcohol sponge (Fig. 9.7).
- *Do not culture the tip of the catheter*. It may be misleading because of contamination with urethral microorganisms when removed.
- The drainage bag should remain attached to the catheter while the patient stands or walks. The bag should be drained to reduce its weight.

- If the patient is being "bladder trained," the tubing may be clamped for a short period of time, but should not be disconnected from the catheter.
- Bags should be drained of urine at 8-hour intervals, with care being taken to avoid contamination of the mouth of the spigot. More frequent drainage is necessary in patients undergoing diuresis.
- Bags may be hung on the sides of beds, chairs, and stretchers, but must never be inverted or raised above the level of the patient's bladder.
- The drainage tube should be fixed to the thigh of females with a Velcro strap device or to the abdomen in males to avoid pressure on the bladder neck by the balloon.
- Perineal care should consist of washing with soap and water one or two times a day. This keeps the periurethral region clean and dry but does not delay infection.
- Catheters should not be irrigated except to clear blood clots. They should be removed or changed if obstruction is suspected. Sterile technique must be maintained during irrigation. *The same syringe should never be used for more than one patient or for the same patient without sterilization between uses.*
- The only reasons to change the bag and catheter are poor flow, leaks, odor, or obstruction.

---

*These recommendations are similar to the Guidelines for Catheter Care developed by The Centers of Disease Control (75).

Features of Good Drainage Systems

Drainage systems vary in configuration, the size of the drainage hoses, and the presence of drip chambers, flutter valves, and vents. Very few have undergone careful clinical evaluation. Flutter valves may obstruct flow and are rarely used. Drip chambers are of doubtful value if the bag is positioned properly. Urine meters nearly double the purchase price and are not needed except for a brief period in intensive care units. Each new system must be evaluated for ease in flow, nursing acceptance, and efficacy in maintaining sterility in the hospital setting. Additional devices are not needed. For example, no difference in the time of onset and incidence of nosocomial urinary infection was found in patients managed with a simple closed drainage bag with an antireflux valve to a more complex system which included a preconnected, coated catheter, a tamper seal at the catheter-drainage junction, a drip chamber, an antireflux valve, a hydrophobic drainage vent, and a povidone-iodine releasing cartridge in line with the outlet tube of the urine collection bag (76).

The features of a good system include the following characteristics:

- Relatively inexpensive
- Minimum number of parts that can be obstructed (flutter valves, drip chambers)
- Can be hung at the foot of the bed and is adaptable for ambulation
- Good flow properties
- Stable construction
- The bag can be drained without splashing or contamination

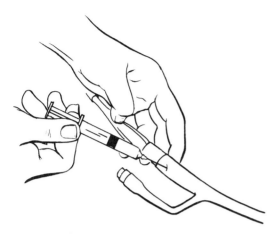

Figure 9.7. Method to obtain urine from the catheter by syringe. Modern drainage tubes have a port for this purpose.

- Urine output can be measured in critically ill patients
- Acceptable to the ward staff compared to other systems

Attempts to Improve Upon Closed Drainage

The Urethral Route Of Infection

Closed drainage systems prevent ascending infection for up to several weeks, but the microorganisms adhere to urothelial cells, proliferate around the urethral meatus, and eventually gain entrance to the bladder by colonizing the sheath of exudate that surrounds the intraurethral portion of the catheter (77–81). Once this occurs, closed drainage is no longer effective except to reduce cross contamination. There is currently no effective means of preventing periurethral colonization. Aseptic closed drainage is ideal for acute general hospitals, but of limited value in long-term facilities other than to prevent cross infection.

A variety of methods have been used to attempt to improve the care of the indwelling catheter. These methods are summarized in Table 9.2 according to the site of attack and efficacy.

Prophylactic Use of Antibiotics

Concomitant use of antibiotics delays infection, but only for the first 4 days (4,7). Prolonged use leads to the emergence of resistant microorganisms and superinfection (9,82).

Meatal Care

Antimicrobial lubricants used at the time of insertion are of marginal or no benefit. Application of povidone iodine or antibiotic ointments or silver

Table 9.2. Attempts To Improve Care of the Indwelling Catheter

Site	Method
Urethra	Aseptic method of insertion[a]
	Antimicrobial lubricants[d]
	Washing the perineum[d]
	Antimicrobial ointments[d]
	Chlorhexidine-soaked sponges[b]
Bladder	Continuous irrigation with antimicrobial solutions[b*]
	Closed drainage[a]
Catheter	New materials (latex versus silicone)[**]
	Impregnation with antimicrobial agents[d]
	The "silver" catheter[d]
	Vented catheters[d]
	The comformable catheter[***]
Drainage tube-junction	Pre-attached collecting systems[b or c]
Drainage bag	Construction (hanging characteristics[a], vents[a], drip chambers[d], valves[d], spigots[d])
Antimicrobial additives to bag	Povidone iodine[d], hydrogen peroxide[d], chlorhexidine[d]
Systemic	Antimicrobial prophylaxis or therapy[d]
Epidemiologic	Geographic separation[a]
General	Handwashing between patients[a]
	Sterilize urine drained from bags[c]
	Disposable irrigation syringes and fluids[a]
	Proper positioning of the drainage system[a]
	Avoid breaking the closed system[a]

Key: a, Effective; b, probably effective; c, possibly effective; d, not effective. *No more effective than closed drainage alone; **silicone catheters tend to be less encrusted during prolonged use; ***, appears to be more comfortable, but there is no evidence that the rate of infection is altered.

sulfadiazine cream to the urethral meatus is ineffective (78,83,84). Even washing the periurethral region has not been shown to add much benefit, although it seems reasonable to clean the area and decrease irritation. Chlorhexidine-saturated sponges abutted to the urethra have been shown to reduce colonization in females (85) (Fig. 9.8).

Prophylactic Irrigation with Antimicrobial Solutions

Continuous irrigation of the bladder with an antimicrobial solution can prevent, but not eradicate, infection. The irrigating solution is contained in a bottle hung by the bedside and instilled through a Y tube or three-way catheter (Fig. 9.9). The solutions contain 0.25% acetic acid, or a mixture of neomycin and polymyxin B (86) or chlorhexidine (87). Acetic acid is no longer used because it can irritate the bladder. Neomycin and polymyxin B solutions are as-

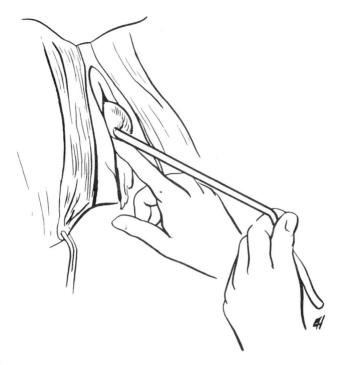

Figure 9.8. Foley catheter fitted with plastic sponges to bathe the urethral meatus with antiseptic solutions. Reproduced with permission from Viant et al. (85).

sociated with emergence of antibiotic-resistant enterococci, yeasts, or gram-negative bacteria and are no more effective than closed drainage (88).

Preconnected Catheters

The junction between the catheter and drainage tube should not be broken. Plastic tape may be applied to the junction to remind the staff not to disconnect the catheter. Preconnected "tamper proof" catheters and drainage bags are marketed vigorously. This promotion is based on a report that preconnected catheters decreased catheter-associated mortality (49). In a recent study, a taped seal applied to the catheter-drainage tubing junction did not significantly lower rates of bacteriuria or mortality in patients undergoing short-term catheterization (89). Preconnected systems are not recommended because they are more expensive and no more effective than separate catheters and drainage bags.

Adding Antimicrobial Compounds to the Drainage Bag

Catheter drainage bags can become contaminated when the bags are emptied or with breaks in technique. It would seem reasonable to try to prevent bacteriuria and cross infection by adding a nontoxic antimicrobial compound to

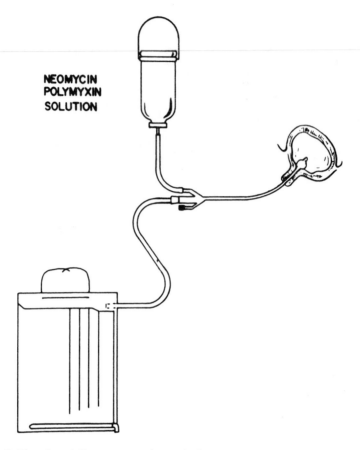

NEOMYCIN
POLYMYXIN
SOLUTION

Figure 9.9. The closed three-way catheter drainage system with neomycin-polymyxin irrigation.

the drainage bag. Initial reports suggested that the addition of povidone io-dine, hydrogen peroxide, or chlorhexidine to the drainage bags might be use-ful (90–92). However, several well-controlled trials have demonstrated conclusively that drainage bag additives do not prevent catheter-associated bladder bacteriuria (93–95). These results are not surprising because catheters and drainage bags become contaminated at about the same time and the peri-urethral route is the major cause of late infections (4,96).

Closed Irrigation

Closed irrigation is designed to permit constant or intermittent flow of wash-ing fluid without the hazard of breaking aseptic technique. This method was devised by Dukes almost 60 years ago. It is commonly used after urologic procedures when there may be considerable bleeding and potential obstruction of the system by blood clots.

Tidal Drainage

Tidal drainage maintains a continuous closed cycle of filling and emptying the bladder. The goal is to "train" or exercise a spastic bladder to prevent irreversible contracted bladders in neurosurgical and paraplegic patients (97). The patient is managed either with a three-way catheter or a Foley catheter attached to a glass Y-tube. One limb of the Y is attached to drainage and the other to a reservoir of fluid suspended from a standard. The rinsing fluid is allowed to flow continuously. The effluent is attached to an inverted U tube. The bladder is emptied by a siphon effect when the intravesical pressure reaches the level of the column of fluid in the tube. The tube can be elevated or lowered to change the pressure required to trip the siphon. A semi-automatic, siphon-pressure, closed drainage system was commercially available some years ago (Cystamat, Leo Pharmaceuticals, Copenhagen, Denmark). This is a beautifully designed system (98). Unfortunately, it was developed about the time intermittent catheterization became popular and may not be available any longer.

Urinary Catheters

Urinary catheters are available in many shapes and forms, depending on the site to be drained and the mode by which they are introduced. They are made of soft rubber, glass, plastic, or silicone and may be coated or impregnated with various materials and chemicals. Size is measured by the external diameter using the French (F) scale. The French size may be converted to millimeters by dividing by three. Thus, a size 18 French catheter is 6 mm in diameter. The larger the F, the greater the outside dimensions. The internal diameter of the lumen may be smaller than indicated by the F size. Latex rubber catheters generally have a thicker wall and smaller internal diameter than silicone catheters, and three-way catheters have even smaller lumens.

A large variety of urinary catheters are available (Fig. 9.10). They usually are identified by the name of the person who designed the instrument. The Foley catheter is kept in the bladder by a retention balloon near the tip. Sizes 16–18 F, fitted with a 5 ml balloon, are commonly used in adults. Larger sizes, combined with a 30 ml balloon, are often used in elderly incontinent females. Smaller sizes are available for children. Special purpose catheters include those with firm, bent tips (Coude), four-winged tips (Malecot), and mushroom tips (de Pezzer).

Catheters are also defined by their site of insertion and duration in place. Examples include the single urethral, indwelling Foley, nephrostomy (inserted into the renal pelvis), suprapubic (inserted into the bladder), and perineal catheters. Attempts to improve the urinary catheter and eliminate it

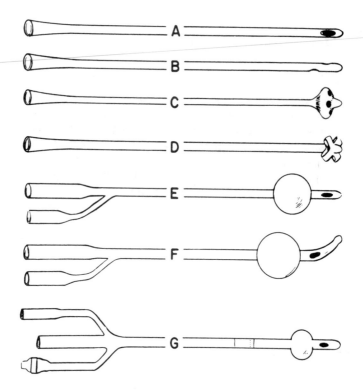

Figure 9.10. Types of commonly used catheters. **A** and **B**, simple urethral catheters. **C**, mushroom or de Pezzer; **D**, winged-tip or Malecot; **E**, Foley with inflated retention bag; **F**, Foley with Coude tip; **G**, 3-way catheter (in this illustration the third lumen opens into the urethra to add lubricants; it ordinarily opens at tip to irrigate the bladder).

entirely by use of the intraurethral spiral and external devices will be discussed later.

The criteria for materials and construction of catheters include the following:

- Urine should flow readily through the lumen
- The material should not irritate the urethra or bladder mucosa
- Microorganism should not adhere to the surface, if possible
- Encrustations should not form on the surface
- Minimal residual urine should be left in the bladder
- Cost should be relatively low

Flow Characteristics

According to Poiseuille's law, the volume of flow in a tube is directly proportional to the pressure drop along the length and to the fourth power of the radius of the tube, and is inversely proportional to the length of the tube and to the viscosity of the fluid. The rate of flow through the standard Foley catheters is proportional to the internal diameter. The larger the bore, the greater the rate of flow (Fig. 9.11). This is one reason why three-way catheters with a small internal diameter should not be used to irrigate blood clots after prostatectomy. Larger sizes may be preferred for patients who may pass blood clots. Large-bore catheters may delay obstruction in patients on long-term drainage. Larger-diameter catheters are more likely to produce pressure on the urethral mucosa, leading to diminished mucosal blood flow and the potential for tissue necrosis. In general, the smallest-sized catheter that will allow free flow of urine is the most desirable. In adults, a commonly used size is 16 French with a 5 ml balloon, but the optimal size needs to be determined in each patient.

Risks

The risk of a foreign material in the urethra and bladder neck include:

- Irritation and urethral ischemia
- Strictures
- Adherence of microorganisms to the surface
- Formation of encrustations and blockage

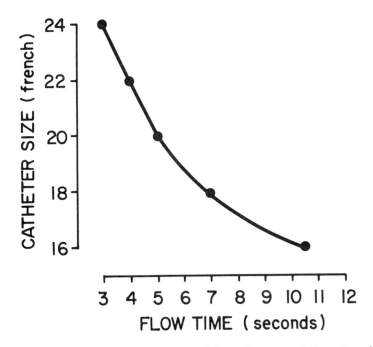

Figure 9.11. The relation between the rate of flow of water and the external diameter (in French units) of standard, latex Foley catheters. Reproduced from Kunin CM, Chin QF, and Chambers S (99).

Irritation and Strictures

Catheters may irritate the urethral mucosa and produce strictures of the urethra, particularly in males. Several outbreaks of urethral strictures have been reported to occur in postoperative patients caused by the lubricating jelly, powder on gloves, and extractable cytotoxic material from the catheter (100). Silicone catheters are least irritating and produce only mild edema of the mucosa in rats (101). This finding has not been substantiated in humans. Anderson (102) examined the appearance of leukocytes and erythrocytes in the urine of patients with latex, silicone-coated latex, and 100% silicone materials. No significant differences in acute cellular reaction were observed among these groups. There also was no advantage of Hydron™-coated latex catheters with latex and polyvinyl chloride catheters. The most important cause appears to be pressure necrosis from "bow-stringing" of an anchored catheter (103) (Fig. 9.12). This is

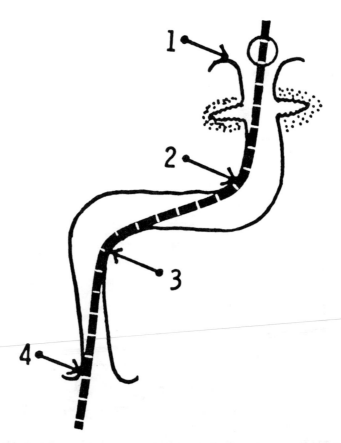

Figure 9.12. The sites in the male urethra most likely to be affected by pressure necrosis and the "bow-stringing" effect of the indwelling catheter. Reproduced with permission from Edwards, Lock, Powell, and Jones (103).

the reason that catheters should be fixed to the abdomen or thigh to prevent excess pressure on the urethra.

Adherence of Microorganisms to Catheters

Adherence of microorganisms as biofilms on the surface of urinary catheters prevents them from being washed away by the urinary stream and irrigation fluids and protects them from antimicrobial drugs. The microbes develop their own microbial ecosystem on the catheter surface (104,105). Tenney and Warren (105) found that concentrations of urease-producing bacteria, Pseudomonas, and group D streptococci fell when the catheter was replaced, whereas the concentrations of *E. coli* and Klebsiella remained unchanged. This finding suggests that different species of bacteria adhere better to the catheter, whereas others adhere more avidly to urothelial cells. We (99) also noted a fall in bacterial counts when the catheter was changed, but found no difference in the distribution of the various microorganisms in the new catheter. *Pseudomonas aeruginosa* becomes imbedded in a biofilm made up of the organisms surrounded with exopolysaccharide on the surface of silicone-latex catheters (106,107). Tritium-labeled gram-negative bacteria adhere less to siliconized rubber than to pure latex or Teflon coated catheters (108).

We developed an *in vivo* method to study adherence of bacteria to urinary catheters (81). Catheters are removed from the patients, cut into segments, and rolled over the surface of plates containing differential agar media. Catheter surfaces were colonized less often in males than females, 16.8 versus 67%, respectively, and yielded correspondingly fewer numbers of bacterial species per catheter. Gram-positive bacteria (mainly *Enterococcus faecalis and Staphylococcus epidermidis*) were isolated more frequently than gram-negative organisms and tended to be more abundant as well. Gram-negative bacteria tended to colonize the catheters the longer the catheters were left in place.

Formation of Encrustations

Encrustations that form within the catheter lumen and on the surface of the balloon are the major cause of obstruction in patients on long-term urinary catheter drainage. Obstruction of the eyelet of the catheter may be sufficient to block flow. Encrustations lead to persistence of infection, obstruction, and irritation of the bladder mucosa. Blocked catheters should be suspected in long-term catheterized patients who become oliguric and who develop leakage, fever, and sepsis. The most important measure is to remove the catheter.

There is no effective method to block the formation of encrustations. Routine irrigation of catheters with saline solutions is ineffective (109). The solution to the problem requires an understanding of exactly how crystals form and aggregate to cause encrustations. The current concept of formation of encrustations on catheters is that struvite (ammonium-magnesium-phosphate) crystals form at alkaline pH and are deposited on the catheters.

Urease-producing bacteria (Proteus, Providencia, and Morganella) are responsible for the alkaline urine because they hydrolyze urea to ammonia. Once the crystals are formed, they aggregate around a matrix glycoprotein and adhere to the surface of the catheter.

Struvite (infection) stones can be prevented from forming by acidifying the urine or by blocking urease production with acetohydroxamic acid. Irrigation of catheters with acid solutions is sometimes used to dissolve encrustations, but the efficacy and hazards of this procedure have not been studied adequately. It is difficult to acidify the urine by oral administration of ascorbic acid or methionine.

We have developed a model to study adherence of struvite crystals to urinary catheters (Fig. 9.13). This system allows urine to be perfused through a catheter for prolonged periods. Variables include pH, flow rate, urine from infected patients or volunteers, catheter materials, and microorganisms. Using this model, we have been able to produce large encrustations on urinary catheters by about 10 to 14 days. It is necessary to use fresh urine each day.

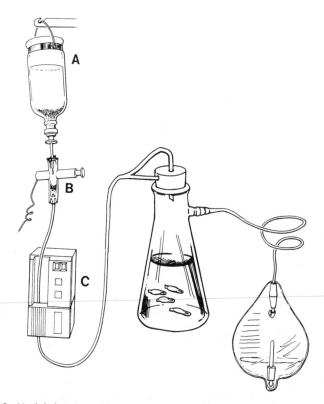

Figure 9.13. Model developed by the author to produce encrustations on catheters in vitro.

In preliminary studies, we observed encrustations to be heavier on latex and Teflon-coated catheters than on silicone or silicone-coated catheters.

Catheter-life
Catheter-life is defined as the duration of time a catheter can be left in place before it becomes blocked, leaks, or is pulled out by the patient (110). The major determinant of catheter-life is formation of encrustations. Encrustations tend to form at the tip of the catheter and portion of the balloon bathed in urine, but not on the side of the balloon pulled against the bladder mucosa. They are distributed within the lumen of the catheter, but not where the surface is in contact with the urethra (Fig. 9.14). Blockers are defined as patients whose catheter becomes encrusted within a week or two after insertion of a fresh catheter (99). Non-blockers do not form encrustations even after several months. Blockers are infected with urease-producing bacteria. We found that about one-third of nursing home patients never formed encrustations, about one-third persistently formed encrustations within 2 weeks or less of a catheter change, and about one-third formed encrustations slowly over time (99).

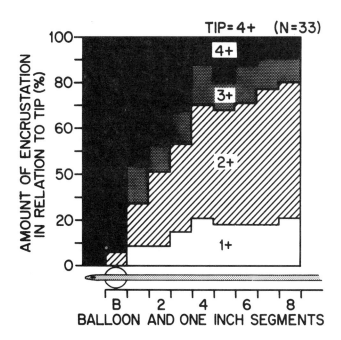

Figure 9.14. Location of encrustations on long-term indwelling catheters in patients infected with urease-producing bacteria and alkaline urine. Reproduced from Kunin CM, Chin QF, and Chambers S (99).

Catheter Materials and Design

Latex Versus Silicone, Teflon, and Teflon-Coated Catheters

Latex catheters are the least expensive and usually sufficient. Silicone catheters do not appear to have a sufficient advantage to be used routinely in acute-care hospitals where catheters are left in place for only a few days. In long-term-care institutions, they may be useful in patients who rapidly form encrustations. In a controlled trial, we found that in "blockers," silicone catheters became clogged less often than latex, Teflon-coated, or silicone-coated catheters (111).

Silver-Coated Catheters

In preliminary studies, catheters coated with silver oxide appeared to delay the onset of bacteriuria (112–114), and short-term use was shown to reduce the occurrence of urinary infections in females not receiving antibiotics (115). In the most recent and largest study, silver-impregnated catheters not only failed to prevent catheter-associated bacteriuria, but also significantly increased the incidence of bacteriuria in male patients and significantly increased the occurrence of staphylococcal bacteriuria (116).

Other Coatings

There is no evidence that "hydrophilic" coated catheters prevent infection. Other approaches to prevent infection and delay formation of biofilms and encrustations on the catheter surface include impregnating catheters with antimicrobial drugs (15), salicylic acid (117), or heparin (118), and irrigating with acidic solutions. Quinolones and protamine sulfate appear to act synergistically against planktonic and biofilm *Pseudomonas aeruginosa* in model systems (119), but recolonization and emergence of resistant strains can be anticipated. Electric currents can kill microbes within the catheter urine, but clinically suitable apparatus has not as yet been developed (120). *Although some of these measures to prevent adherence of microorganisms to catheters may eventually be effective, it is much simpler and probably more cost-effective to simply change the catheter or remove it entirely.*

The Conformable Catheter

The comfortable catheter is a novel and potentially valuable approach to catheter care. The urethral segment of the "conformable" catheter consists of a flexible, thin rubber rather than more rigid latex or silicone (121). It is reported to be more comfortable, to stay in place several more days, and to be obstructed less often by struvite. It does not appear to prevent acquisition of infection, but this point needs to be studied further.

Lubricating Catheters

The concept is that the urethra becomes dry, irritated, and inflamed with continuous catheterization. There might be less irritation if the catheter could be continuously lubricated. A prototype "lubricating catheter" was developed by Kunin and Finkelberg (122). The lubricant is delivered through an additional channel within the catheter and extruded intermittently into the urethra. In a controlled trial, methyl cellulose gel or polymyxin B lubricant was inserted once daily and the rate of acquisition of bacteriuria was compared with catheters that were not lubricated. Significant protection was demonstrated in females who received lubricant with or without polymyxin B. No differences were found in males. A mechanical delivery system needs to be devised to provide constant flow of lubricant. An improved system should have considerable promise.

Vented Catheters
Closed drainage bags ordinarily are vented to allow displacement of air as urine flows into the bag. In a properly flowing system, the drainage tube will contain urine only in the horizontal segments or portion of loops. When a solid column of urine is noted, the vent is not functioning properly. This can be demonstrated at the bedside by puncturing the end of the catheter with a needle. Air will flow through the needle into the collecting tube and it will empty promptly. In my experience, it is rare to find a standing column of urine in a catheter. When this does occur, however, it may produce a negative pressure within the system, causing the bladder mucosa to be sucked into the catheter eyelets. We have not found vented catheters to improve emptying of the bladder (123,124).

Intraurethral Devices

Patients with prostatic hypertrophy need to be decompressed at the level of the prostatic urethra. The remaining portions of the indwelling catheter serve no useful function other than as a channel for urine. The prostatic channel can be opened by use of an intraprostatic spiral (125) or a self-retaining intraurethral catheter (126). Satisfactory voiding can be achieved for 6 to 12 months without the development of urethral strictures or the need for a drainage bag. The devices appear to be most useful for high-risk patients. More studies need to be done to determine the rate of infection and other complications.

The Retention Balloon

The balloon is a necessary "evil" required to retain the catheter in the bladder. It serves as a nidus of infection, allows puddling of residual urine, and exerts tension on the bladder neck. Erosion and ulceration of the neck of the bladder are found at autopsy in patients on long-term drainage.

Five-ml balloons are ordinarily sufficient to keep the catheter in place and retain less residual urine than the 30-ml size. Larger balloons may produce more bladder irritation (127). Insufficient filling of the larger balloon may cause mucosal ulceration due to pressure of the catheter tip against the bladder wall. This ulceration can perforate the wall of the urinary bladder. A 30-ml balloon may be of special value in certain circumstances. I encountered an elderly male patient in whom the balloon prolapsed into the urethra and caused acute retention and bacteremia. The situation was corrected by substituting a 5-ml with a 30-ml balloon.

The balloon may also inadvertently be inflated in the urethra (128). Automatic deflating catheters allow the balloon to collapse into a second balloon positioned on the other end of the catheter. These devices may be of particular value for the confused patient who attempts to pull out his catheter.

Minimizing Residual Urine in the Bladder

The urine drainage hole is placed near the tip of the standard Foley catheter. This allows residual urine to accumulate below the balloon. Residual urine can be reduced by placing a hole 2 to 3 cm below the base of the retaining balloon (129). Positioning of the hole below the balloon does not eliminate the film of urine adherent to the surface of the balloon or bacteria that might become enmeshed on the surface.

Removal of the Catheter When the Balloon Fails to Deflate

Catheters are removed from the patient by aspirating fluid or air from the balloon by syringe at the filling port or by cutting off the end of the catheter. On rare occasions, the balloon may fail to deflate. The major reason is obstruction at some point along the channel leading to the balloon. This obstruction may be bypassed when the catheter is cut at a point close to the urethral meatus. If this step is unsuccessful, the channel may be cleared with a catheter guide wire. Other procedures include injecting light weight mineral oil into the inflating lumen of the catheter to dissolve the balloon (130), using a snail-headed retriever (131), or inserting a fine lumbar puncture needle into the balloon through the urethra using ultrasound guidance (132). Ether is not recommended to rupture the balloon because it is inflammable and may cause cystitis.

Questions About the Urinary Catheter

Definition of "Significant" Bacteriuria in the Catheterized Patient

Most patients with indwelling urinary catheters will either have $> 10^5$ cfu/ml or sterile urine. Bacterial counts $< 10^5$ cfu/ml may be encountered just as the bladder begins to be colonized (133). The counts will be $> 10^5$ cfu/ml within a day or so thereafter. The end-point is not the absolute bacterial count, but the finding that a previously sterile urine contains bacteria. For epidemiologic studies, it is useful to select a reasonable criterion for colonization. Because the growth rate of bacteria is rapid, it makes little difference whether the endpoint used is 1,000, 10,000, or 100,000 or more, provided that the methodology and criteria are clearly defined.

How Often Should the Catheter and Drainage Bag be Changed?

There is no need to change a catheter in patients in acute general hospitals when the urine is flowing freely, the catheter is not encrusted, and the drainage bag is functioning well. Frequent catheter changes may introduce bacteria and may cause bacteremia. Catheters should not be irrigated routinely. This breaks the closed system and is of no value. Some nursing home patients rapidly form encrustations and develop blocked catheters. Each patient needs to be evaluated for the optimal time to change his or her catheter. A reasonable approach is to remove the catheter after 1 to 2 weeks and observe it for encrustations. If none are present, the catheter may be left in place for several more weeks and observed again. Once marked encrustations are noted, the catheter should be changed about a week before heavy encrustations are expected.

Polymicrobial Bacteriuria and Susceptibility Tests

Patients with long-term indwelling urethral or suprapubic catheters are often colonized with three or more bacterial species. No useful purpose is served by routine culture and susceptibility tests because antimicrobial therapy is ineffective unless the catheter is removed. Urine for culture should never be obtained from the drainage bag, but from the tubing or catheter. Culture and susceptibility tests should be reserved for patients with sepsis. The laboratory must be notified that the urine was obtained from a catheterized patient, otherwise the technicians may consider the microorganisms to be contaminants.

Purple Drainage Bags

Purple-red discoloration of the drainage tubing and bag is sometimes observed in patients on long-term catheter drainage. The pigment contains a mixture of indirubin dissolved in the plastic and indigo on its surface (134). Some stains of *Providencia stuartii*, *Klebsiella pneumoniae*, and *Enterobacter agglomerans* produce indigo on agar containing indoxyl sulfate (135). It is thought that tryptophane is metabolized to indoxyl sulfate in the gut and then the product is absorbed and excreted in the urine. It is then converted to insoluble indigo by bacterial enzymes and contact with air in the collecting bag and tubing.

Audit of Quality of Catheter Care

Hospitals need to develop guidelines for catheter care and provide assurance that they are being followed. Periodic surveys should be conducted to evaluate the indications for insertion of catheters, how well they are managed, and whether they are removed when no longer needed. The survey should be designed to identify issues that need to be resolved at a hospital policy level and detect specific problems that can be corrected by education of the staff. A sample process audit is presented for this purpose.

Spot Audit of Catheter Care

Purpose:
1. To identify the reasons why catheters are ordered by physicians.
2. To evaluate how well urinary drainage devices are being managed by the nursing staff.
3. To consider alternate methods of care.

Method:
Representative nursing units are identified in general medicine, pediatrics, surgical specialties (orthopedic, urology, cardiovascular, neurosurgery, obstetrics/gynecology), intensive care units, and the recovery room. The survey is conducted by a Catheter Care Evaluation Team appointed by the Hospital Infection Control Committee. One of the members should be a physician interested in the problem of catheter care. Members of the survey team should not have worked on the units to be surveyed. The survey is conducted without prior notice to the staff.

1. Identification of the population at risk (denominator).

A list should be prepared of all patients on the unit and each patient should be seen. The following information should be obtained for all patients:

- Name and hospital number
- Age and sex
- Major diagnoses
- Current antimicrobial therapy
- Use of a urine drainage device

The device should be identified by inspection at the bedside as:

Indwelling urethral
Suprapubic
Nephrostomy
Intermittent
Condom
Other

The prevalence of urinary drainage devices according to type of device is then calculated for each unit and for all units according to age, sex, and underlying disease.

2. Characterization of patients using urinary drainage devices (numerator).

The following information is collected for each individual on urinary drainage according to the type of drainage being used.

- Indications for use of the device
- Duration the device has been in place
- Time when the device will be removed or changed to another type of drainage
- Necessity of the device
- Availability of safer methods of drainage

3. Care of the System

For patients with indwelling or condom catheters.

- Is the device attached to closed drainage?
- Is the bag hung properly?
- Is drainage tube positioned properly and fixed to the thigh or abdomen?
- Has the catheter been irrigated during the previous 24 hours?
  If so, what solution was used and how was it administered?
- Who ordered the irrigation?
- Was the periurethral area washed during the past 24 hours?
- How many times was the bag emptied in the past 24 hours?
- What type of collection device was used for emptying the drainage device?
  Who empties the bag?
  How is the urine disposed?
  Are urine containers cleaned or sanitized between uses?
  Is residual urine left in the container?
  Are they used for more than one patient?
  Are hands washed before or after emptying the drainage bag?
  Are gloves used?
- When was the latest urine culture obtained?
  Are cultures done routinely or on specific orders from the physician?
- How are specimens obtained from the system?
  Aspiration from catheter or drainage port?
  By breaking the junction of the catheter and drainage bag tubing?
  Was the catheter clamped to help collect urine?
  Is urine from the drainage bag used to measure glucose or for other tests?
- Is there urine on the bed or floor?
- What type of catheter is being used (Latex, Teflon-coated, silicone, silicone-coated, other)?
- Has the catheter or drainage bag been changed since the patient arrived on the unit?
  If so, when?
- Is the date the catheter was inserted recorded on the chart?
- Describe the appearance of the bag for blood, sediment, odor.
- Is urine present in the drainage tube?

If so, is this limited to looped areas only?
- How well is urine flowing into bag?
- Is the patient receiving systemic antimicrobial drugs for treatment of a urinary tract infection?
  If so, what drugs are being used?

For patients on intermittent catheterization.

- Describe the technique being used for each patient
  Frequency
  Lubricant
  Size and type of catheter
  Preparation of the meatus
  Who performs the catheterization?
- Are antimicrobial irrigations used after the urine is drained from the bladder?
  If so, what solutions are being used?
- Are systemic antimicrobial agents being used to treat a urinary tract infection?
  If so, what drugs are being used?

For patients managed with condom catheters.

- Describe the system being used
  Describe type (brand) used.
  How is it held in place?
  How often is it changed?
  What care is given to the penis?
  Twisting?
  Excoriation of penis?
  Has the patient pulled it off in the past 24 hours?
- Are systemic antimicrobial agents being used to treat a urinary tract infection?
  If so, what drugs?

Analysis of Data

The data should be tabulated for each unit according to specialty service and summarized for the entire institution. The results should be reviewed by the Infection Control Committee. Recommendations for change should be made to the hospital staff and administration.

How to Determine the Efficacy of Drainage Systems

Efficacy studies of catheter drainage systems must be conducted as stratified, prospective, controlled clinical trials. The end-point is acquisition of bacteriuria. It is not appropriate to evaluate systems based on the number of patients who are symptomatic or have infected urine over a specific period of time. This number is misleading because some patients may have acquired their infection outside the hospital, patients with serious illness tend to remain in the hospital longer, and postoperative patients may only have the catheter in place for a few days.

Sample Protocol

All patients on catheter drainage should be monitored daily by culture obtained as soon as possible after the catheter is inserted. Needle aspiration of the catheter or tubing port should be performed each day, preferably by a technician from the clinical bacteriology laboratory or the nurse epidemiologist. Urine specimens should be cultured within a few hours after collection or promptly refrigerated until cultured. All patients with an initial positive culture are excluded from the study. All patients with an initially negative culture should be observed daily until the bacterial count exceeds 10^4 to 10^5 cfu/ml. They are considered positive on the day these counts are reached. All patients should be identified by age, sex, service, underlying disease, and receipt of antimicrobial therapy. Each group should be analyzed separately and collectively. The calendar day the catheter is inserted is designated as day 0. Day 1 begins at the time of routine monitoring on the following day, regardless of the number of hours that elapsed between time of insertion of the catheter and collection. Sometimes the patient will not be on the ward when monitoring is to be done. If the patient enters the study on day 2 or later and is found to be positive, he or she is excluded from the study. If negative, he or she is considered to have been negative from day 0.

The cumulative risk of *acquiring* infection on each day after insertion of the catheter is calculated as follows:

$$\text{Cum. \% positive by given day } (\times) = \frac{\text{Cum. no. positive on day X}}{\text{Cum. no. positive on day X} + \text{no. negative on day X}} \times 100$$

The major problem in analysis is loss of negatives in the denominator. Catheters may be removed or the patient may have been discharged before they developed a positive culture. One way to get around this problem is to choose an arbitrary cut-off day and retain for analysis only those patients who have been followed for the entire period. Unfortunately, many patients will be lost to the study. A better approach is to use the life table method to deal with patients lost to the study.

Promotion of Untested Equipment by Manufacturers

Medical devices, as seemingly simple as catheters and drainage bags, are not regulated by the FDA with the same zeal as drugs. Devices are often marketed without adequate clinical trials. For example, equipment to instill hydrogen peroxide into drainage bags was marketed solely on the basis of one small trial. Some manufacturers apply iodine to the external portion of catheters based on conjecture that this will prevent infections. Sterile gloves are sufficient. Silicone catheters are heavily promoted to hospitals even though their major advantage is to delay formation of encrustations in nursing home patients. Preconnected catheters and extra devices added to a sturdy drainage bag offer little advantage and are more expensive. Decisions to purchase new urinary drainage equipment should be based on the advice of well-informed hospital infection control practitioners and nurses who have practical experience in this field.

Historical Perspective

The evolution of our understanding of catheter-associated infections and their prevention are traced in Table 9.3. Sir Andrew Clark described "catheter fever" in men with prostatic obstruction treated with catheters in 1883 (136). Sir Cuthbert Dukes reported the occurrence of fever and pyuria associated with the use of indwelling catheters and introduced closed drainage in 1928 (74). In 1930, Barrington and Wright demonstrated that catheterized patients developed bacteremia (137). Miller, Gillespie, Linton, Slade, and Mitchell reintroduced the closed drainage method in 1958 (138).

Paul Beeson published his landmark editorial entitled *The Case Against the Catheter* in 1958 (139). Beeson's concluding remarks are as apt today as then. "At times the catheter is indispensable for therapy, and there are many good indications for its use. Nevertheless the decision to use this instrument should be made with the knowledge that it involves risk of producing a serious disease which is often difficult to treat. The procedure does not seem warranted merely to obtain a clean specimen for urinalysis. It is not required even for bacteriologic study, since with proper precautions clean-voided specimens can be used for this purpose. The indication should be especially clear when the decision is made to employ an indwelling catheter. Convenience of the attending doctors and nurses is surely not acceptable. Its use in the management of diabetic ketoacidosis is especially risky since patients with diabetes are notably subject to urinary tract infections and the severest forms of pyelonephritis."

Introduction of Closed Drainage Methods

Beeson was unaware at the time this editorial was written that a major advance had already been made to prevent catheter-associated infections. Thirty years earlier, Cuthbert Dukes, a pathologist at St. Mark's Hospital in London, became concerned about the problem (74). He noted the inevitable

Table 9.3. Important Landmarks That Led to Improved Catheter Care

Year	Author(s)	Observation
1883	Clark (136)	Remarks on catheter fever.
1928	Dukes (74)	Established the value of closed drainage in preventing tract infections in patients undergoing colorectal surgery.
1930	Barrington and Wright (137)	Demonstrated catheter-associated bacteremia.
1954	Guttmann (25)	Developed sterile intermittent catheterization for patients with spinal cord injury.
1957	Kass and Schneiderman (77)	Demonstrated the periurethral route of infection.
1958	Beeson (139)	Alerted the medical profession to the risks of catheterization.
1958	Miller et al. (138)	Established the value of closed drainage in patients undergoing prostatectomy.
1960	Desautels (140)	Demonstrated efficacy of aseptic management of the catheter.
1962	Martin and Bookrajian (86)	Introduced bladder irrigation with antibiotic solutions.
1966	Kunin and McCormack (4)	Established the value of plastic closed drainage bags in preventing infection in hospitals.
1972	Lapides et al. (27)	Demonstrated the value of clean intermittent self-catheterization in treatment of the neurogenic bladder.
1973	Maki et al. (52)	Demonstrated cross infection among patients.
1980	Garibaldi et al. (142)	Established that the major pathway is by the periurethral route.
1982	Platt et al. (49)	Found that catheter-associated bacteriuria increased mortality threefold in hospitalized patients.
1982	Warren et al. (5)	Studies of catheter-associated infections in nursing homes.
1983	Burke et al. (78)	Local application of antiseptics does not prevent infection.
1983	Marron et al. (72)	Nonuse of catheters in nursing homes.
1984	Nordqvist et al. (71)	Catheter free geriatric care.
1984	Thompson et al. (93)	Additives to the drainage bag are ineffective.
1992	Kunin, Douthitt et al. (6)	Mortality is increased threefold in long-term catheterized patients in nursing homes.
1995	Ouslander & Schnelle (73)	Methods to manage incontinence in nursing homes with catheters.

occurrence of urinary infections in patients managed with indwelling catheters after excision of the rectum for cancer. Using a quantitative count of pus cells, he found that the urine was free of infection until the second or third postoperative day. Thereafter, large number of leukocytes appeared in the urine. A "stream of pus" occurred by the sixth to eighth day. He suspected that infection was caused by contamination of a wooden peg used to seal the catheter and drainage into open bottles. These assumptions proved to be correct. Dukes substituted a sterile collection bottle and intermittently irrigated the closed system with a solution of oxycyanide of mercury (Fig. 9.15). In addition, the catheter was fixed in place by gauze dressings around the penis in males and by glycerin-soaked sponges abutting the vulva in females. These measures prevented infection during the postoperative period. Unfortunately, his work was soon forgotten.

Interest in finding a solution to preventing infection arising from the indwelling urinary catheter waned until the early 1960s when Gillespie, Linton, Slade, and Miller in Bristol, England (138) introduced closed drainage. Methods to develop closed systems by English workers were simple but effective (Fig. 9.16). A rubber stopper was placed in the neck of a tall collec-

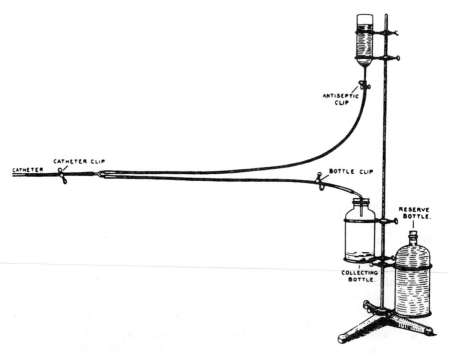

Figure 9.15. Illustration of the closed irrigation method devised by Dukes in 1928. Reproduced with permission from (74).

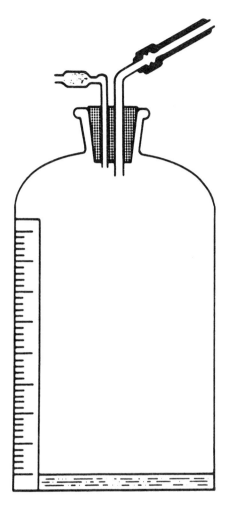

Figure 9.16. Closed drainage bottle described by Gillespie and co-workers used to demonstrate efficacy of the method in England. Solution at bottom is formalin. Bottle is emptied by removing plug at the top. Reproduced with permission from (138).

tion bottle. An air vent was provided, and the tubes were not permitted to be in contact with urine in the bottle. Formalin was added to the bottle to maintain sterility of the voided urine. This system, although remarkably successful in reducing infection, was not readily transferable to the busy American hospital. Open drainage bottles were used when I was a house-officer in the 1950s. The collecting tubes, placed at the bottom of the bottle, offered a direct pathway for contaminated urine to ascend to the bladder. The tubes often fell out, leaving a puddle of urine by the bedside. Sometimes the bottles were kicked over and we had to step around broken glass mixed with spilled urine while making rounds. No one seemed particularly concerned.

Several American urologists, primarily Desautels and Ansell (140,141), began to reexplore the concept of closed drainage and met with considerable success. Plastic closed drainage systems were developed a few years later (4), but did not become widely available until the 1970s. Closed drainage systems are highly effective in delaying the onset of catheter-associated infections for up to several weeks (Fig. 9.1). Despite considerable effort, progress in improving upon closed drainage has met with very limited success. Most of the subsequent studies continue to document the need to develop better methods to improve or avoid urinary drainage.

Can We Develop a Better Urinary Catheter?

The bladder is a smooth-walled, distensible structure that contracts when the internal pressure exerted by the expanding volume of urine reaches a critical point. The detrusor activity is synchronized with a combination of voluntary and involuntary relaxation of the external sphincter. The flow of urine then distends the normally collapsed urethral passage, allowing virtual complete emptying of the bladder. This cyclic process is the bladder's major mechanism of defense against infection. Microorganisms may be introduced into the bladder during a single catheterization, but they are usually washed out by the flow of urine. The indwelling catheter violates the bladder defense altogether. The cycle of filling, expansion, and emptying of the bladder is converted to a continuous flow of urine. The bladder cannot empty completely because of the retention balloon. The balloon erodes the smooth mucosal surface as it is pulled down to block the outflow of urine. The urethra is distended, its blood supply is attenuated by lateral pressure, and the lubricating periurethral glands are blocked. An open channel exists that permits microorganisms to flow upstream into the bladder and a stressed periurethral surface, offering a second channel for bacterial colonization around the catheter. The indwelling catheter acts as a foreign body that converts a dynamic system to a static state (143).

The challenge for the future is to produce an instrument that matches as closely as possible the normal physiologic and mechanical characteristics of the voiding system. It seems to me that this will require the construction of a thin-walled, continuously lubricated, collapsible catheter to restore the integrity of the urethra; a system to hold the catheter in place without a balloon; and one that imitates the intermittent washing of the bladder urine. The most interesting advances are use of intraprostatic devices without catheters, small percutaneous suprapubic catheters, and the conformable catheter. The efficacy of each component of the system will need to be evaluated in carefully conducted, controlled clinical trials. There is also a major need for better fitting male condom catheters and for external urine collection devices for incontinent females (144). Catheters of the future may be more expensive, but should be well worth the investment.

References

1. Turck M, Goffe B, Petersdorf RG. The urethral catheter and urinary tract infection. J Urol 1962;88:834–837.
2. Brumfitt W, Davies BI, Rosser E. Urethral catheter as a cause of urinary-tract infection in pregnancy and puerperium. Lancet 1961;2:1059–1062.
3. Gillespie WA, Lennon GG, Linton KB, et al. Prevention of urinary infection in gynaecology. Br Med J 1964;2:423–425.
4. Kunin CM, McCormack RC. Prevention of catheter-induced urinary-tract infections by sterile closed drainage. N Engl J Med 1966;274:1155–1161.
5. Warren JW, Steinberg L, Hebel JR, et al. The prevalence of urethral catheterization in Maryland nursing homes. Arch Intern Med 1989;149:1535–1537.
6. Kunin CM, Douthitt S, Dancing J, et al. The association between the use of urinary catheters and morbidity and mortality among elderly patients in nursing homes. Am J Epidemiol 1992;135:291–301.
7. Garibaldi RA, Burke JP, Dickman ML, et al. Factors predisposing to bacteriuria during indwelling urethral catheterization. N Engl J Med 1974;291:215–219.
8. Kass EH. Asymptomatic infections of the urinary tract. Trans Assoc Am Physicians 1956;69:56–63.
9. Warren JW, Hoopes JM, Muncie HL, et al. Ineffectiveness of cephalexin in treatment of cephalexin-resistant bacteriuria in patients with chronic indwelling urethral catheters. J Urol 1983;129:71–73.
10. Vollaard EJ, Clasener HAL, Zambon JV, et al. Prevention of catheter-associated gram-negative bacilluria with norfloxacin by selective decontamination of the bowel and high urinary concentration. J Antimicrob Chemother 1989;23:915–922.
11. Van der Wall E, Verkooyen RP, Oostinga J, et al. Prophylactic ciprofloxacin for catheter-associated urinary-tract infection. Lancet 1992;339:946–951.
12. Ena J, Amador C, Martinez C, et al. Risk factors for acquisition of urinary tract infections caused by ciprofloxacin resistant *Escherichia coli*. J Urol 1995;153:117–120.
13. Fraimow HS, Jungkind DL, Lander DW, et al. Urinary tract infection with an *Enterococcus faecalis* isolate that requires vancomycin for growth. Ann Intern Med 1994;121:22–26.
14. Morck DW, Olson ME, McKay SG, et al. Therapeutic efficacy of fleroxacin for eliminating catheter-associated urinary tract infection in a rabbit model. Am J Med 1993;94:23S-30S.
15. Reid G, Sharma S, Advikolanu K, et al. Effects of ciprofloxacin, norfloxacin, and ofloxacin on in vitro adhesion and survival of *Pseudomonas aeruginosa* AK1 on urinary catheters. Antimicrob Agents Chemother 1994;38:1490–1495.
16. Harding GKM, Nicolle LE, Ronald AR, et al. How long should catheter-acquired urinary tract infection in women be treated? Ann Intern Med 1991;114:713–719.
17. Taylor BD, Nickel JE. Suprapubic cystostomy and the use of polyethylene tubing. J Obstet Gynecol 1966;28:854–856.
18. Hodgkinson CP, Hodari AA. Trocar suprapubic cystostomy for postoperative bladder drainage in the female. J Obstet Gynecol 1966;96:773–783.
19. Hirsch DD, Fainstein V, Musher DM. Do condom catheter collecting systems cause urinary tract infection? JAMA 1979;242:340–341.
20. Fierer J, Ekstrom M. An outbreak of *Providencia stuartii* urinary tract infections. JAMA 1981;245:1553–1555.
21. Montgomerie JZ, Morrow JW. Long-term Pseudomonas colonization in spinal cord injury patients. Am J Epidemiol 1980;112:508–517.
22. Ouslander JG, Greengold BA, Silverblatt FJ, et al. An accurate method to obtain urine for culture in men with external catheters. Arch Intern Med 1987;147:286–288.
23. Nicolle LE, Harding GKM, Kennedy J, et al. Urine specimen collection with external devices for diagnosis of bacteriuria in elderly incontinent men. J Clin Microbiol 1988;26:1115–1119.
24. Ouslander JG, Greengold B, Chen S. External catheter use and urinary tract infections among incontinent male nursing home patients. J Am Geriatr Soc 1987;35:1063–1070.
25. Guttman L, Frankel H. The value of intermittent catheterization in the early management of traumatic paraplegia and tetraplegia. Paraplegia 1966;4:63–83.
26. Tribe CR, Silver JR. Renal failure in paraplegia. London: Pitman, 1969.

27. Lapides J, Diokno AC, Silber SJ, et al. Clean, intermittent self-catheterization in the treatment of urinary tract disease. J Urol 1972;107:458–461.
28. Koleilat N, Sidi AA, Gonzalez R. Urethral false passage as a complication of intermittent catheterization. J Urol 1989;142:1216–1217.
29. Mohler JL, Cowen DL, Flanigan RC. Suppression and treatment of urinary tract infection in patients with an intermittently catheterized neurogenic bladder. J Urol 1987;138: 336–340.
30. Anderson R. Prophylaxis of bacteriuria during intermittent catheterization of the acute neurogenic bladder. J Urol 1980;123:364–366.
31. Rhame FS, Perkash I. Urinary tract infections occurring in recent spinal cord injury patients on intermittent catheterization. J Urol 1979;122:669–673.
32. Kevorkian CG, Merritt J, Ilstrup D. Methenamine mandelate with acidification: an effective urinary antiseptic in patients with neurogenic bladder. Mayo Clin Proc 1984;59: 523–529.
33. Haldorson AM, Keys TF, Maker MD, et al. Nonvalue of neomycin installation after intermittent urinary catheterization. Antimicrob Agents Chemother 1978;14:368–370.
34. Waller L, Jonsson O, Norlen L, et al. Clean intermittent catheterization in spinal cord injury patients: long-term follow-up of a hydrophilic low friction technique. J Urol 1995;153: 345–348.
35. Diokno AC, Mitchell BA, Nash AJ, et al. Patient satisfaction and the lofric catheter for clean intermittent catheterization. J Urol 1995;153:349–351.
36. Silbar EC, Cicmanec JF, Burke BM, et al. Microwave sterilization: a method for home sterilization of urinary catheters. J Urol 1989;141:88–90.
37. Kass EH, Koff SA, Kiokno AC. Fate of vesicoureteral reflux in children with neuropathic bladders managed by intermittent catheterization. J Urol 1980;125:63–64.
38. Perkash I, Giroux J. Clean intermittent catheterization in spinal cord injury patients: a follow-up study. J Urol 1993;149:1068–1071.
39. DeWire DM, Owens RS, Anderson GA, et al. A comparison of the urologic complications associated with long term management of quadriplegics with and without chronic indwelling catheters. J Urol 1992;147:1069–1072.
40. Michelson JD, Lotke PA, Steinberg ME. Urinary-bladder management after total joint-replacement surgery. N Engl J Med 1988;319:321–326.
41. Irani J, Fauchery A, Dore B, et al. Systematic removal of catheter 48 hours following transurethral resection and 24 hours following transurethral incision of prostate: a prospective randomized analysis of 213 patients. J Urol 1995;153:1537–1539.
42. Centers for Disease Control. Public health focus: surveillance, prevention and control of nosocomial infections. MMWR Morb Mortal Wkly Rep 1992;41:783–787.
43. Haley RW, Culver DH, White JW, et al. The nationwide nosocomial infection rate: a need for vital statistics. Am J Epidemiol 1985;121:159–167.
44. Bronsema DA, Adams JR, Pallares R, et al. Secular trends in rates and etiology of nosocomial urinary tract infections at a university hospital. J Urol 1993;150:414–416.
45. Libow LS, Starer P. Care of the nursing home patient. N Engl J Med 1989;321:93–96.
46. Pittet D, Wenzel RP. Nosocomial bloodstream infections. Secular trends in rates, mortality, and contribution to total hospital deaths. Arch Intern Med 1995;155:1177–1184.
47. Spengler RF, Greenough WB III. Hospital costs and mortality attributed to nosocomial bacteremias. JAMA 1978;240:2455–2458.
48. Filice GA, Van Etta LL, Darby CP, et al. Bacteremia in Charleston County, South Carolina. Am J Epidemiol 1986;123:128–136.
49. Platt R, Polk BF, Murdock B, et al. Mortality associated with nosocomial urinary-tract infection. N Engl J Med 1982;307:637–642.
50. Givens CD, Wenzel RP. Catheter-associated urinary tract infections in surgical patients: a controlled study on the excess morbidity and costs. J Urol 1980;124:646–648.
51. Whitby JL, Blair JN, Rampling A. Cross-infection with Serratia marcescens in an intensive-therapy unit. Lancet 1972;2:127–128.
52. Maki DG, Hennekens CG, Phillips CW, et al. Nosocomial urinary tract infection with Serratia marcescens: an epidemiologic study. J Infect Dis 1973;128:579–587.
53. Schaberg DR. Epidemics of nosocomial urinary tract infection caused by multiply resistant gram-negative bacilli: epidemiology and control. J Infect Dis 1976;133:363–366.
54. Turck M, Stamm W. Nosocomial infection of the urinary tract. Am J Med 1981;70:651–654.

55. Zervos MJ, Kauffman CA, Therasse PM, et al. Nosocomial infection by gentamicin-resistant *Streptococcus faecalis*. An epidemiologic study. Ann Intern Med 1987;106:687–691.
56. Maki DG, Hennekens CG, Bennett JV. Prevention of catheter-associated urinary tract infection. JAMA 1972;221:1270–1271.
57. Jain P, Parada JP, David A, et al. Overuse of the indwelling urinary catheter in hospitalized medical patients. Arch Intern Med 1995;155:1425–1429.
58. Lichtenstein MJ, Federspiel CF, Schaffner W. Factors associated with early demise in nursing home residents: a case control study. J Am Geriatr Soc 1985;33:315–319.
59. Garibaldi RA, Brodine S, Matsumiya S. Infections among patients in nursing homes, policies, prevalence and problems. N Engl J Med 1981;305:731–735.
60. Scheckler WE, Peterson PJ. Infections and infection control among residents of eight rural Wisconsin nursing homes. Arch Intern Med 1986;146:1981–1984.
61. Farber BF, Brennen C, Puntereri AJ, et al. A prospective study of nosocomial infections in a chronic care facility. J Am Geriatr Soc 1983;32:499–502.
62. Jackson MM, Fierer J, Barrett-Connor E, et al. Intensive surveillance for infections in a three-year study of nursing home patients. Am J Epidemiol 1992;135:685–696.
63. Irvine PW, Van Buren N, Crossley K. Causes for hospitalization of nursing home residents: the role of infection. J Am Geriatr Soc 1984;32:103–107.
64. Katz PR, Beam Jr TR, Brand F, et al. Antibiotic use in the nursing home. Physician practice patterns. Arch Intern Med 1990;150:1465–1468.
65. Jones SR, Parker DF, Liebow ES, et al. Appropriateness of antibiotic therapy in long-term care facilities. Am J Med 1987;83:499–502.
66. Warren JW, Damron D, Tenney JH, et al. Fever, bacteremia, and death as complications of bacteriuria in women with long-term urethral catheters. J Infect Dis 1987;155:1151–1158.
67. Orr PH, Nicolle LE, Duckworth H, et al. Febrile urinary infection in the institutionalized elderly. Am J Med 1996;100:71–77.
68. Jewes LA, Gillespie WA, Leadbetter A, et al. Bacteriuria and bacteraemia in patients with long-term indwelling catheters—a domiciliary study. J Med Microbiol 1988;26:61–65.
69. Warren JW, Muncie Jr HL, Hall-Craggs M. Acute pyelonephritis associated with bacteriuria during long-term catheterization: a prospective clinicopathological study. J Infect Dis 1988;158:1341–1346.
70. Kunin CM, Chin QF, Chambers ST. Morbidity and mortality associated with indwelling urinary catheters in elderly patients in a nursing home—Confounding due to the presence of associated diseases. J Am Geriatr Soc 1987;35:1001–1006.
71. Nordqvist P, Ekelund P, Edouard L, et al. Catheter free geriatric care. J Hosp Infect 1984;5:298–304.
72. Marron KR, Fillit H, Peskowitz M, et al. The nonuse of urethral catheterization in the management of urinary tract incontinence in the teaching nursing home. J Am Geriatr Soc 1983;31:278–281.
73. Ouslander JG, Schnelle JF, Uman G, et al. Predictors of successful prompted voiding among incontinent nursing home residents. JAMA 1995;273:1366–1370.
74. Dukes C. Urinary infections after excision of the rectum: their cause and prevention. Proc Royal Soc Med 1928;22:1–11.
75. Wong ES. Guidelines for prevention of catheter-associated urinary tract infections. Am J Infect Control 1983;11:28–33.
76. Wille JC, Blusse van Oud Alblas A, Thewessen EAPM. Nosocomial catheter-associated bacteriuria: a clinical trial comparing two closed urinary drainage systems. J Hosp Infect 1993;25:191–198.
77. Kass EH, Schneiderman LJ. Entry of bacteria into the urinary tracts of patients with inlying catheters. N Engl J Med 1957;256:556–557.
78. Burke JP, Jacobson JA, Garibaldi RA, et al. Evaluation of daily meatal care with poly-antibiotic ointment in prevention of urinary catheter-associated bacteriuria. J Urol 1983;129:331–334.
79. Daifuku R, Stamm WE. Bacterial adherence to bladder uroepithelial cells in catheter-associated urinary tract infection. N Engl J Med 1986;314:1208–1213.
80. Schaeffer AJ, Chmiel J. Urethral meatal colonization in the pathogenesis of catheter-associated bacteriuria. J Urol 1983;130:1096–1099.
81. Kunin CM, Steele C. Culture of the surface of urinary catheters to sample the urethral flora and study the effect of antimicrobial therapy. J Clin Microbiol 1985;21:902–908.

82. Britt MR, Garibaldi RA, Miller WA, et al. Antimicrobic prophylaxis for catheter-associated bacteriuria. Antimicrob Agents Chemother 1977;11:240–243.
83. Butler HK, Kunin CM. Evaluation of polymyxin catheter lubricant and impregnated catheters. J Urol 1968;100:560–566.
84. Huth TS, Burke JP, Larsen RA, et al. Randomized trial of meatal care with silver sulfadiazine cream for the prevention of catheter-associated bacteriuria. J Infect Dis 1992;165:14–18.
85. Viant AC, Linton KB, Gillespie WA. Improved method for preventing movement of indwelling catheters in female patients. Lancet 1971;1:736–737.
86. Martin CM, Bookrajian EN. Bacteriuria prevention after indwelling urinary catheterization: a controlled study. Arch Intern Med 1962;110:703–711.
87. Kirk D, Dunn M, Bullock DW, et al. Hibitane bladder irrigation in the prevention of catheter-associated urinary infection. Br J Urol 1979;51:528–531.
88. Warren JW, Platt R, Thomas RJ, et al. Antibiotic irrigation and catheter-associated urinary tract infections. N Engl J Med 1978;299:570–573.
89. Huth TS, Burke JP, Larsen RA, et al. Clinical trial of junction seals for the prevention of urinary catheter-associated bacteriuria. Arch Intern Med 1992;152:807–812.
90. Evans AT, Cicmanec JF. The role of betadine microbicides in urine bag sterilization. In: Proceedings Second World Conference on Antisepsis. New York: HP Publishing Co., 1980:85–86.
91. Maizels M, Schaeffer AJ. Decreased incidence of bacteriuria associated with periodic installations of hydrogen peroxide into the urethral catheter drainage bag. J Urol 1980;123:841–845.
92. Southampton Infection Control Team. Evaluation of aseptic techniques and chlorhexidine of the rate of catheter-associated urinary-tract infection. Lancet 1982;1:89–91.
93. Thompson RL, Haley CE, Searcy MA, et al. Catheter-associated bacteriuria. Failure to reduce attack rates using periodic instillations of a disinfectant into urinary drainage systems. JAMA 1984;251:747–751.
94. Gillespie WA, Jones JE, Teasdale C, et al. Does the addition of disinfectant prevent infection in catheterized patients? Lancet 1983;2:1037–1039.
95. Sweet DE, Goodpasture HC, Holl K, et al. Evaluation of H_2O_2 prophylaxis of bacteriuria in patients with long-term indwelling foley catheters: a randomized controlled study. Infect Control 1985;6:263–266.
96. Kunin CM. The drainage bag additive saga. Infect Control 1985;6:261–262.
97. Talbot HS. Care of the bladder in neurological disorders. JAMA 1956;161:944–947.
98. Holm HH, Egeblad K. Disposable apparatus for closed bladder tidal drainage. J Urol 1970;104:753–754.
99. Kunin CM, Chin QF, Chambers ST. Indwelling urinary catheters in the elderly. Relation of "catheter life" to formation of encrustations in patients with and without blocked catheters. Am J Med 1987;82:405–411.
100. Wilksch J, Vernon-Roberts B, Garrett R, et al. The role of catheter surface morphology and extractable cytotoxic material in tissue reactions to urethral catheters. Br J Urol 1983;55:48–52.
101. Edwards L, Trott PA. Catheter-induced urethral inflammation. J Urol 1973;110:678–681.
102. Anderson RU. Response of bladder and urethral mucosa to catheterization. JAMA 1979;242:451–453.
103. Edwards LE, Lock R, Powell C, et al. Post-catheterization of urethral strictures. A clinical and experimental study. Br J Urol 1983;55:53–56.
104. Rubin M, Berger SA, Zodda FN, et al. Effect of catheter replacement on bacterial counts in urine aspirated from indwelling catheters. J Infect Dis 1980;142:291.
105. Tenney JH, Warren JW. Bacteriuria in women with long-term catheters: paired comparison of indwelling and replacement catheters. J Infect Dis 1988;157:199–202.
106. Nickel JC, Downey J, Costerton JW. Movement of *Pseudomonas aeruginosa* along catheter surfaces. Urol 1992;39:93.
107. Ladd TI, Schmiel D, Nickel JC, et al. Rapid method for detection of adherent bacteria on foley urinary catheters. J Clin Microbiol 1985;21:1004–1006.
108. Sugarman B. Adherence of bacteria to urinary catheters. Urol Res 1982;10:37–40.
109. Muncie HL Jr, Hoopes JM, Damron DJ, et al. Once-daily irrigation of long-term urethral catheters with normal saline. Arch Intern Med 1989;149:441–443.

110. Norberg B, Norberg A, Parkhede U. The spontaneous variation of catheter life in long-stay geriatric inpatients with indwelling catheters. Gerontology 1983;29:332–335.

111. Kunin CM, Chin QF, Chambers ST. Formation of encrustations on indwelling urinary catheters in the elderly: A comparison of different types of catheter materials in 'blockers' and 'nonblockers.' J Urol 1987;138:899–902.

112. Akiyama H, Okamoto S. Prophylaxis of indwelling urethral catheter infection: clinical experience with a modified Foley catheter and drainage system. J Urol 1978;121:40–42.

113. Schaeffer AJ, Story KO, Johnson SM. Effect of silver oxide/trichloroisocyanuric acid antimicrobial urinary drainage system on catheter-associated bacteriuria. J Urol 1988;139: 69–72.

114. Lundeberg T. Prevention of catheter-associated urinary-tract infections by use of silver-impregnated catheters. Lancet 1986;2:1031.

115. Johnson JR, Roberts PL, Olsen RJ, et al. Prevention of catheter-associated urinary tract infection with a silver oxide-coated urinary catheter: Clinical and microbiologic correlates. J Infect Dis 1990;162:1145–1150.

116. Riley DK, Classen DC, Stevens LE, et al. A large randomized clinical trial of a silver-impregnated urinary catheter: lack of efficacy and staphylococcal superinfection. Am J Med 1995;98:349–356.

117. Farber BF, Wolff AG. The use of salicylic acid to prevent the adherence of *Escherichia coli* to silastic catheters. J Urol 1993;149:667–670.

118. Fuse H, Ohkawa M, Nakashima T, et al. Crystal adherence to urinary catheter materials in rats. J Urol 1994;151:1703–1706.

119. Soboh F, Khoury AE, Zamboni AC, et al. Effects of ciprofloxacin and protamine sulfate combinations against catheter-associated *Pseudomonas aeruginosa* biofilms. Antimicrob Agents Chemother 1995;39:1281–1286.

120. Davis C, Shirtliff M, Trieff N, et al. Quantification, qualification, and microbial killing efficiencies of antimicrobial chlorine-based substances produced by iontophoresis. Antimicrob Agents Chemother 1994;38:2768–2774.

121. Brocklehurst C, Hickey DS, Davies I, et al. A new urethral catheter. Brit Med J 1988;296: 1691–1693.

122. Kunin CM, Finkelberg Z. Evaluation of an intraurethral lubricating catheter in prevention of catheter-induced urinary tract infections. J Urol 1971;106:928–930.

123. Tupasi T, Kunin CM. A top-vented urinary closed drainage system. J Urol 1971;106: 416–417.

124. Monson TP, Macalalad FV, Hamman JW, et al. Evaluation of a vented drainage system in prevention of bacteriuria. J Urol 1977;117:216–219.

125. Nielsen KK, Klarskox P, Nordling J, et al. The intraprostatic spiral. New treatment for urinary retention. Brit J Urol 1990;65:500–503.

126. Nissenkorn I. Experience with a new self-retaining intraurethral catheter in patients with urinary retention: a preliminary report. J Urol 1989;142:92–94.

127. Kelly TWJ, Griffiths GL. Balloon problems with foley catheters. Lancet 1983;2:1310.

128. Sellett T. Iatrogenic urethral injury due to preinflation of a foley catheter. JAMA 1971;217:1548–1549.

129. Rubino SM, Scialabba MA. A clinical evaluation of a modified foley catheter. Am J Obstet Gynecol 1983;146:103–104.

130. Murphy GF, Wood DP Jr. The use of mineral oil to manage the nondeflating foley catheter. J Urol 1993;149:89–90.

131. Yu DS, Yang TH, Ma CP. Snail-headed catheter retriever: a simple way to remove catheters from female patients. J Urol 1995;154:167–168.

132. Moffat LEF, Teo C, Dawson I. Ultrasound in management of undeflatable foley catheter balloon. J Urol 1985;26:79.

133. Stark R, Maki D. Bacteriuria in the catheterized patient. What quantitative level of bacteriuria is relevant? N Engl J Med 1984;311:560–564.

134. Dealler SF, Belfield PW, Bedford M, et al. Purple urine bags. J Urol 1989;142:769–770.

135. Dealler SF, Hawkey PM, Millar MR. Enzymatic degradation of urinary indoxyl sulfate by *Providencia stuartii* and *Klebsiella pneumoniae* causes the purple urine bag syndrome. J Clin Microbiol 1988;26:2152–2156.

136. Clark A. Remarks on catheter fever. Lancet 1883;2:1075–1077.

137. Barrington FJF, Wright HD. Bacteremia following operations on the urethra. J Path Bact 1930;33:871–888.
138. Miller A, Gillespie WA, Slade N, et al. Prevention of urinary infection after prostatectomy. Lancet 1960;2:886–888.
139. Beeson PB. The case against the catheter. Am J Med 1958;24:1–3.
140. Desautels RE. Aseptic management of catheter drainage. N Engl J Med 1960;263: 189–191.
141. Ansell J. Some observations on catheter care. J Chronic Dis 1962;15:675–682.
142. Garibaldi RA, Burke JP, Britt MR, et al. Meatal colonization and catheter-associated bacteriuria. N Engl J Med 1980;303:216–318.
143. Kunin CM. Can we build a better urinary catheter? N Engl J Med 1988;319:365–366.
144. Johnson DE, O'Reilly JL, Warren JW. Clinical evaluation of an external urine collection device for nonambulatory incontinent women. J Urol 1989;141:535–537.

10

Pathogenesis of Infection: The Invading Microbes

Overview

The pathogenesis of urinary tract infections involves a series of complex, interdependent host-parasite interactions. The invading microorganisms are generally part of the endogenous flora of the host. They compete for survival with other normal flora and must overcome powerful host defense mechanisms. To produce ascending infection they need to colonize the urethra, adhere to the urothelium, grow in the urine, ascend the ureters, and enter the kidney. To produce hematogenous infections and invade the kidney, they must overcome humoral immunity and phagocytic defense mechanisms. Microorganisms that cause urinary tract infections are commonly referred to as uropathogens. Those with special virulence properties are referred to as uropathogenic or invasive strains. Each virulence factor has a special role depending on the stage of infection. Fimbriae and other adhesins are important in the early stages. They permit the microbe to adhere to host cells, resist wash out by the urinary stream, and invade cells. Capsules resist phagocytosis; hemolysins and endotoxin cause tissue injury; and aerobactin scavenges for iron. Urease-producing microbes are particularly virulent because ammonia is cytotoxic and a high urinary pH favors the formation of struvite stones. Relatively virulent microorganisms are required to produce uncomplicated infections in the normal host. Less virulent microorganisms produce complicated infections in the compromised host.

The wide variety of microbial species that cause uncomplicated and complicated infections are listed in Tables 1.3, 1.4, and 1.5. Urinary tract infections are most often caused by facultative anaerobic, gram-negative enteric bacteria of the family *Enterobacteriaceae*. *Escherichia coli* is the most important member. Obligate anaerobes, although 100 to 1000 times more abundant than *E. coli* in the stool, do not grow well in urine and rarely cause urinary infections. Anaerobes are occasionally a component of polymicrobial infections in patients with long-standing urolithiasis, renal and perirenal abscesses, and Fournier's disease (necrotizing fasciatus). Gram positive bacteria colonize the gut, skin, and mucosal surfaces. Certain species, such as *Staphylococcus aureus, Staphylococcus saprophyticus,* enterococci, and *Corynebacterium urealyticum,* have special urovirulence. Candida and other yeasts are usually acquired from the gut under the selective pressure of antibacterial therapy. They may produce hematogenous infections in compromised hosts. Pseudomonas, Serratia, and Acinetobacter are acquired from the aqueous environment. Mycobacteria and systemic fungi produce local and metastatic infections of the urinary tract.

This chapter will describe the microbes that cause urinary tract infections and discuss the factors that determine their virulence. The immune response to infection and the potential for development of a vaccine to prevent urinary tract infections and pyelonephritis will also be examined.

The *Enterobacteriaceae*

The *Enterobacteriaceae* are the most common invaders of the urinary tract. They include *E. coli* and species of Klebsiella, Enterobacter, Proteus, Providencia, Morganella, Serratia, Salmonella, and Shigella. They share a common antigen (1) and have similar DNA domains. They can be differentiated by biochemical, serologic, and genetic methods. Many of the species have numerous serovars. Individual strains can be identified further by their outer membrane proteins, fimbriae, flagella, production of hemolysin, iron siderophores, DNA fingerprinting, genetic probes, ribotyping, and antibiograms. Strains of Proteus can be differentiated by the Dienes phenomenon.

The outer membrane of the cell wall of *Enterobacteriaceae* contains complex polysaccharide polymers (Fig. 10.1). The terminal sugars are highly varied both in structure and linkage. These are the O antigen determinants. Strains possessing O antigens are termed smooth and are typeable with suitable panels of antisera. Strains that do not possess O antigens are described as rough or serum agglutinable strains. These strains lack galactose or other sugars needed to confer O antigenicity. Rough strains tend to be more susceptible to phagocytosis and less virulent. Capsular (K) antigens are complex surface polysaccharides that resist phagocytosis. The flagella (H antigens) are tubular protein structures responsible for motility. Strains that do not possess flagella are nonmotile and H-antigen negative.

Endotoxin

The toxic constituent of gram-negative bacteria (endotoxin or core lipopolysaccharide) is located deeper in the outer membrane cell wall as shown in the diagram. It is linked to other portions of the membrane through 2 keto-

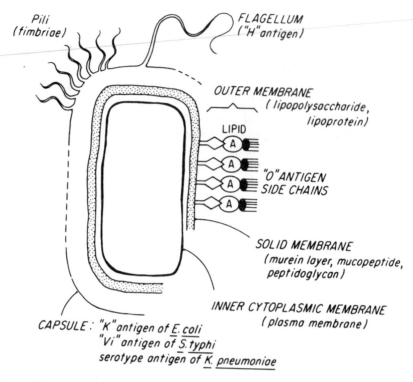

Figure 10.1. Schematic presentation of the antigenic structure of gram-negative enteric bacteria. Reproduced with permission from Young (2).

3-deoxyoctonate trisaccharides. The most purified form is known as lipid A (Fig. 10.2). Lipid A is a polymer containing glucosamine disaccharide units linked through pyrophosphate bridges and esterified with lauric, palmitic, and myristic acids. Endotoxin damages cell membranes, releases lysosomal enzymes, stimulates the production of nitrous oxide, and activates the complement and clotting cascades. When inoculated intravenously it causes fever, leukopenia, circulatory collapse, capillary hemorrhages, necrosis of tumors, and the Shwartzman phenomenon. Small doses of endotoxin produce fever. Large doses produce fever, shock, profound metabolic acidosis, reduction in serum complement, and disseminated intravascular clotting (DIC). Endotoxin tolerance may explain the remarkable tendency of the symptoms of pyelonephritis to subside spontaneously (4).

The core lipopolysaccharides share common antigenic determinants which cross taxonomic lines with a wide variety of gram-negative bacteria. Monoclonal antibodies against endotoxin epitopes are not considered sufficiently effective to be licensed for human use at this time (5). Endotoxin has several important roles in urinary tract infection. It decreases ureteral peri-

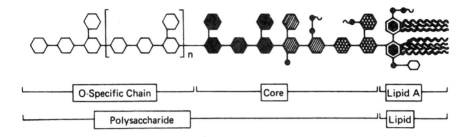

: Monosaccharide, ● : Phosphate, ~ : Ethanolamine
~~~ : Long Chain (Hydroxy) Fatty Acid

Figure 10.2. The three regions in gram negative bacterial lipopolysaccharide. The lipid A region corresponds to endotoxin. Reproduced with permission from Westphal, Jann, and Himmelspach (3).

staltic tone (6,7) and contributes to renal damage in pyelonephritis. It stimulates a vigorous polymorphonuclear (PMN) response by urothelial cells (8) and shedding of epithelial cells into the urine (9). PMNs are also recruited locally by an independent mechanism induced by adhesion of P-fimbriae to urothelial cells (10). This activates a local mucosal cytokine network and release of interleukins IL- 6 and IL-8 (11,12). Shedding of cells and rapid mobilization of leukocytes enhance clearance of the microorganisms from the urine in experimental animals and humans (13). This early response to invading microorganisms is considered to be an important host defense mechanism.

The Enterobacterial Common Antigen (ECA)

Enterobacteriaceae share a common antigen (ECA) (1). It is composed of a trisaccharide repeating unit of N-acetyl-D-glucosamine, N-acetyl-D-mannosaminuronic acid, and 4-acetamido-4,6-dideoxy-D galactose. It is linked closely to the outer membrane structures of the cell wall and found in the ribosomal cytoplasm (14). ECA occurs in a haptenic and an immunogenic form. An antibody response is elicited by *E. coli* O14 and several other O groups. The antibody is cross reactive with all other *Enterobacteriaceae*. Aside from its taxonomic interest, the role of this antigen in the pathogenesis of infections is not entirely clear (15). Several groups of investigators have sought to determine whether immunization with *E. coli* O14 or with ECA is protective against experimental pyelonephritis and other gram negative bacterial infections. Protection has been described by some investigators (16) but not by others (17). The level of anti-ECA does not correlate with prognosis in patients with gram negative bacteremia (18). Antibody response to ECA has been described in acute and chronic urinary tract infection, shigellosis, and peritonitis.

Antibodies directed against ECA are useful to localize bacterial products in human renal tissue and in experimental pyelonephritis. Cross-reactions of mammalian tissues to the antigen may have a role in the pathogenesis of inflammatory bowel disease and pyelonephritis. An antigen derived from the colon of germ-free rats cross-reacts with sera of patients with ulcerative colitis (19). Absorption of the patient's serum with *E. coli* O14 inhibits its binding to colon tissue extracts. Cross-reactions between human kidney tissue and *E. coli* have been noted, suggesting that ECA may have a role in the pathogenesis of pyelonephritis (20). The role of ECA in protection from infection and in the pathogenesis of pyelonephritis remains to be determined.

Escherichia coli

E. coli is the most common cause of urinary tract infections. There are over 170 different O or cell-wall antigen groups, over 80 capsular (K) groups, and over 50 flagellar (H) antigen groups. Only a limited number of O antigen groups are associated with human infection. Flagellar antigens are useful for identification, but do not appear to be related to virulence in *E. coli*. The outer membrane proteins or porins permit the flow of solutes into the bacterial cell. The major porins in *E. coli* are Omp F, Omp C and Omp A. There are several types of fimbriae (pili) and adhesins. The sex pili transmit genetic material by means of bacterial conjugation (Fig. 10.3). Other fimbriae, such as type 1 and P and S-fimbriae, attach to host cells and will be discussed later.

O, K, and H Antigens

Uropathogenic E. coli

A relatively smaller number of O groups and combinations of O, K, and H serotypes are found in patients with cystitis, pyelonephritis, and bacteremia than can be accounted for by their abundance in the stool (21) (Table 10.1). These serotypes represent clones that often carry additional virulence factors. Some clones, such as O18:K1:H7, are associated with neonatal meningitis and sepsis (22), whereas others are associated with nursery outbreaks. Individual clones can be identified further by phenotypic and molecular markers (Table 10.2). The clonal markers are useful to identify epidemic strains and trace migration of strains from the colon to the urethra. The O and K antigens confer urovirulence, but are too numerous and geographically variable to be the sole markers of virulence. Community-acquired cystitis, pyelonephritis, and bacteremia are caused by a wide variety of serotypes often without a discernible clonal pattern (23, 24). Accordingly, uropathogenic strains are identified more commonly by the presence of several virulence

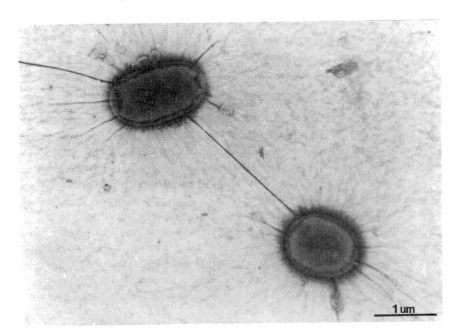

Figure 10.3. Electron micrograph showing conjugation between *E. coli* by means of sex fimbriae (pili). Note the smaller adhesive fimbriae that surround the surface of the cell. Courtesy of Lauren O. Bakaletz.

Table 10.1. Serologic Markers of *E. coli*

O, K, and H Antigens	
Marker	Commonly Found in Urinary Tract Infections
O Antigens	1, 2, 4, 6, 7, 16, 18, 25, 50, and 75.
Serogroups*	O1:K1:H7, O2:K1:H4, O4:K12:H1, O16:K1:H6 and O18ac:K5:H, O18:K5:H7

*These clones are more frequent in patients with cystitis, pyelonephritis, and bacteremia than can be accounted for by their abundance in the stool.

Table 10.2. Molecular Markers for Individual Clones

Ribotyping
Outer membrane proteins (OMPs)
Pulse-field electrophoresis of genomic DNA
Genetic probes for virulence factors
Biochemical fingerprinting
Nicotinamide requirement
B2 carboxyesterase electrophoretic pattern

factors; these include P-fimbriae, hemolysin, aerobactin, as well as the O and K polysaccharides (25–27).

Enteropathic E. coli

Enteropathic *E. coli* can also be identified for epidemiologic purposes by their O and H antigens, but they rarely, if ever, cause urinary infections. *E. coli* O157:H7 causes hemorrhagic colitis, the hemolytic uremic syndrome, and thrombotic thrombocytopenic purpura (28). Enteropathogenicity is conferred by several Shiga-like toxins. Strains of *E. coli* other than O157:H7 can produce Shiga-like toxins and cause similar illnesses. Other enteropathic strains produce heat labile and heat stabile enterotoxins. Theoretically, any *E. coli* could become uropathogenic or enteropathogenic once it receives the appropriate genetic material by plasmid mediated or other genetic transfer mechanisms. Enteric pathogens, such as Salmonella and Shigella, can cause urinary tract infections. It appears to be only a matter of time for reports to appear that a uropathogenic *E. coli* is found to be enteropathic and vice versa. There are already reports of neonatal colitis caused by non-toxigenic, P-fimbriated, pyelonephritic strains of *E. coli* (29) and of P-fimbriated bacteria in gallstones (30).

Possible Explanations Why Enteropathic *E. coli* Do Not Cause Urinary Infections

- They are food-borne and not part of the resident flora of the gut.
- They attach to intestinal cells by colonization factor antigen (CFA) adhesins rather than type 1 or P-fimbriae.
- They lack the adhesins and other virulence factors of uropathogenic strains.
- Enterotoxins may interfere with colonization of the urinary tract.

Serotyping and Molecular Markers to Study Acquisition of Urinary Tract Infection

Serotyping and molecular markers permit strains of *E. coli* to be traced as they emerge from the gut, colonize the periurethral zone, and produce infection. Uncomplicated infections are almost always caused by a single strain (31) although dual infection with *Staphylococcus saprophyticus* is occasionally reported. When two strains of *E. coli* are inoculated in the bladder of mice, one soon becomes predominant (32). Dominance by one strain is also observed when mixed cultures of *E. coli* are grown in broth. The "fitter" type, with a slight growth advantage, rapidly takes over the population (33). Superinfection with a new microorganism does not occur in uncomplicated infections unless the established strain is eradicated by antimicrobial therapy. Attempts to replace the established strain by instillation of a new strain into the human bladder have not been successful.

It is commonly held that urinary tract infections are caused by fecal contamination of the periurethral zone. Women are often advised to wipe themselves from front to back. This notion remains unproved. Cultures of the periurethral zone and serotyping have helped to clarify this issue. If urinary tract infections were caused by fecal contamination, one would expect to find multiple strains of *E. coli* in the vaginal introitus and periurethral zone. Stamey and others have shown that few or no *E. coli* colonize the periurethral zone and vagina of healthy females (34); that these zones are colonized by a single uropathogen in females prone to recurrent infections; and that the same strain often persists and may cause recurrent infections in susceptible individuals (34–41).

Evidence Against the Notion That Urinary Tract Infections in Females Are Caused by Gross Fecal Soilage

- The vaginal introitus and periurethral zone are usually free of *E. coli* in most women.
- Most women do not have urinary tract infections or suffer only a few scattered episodes.
- Women prone to recurrent infection carry a single strain in the periurethral zone for prolonged periods of time.
- A limited number of serotypes with the same markers tend to colonize the periurethral zone for prolonged periods of time.
- A single strain is almost always isolated in uncomplicated urinary tract infection.

Differentiation Between Persistence, Relapse, and Reinfection

Recurrent infections may be caused by the same or a different microorganism. *Persistence* is defined as the continued presence of the same serotype of *E. coli* or the same microorganism despite therapy. *Relapse* is defined as the appearance of the same strain of *E. coli* or the same microbial species soon after it was apparently eradicated from the bladder urine. *Reinfection* is defined as colonization of the urine with a new serotype of *E. coli* or a new microbial species. It may be difficult at times to distinguish relapse from reinfection using O antigen typing alone. Rough or untypeable strains are found in about half of females with asymptomatic bacteriuria and cystitis. These need to be characterized by molecular markers. The causative microbe may be eradicated from the bladder urine but persist on the periurethral zone or feces and produce reinfection many months later (34–41). Some otherwise healthy females are colonized persistently with the same strain even without developing infection (36). Examples of persistent colonization of the same serotype of *E. coli* without infection are shown in Figures 10.4 and 10.5.

Recurrent infections in girls are most often caused by reinfection with a new strain (42–44). After successful treatment, about 80% of recurrences are caused by a new serologic type of *E. coli* or a new bacterial species. This finding is illustrated in children with recurrent infections (Fig. 10.6). Note the change in serotype with each course of therapy. Recurrent infections in adult women are also caused by reinfection, but in approximately one-third to

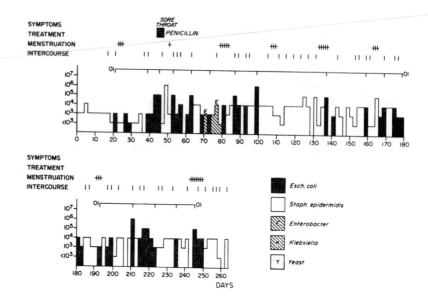

Figure 10.4. Sequential alternate-day cultures in an otherwise healthy woman in relation to frequency of sexual intercourse, menstruation, and urinary tract symptoms. Note the intermittent colonization with small numbers of *E. coli* 01 without development of significant bacteriuria. Each isolation of *E. coli* 01 is marked by a short vertical line. Reproduced with permission from Kunin, Polyak, and Postel (36)

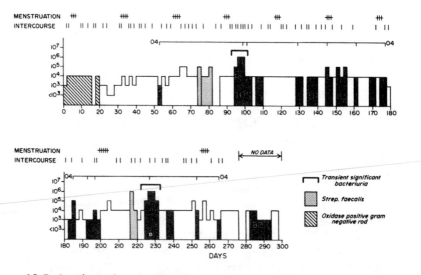

Figure 10.5. Another otherwise healthy woman, studied as in Figure 10.4. Note two periods of transient significant bacteriuria with *E. coli* 04 and continued intermittent colonization with this strain. Reproduced with permission from Kunin, Polyak, and Postel (36).

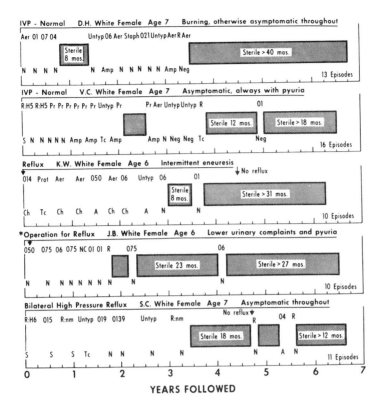

Figure 10.6. The natural history of recurrent urinary tract infection in girls followed for seven years. The numbers refer to *E. coli* O serotypes. R means a "rough" strain; Aer means *Enterobacter aerogenes,* Pr means *Proteus mirabilis,* and NC means not cultured. N, Amp, Tc, Ch, and S indicate therapy with nitrofurantoin, ampicillin, tetracycline, chloramphenicol, and sulfonamide. Note the tendency for *E. coli* serotypes to change with each recurrence after successful eradication of a preceding infection. The recurrent episodes tended to become more widely spaced over time and stop. Reproduced with permission from Kunin (45).

one-half of cases the same strain is reintroduced from an extraurinary-tract reservoir (37,39–41). Recurrent infections in men tend to be caused by relapse with the same microorganism in a prostatic focus.

Examples of Spontaneous Cure and Low-Count Bacteriuria

Spontaneous Cure
Serotyping of *E. coli* can also be used to document the occurrence of *spontaneous cure* (Fig. 10.7). In the cases shown in the figure the same *E. coli*

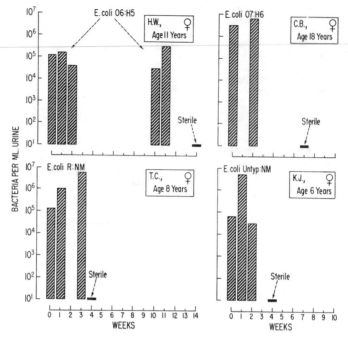

Figure 10.7. Four documented cases of "spontaneous cure" of bacteriuria in school girls. Colonization is considered to be significant because of the recovery of the same serologic type of *E. coli* on multiple occasions. Reproduced with permission from Kunin, Deutscher, and Paquin (42).

Key Lessons Learned from Serotyping and Molecular Markers in *E. coli*

- The bacterial flora of the gut contains a variety of different serotypes of *E. coli* that are constantly changing.
- Certain clones tend to produce cystitis, pyelonephritis, and bacteremia more often than can be accounted for by their abundance in the stool.
- Urinary tract infection is preceded by colonization of the periurethral zone by the strain that eventually causes the infection.
- Urinary tract infections in females are not caused by gross fecal contamination.
- A single strain causes uncomplicated urinary tract infections. The same strain tends to persist if the patient is not treated, but it may clear spontaneously.
- The vaginal introitus of females prone to recurrent urinary tract infections tends to be persistently colonized with the same strain of *E. coli*.
- Persistent colonization of the periurethral zone with the same strain need not cause infection.
- Relapse is defined as recurrence with the same strain.
- Reinfection is defined as recurrence with a new strain or microorganism.
- Periurethral or fecal colonization with the same strain may continue after the infection is eradicated and account for the next infection. It may be difficult to distinguish reinfection from relapse unless periurethral and fecal cultures are obtained between episodes.

serotype was present in the urine repeatedly and then disappeared spontaneously without therapy.

Low-Count Bacteriuria

The standard criterion for significant bacteriuria is $>10^5$ cfu/ml. Lower
counts are found in women with the pyuria-dysuria syndrome and with
high fluid intake and frequent voiding. Serologic typing and other epidemiologic markers can be used to demonstrate the persistence of low or
borderline counts of the same strain. The first documentation, to my
knowledge, of persistent low-count bacteriuria with urinary tract infection is shown in Figure 10.8. This girl had counts as low as 10^3 cfu/ml with
the same strain of *E. coli* for over a year.

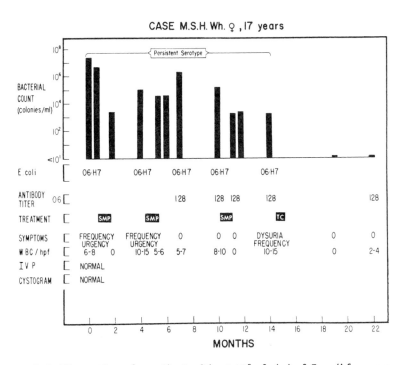

Figure 10.8. Illustration of a patient with $< 10^5$ cfu/ml of *E. coli* for more
than a year. The same serogroup was recovered repeatedly. Several episodes of
symptomatic infection did not respond to sulfonamide therapy, but finally
responded to tetracycline. This is an example of persistent low-count
bacteriuria in a child. Reproduced with permission from Kunin, Deutscher, and
Paquin (42).

E. coli Virulence Factors

Uropathogenic *E. coli* exhibit several distinct virulence factors (Table 10.3). The contribution of each factor to the pathogenesis of urinary tract infection is based on their frequency in the fecal flora, association with asymptomatic bacteriuria, cystitis, and pyelonephritis, and virulence in experimental animal models of infection. The distribution of virulence factors obtained from a large number of studies in humans is summarized in Table 10.4. Because of differences in study design, definitions and populations studied, these results must be interpreted with caution. It also must be emphasized that many uropathogenic clones carry multiple virulence factors. All of the factors listed in Table 10.4, other than type 1 fimbria, are found more often in clinical isolates than would be expected from their abundance in the feces. This indicates epidemic virulence. P-fimbria, aerobactin, hemolysin, and O groups are more often associated with pyelonephritis than cystitis or asymptomatic bacteriuria. This indicates urovirulence. Note that type 1 fimbria are found more often in cystitis than in pyelonephritis.

Fimbria and Other Adhesins in the Pathogenesis of Urinary Tract Infection

The first stage of infectious processes involves the recognition and binding of the invading microbe to the host cell. This is a highly specific step in which a specialized organelle located on the surface of the microbe attaches to a specific surface component of the host cell. For example, the host specificity of bacteriophage depends on the recognition of the molecular configuration of its tail protein by receptors on the bacterial cell wall. Similarly, the infectivity of the influenza viruses depends on hemagglutinins in their capsid, and the specificity and tissue tropism of enteroviruses are dependent on specific surface binding substances. Bacteria adhere to host cells or surfaces in a specific manner. An *adhesin* on the bacterial surface binds to a *receptor* on the host cell. Bacterial adherence allows the invading microorganisms to do the following:

Table 10.3. Virulence Factors Associated with Uropathogenic *E. coli*

Factor	Associated Characteristic
Adhesins	Fimbriae (Type 1, P, and S)
	Dr and other nonfimbrial adhesins
Serum Resistance	O antigen groups
	Colicin production (ColV), K1 and OmpA
Extracellular proteins	Hemolysin, Aerobactin, OmpT protease
	Soluble virulence factor
Resistance to Phagocytosis	Capsular polysaccharides

*Based on the reviews by Johnson (27) and Donnenberg and Welch (46).

Table 10.4. Association of Virulence Factors Among Clinical Isolates of *E. coli**

	Proportion (%) of Strains			
Virulence Factor	Pyelonephritis	Cystitis	Asymptomatic Bacteriuria	Fecal
Type 1 fimbria	60	71	58	60
P-fimbria	70	36	24	19
Aerobactin	73	49	38	41
Hemolysin	49	40	20	12
K1	32	14	22	23
Serum resistance	61	63	25	52
O group present	74	64	38	38

*Summarized from Johnson JR (27).

- Resist removal from mucosal surfaces by tears, saliva, and urine.
- Deliver toxins to receptors on cell membranes.
- Attach to target tissues distant from the point of entry.

Bacterial adherence can also be viewed as a mechanism whereby the host recognizes invading microbes and mobilizes scavenger cells to remove them before they can initiate infection. The microbe can counter this defense by turning off production of the adhesin (phase variation) and no longer be recognized by host cells.

Adhesion is determined by incubating host cells with bacteria, washing away nonadherent microbes, and counting the number that adhere per cell and the number of cells to which they adhere. Radiolabeled bacteria can also be used in a similar manner. The ability of the microbe to adhere to cells from the urothelium, intestine, mouth, vagina, or other organs provides clues concerning tissue tropisms. Bacteria-host cell interactions are determined even more readily by hemagglutination tests. Red blood cells obtained from people with different blood groups or animals provide important clues to the nature of the binding sites. The chemical configuration of the adhesins and receptors can be inferred by adding compounds that block hemagglutination.

Type 1, Mannose Sensitive Fimbria

Type 1 fimbriae are commonly found on *E. coli*. They appear to have a role in the initial colonization of the urethral and bladder. They are said to be mannose sensitive because D-mannose blocks hemagglutination and attachment to target cells (47,48). They agglutinate mannan-containing yeast and guinea pig erythrocytes and adhere to human buccal and urothelial cells. They are recognized, ingested, and killed by polymorphonuclear leukocytes (49–52). They also bind to and are inactivated by uromucoid or Tamm-Horsfall protein (THP) (53–57). THP is produced by the cells of the ascending loop of Henle and the distal convoluted tubule and contains mannose in its carbohydrate chain. Type 1 fimbria also bind to a component of vaginal mucus (58) and to constituents of cranberry and blueberry juices (59,60).

Type 1 fimbria are expressed preferentially in liquid media and undergo a process called phase-variation during which they lose their fimbria in response to changes in their environment (61). Phase variation occurs in the urine (62,63) in response to urea (64) and hypertonic conditions (65). *E. coli* rarely express type 1 fimbria in infected urine, but they appear in broth cultures. It is thought that type 1 fimbria initiate urinary tract infections by binding to urothelial cells. Once the infection is established, they shed their fimbria to avoid being recognized by THP and PMNs.

The evidence that type 1 fimbria plays an important role in initiation of urinary tract infections is based on several lines of evidence. These lines include the observations that D-mannose and related compounds block ascending infection of mice and rats by type I fimbriated *E. coli* (66), and passive immunization with monoclonal antibodies prevents ascending infection in mice (67).

Key Points About Type I Fimbria

- They are commonly present on *E. coli* found in the gut and in urinary tract infections.
- They appear to have a role in initiation of urinary tract infection by binding to urothelial cells.
- They bind to Tamm-Horsfall protein in the urine and phagocytosed by PMNs.
- They undergo phase variation and lose their fimbria in urine presumably to escape recognition.
- They bind to constituents in cranberry and blueberry juices.
- They do not appear to have special virulence for the kidney.

P-Fimbria

P-fimbria are so-named because they bind to P-blood group substances. The structures of P-fimbria as observed under the electron microscope are shown in Figures 10.9 and 10.10. They differ from type 1-fimbria in being mannose-resistant and expressed on solid rather than liquid media. The tip of P-fimbria recognizes receptors bearing Galα1→4Galβ- and GalNacβ1→3Galα1→4Galβ1- containing oligosaccharide sequences of glycolipids (Gal-Gal adhesins). They agglutinate humans' erythrocytes and bind to uroepithelial cells that possess P1 and P2 blood group substances. The p blood group is very rare and does not bind Gal-Gal fimbria. PMNs express only a trace of Gal-Gal and do bind to THP.

Expression

P-fimbria are less likely to undergo phase extensive variation in urine than are type 1 fimbria (62). The phenotypic expression of P-fimbria is blocked

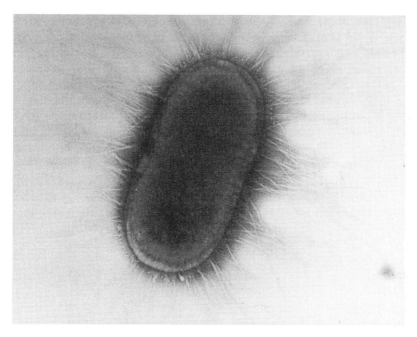

Figure 10.9. Illustration of *E. coli* P-fimbria as seen by electron microscopy. Courtesy of Lauren O. Bakaletz.

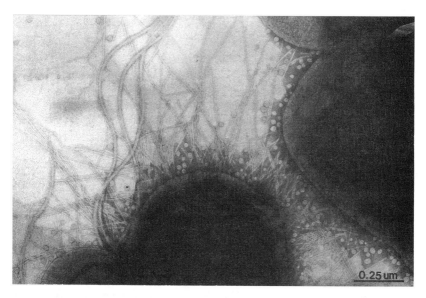

Figure 10.10. More detailed view of the tubular structure of P-fimbria on electron microscopy. The larger and longer tubular structures are flagella. Courtesy of Lauren O. Bakaletz.

by salicylate, hypertonic media, and Mar (multiple-antibiotic resistant) mutants of *E. coli* (65). The mechanism appears to be mediated through OmpF and other outer membrane proteins that are involved in osmoprotective mechanisms. *E. coli* often express both type 1 and P-fimbriae phenotypes, and mannose-resistant hemagglutination may be due to other adhesins. Therefore, specific identification requires use of specific antibodies, latex particles covalently bound to α-D-Gal(-4)- β-D-Gal-disaccharide (68) (PF TEST; Orion Diagnostica, Espoo, Finland), or hemagglutination inhibition with extracts of pigeon or cockatiel egg white (69). A remarkable amount of information is available about the synthesis, structure, and genetic control of P-fimbria (70) but is beyond the scope of this book. When reading the literature in this field, the reader is cautioned that the presence of an adhesion gene, such as *pap*G which encodes for PapG on the tip of the P-fimbria, does not necessarily mean that the PapG phenotype is expressed.

Uncomplicated Pyelonephritis
P-fimbriae are major virulence factors for acute, uncomplicated pyelonephritis in boys, girls, and adult women (Table 10.4). The elucidation of their role in the pathogenesis of urinary tract infections is the result of the work of a remarkable group of investigators in Sweden. This group includes Svanborg-Edén, Hanson, Källenius, and Winberg. Other early contributors to this field are the Ørskovs in Denmark, and O'Hanley, Schoolnik, Falkow, Hull, and Roberts in the United States. The evidence that P-fimbriae are of critical importance in the pathogenesis of uncomplicated urinary tract infections is based on elegant studies of the specificity of adherence of these strains to urothelial cells (71), the relation of the antigen to the P blood group in man (72,73), clinical-epidemiologic correlations (Table 10.4), and experimental infections in animal models (74,75). Further support for the notion that P-fimbria cause pyelonephritis is based on the finding of receptors to *E. coli* adhesins in Bowman's capsule, the glomerulus, renal tubules, and the bladder (76,77). Strains isolated from patients with pyelonephritis are internalized into human renal proximal tubular cells and enclosed in membrane-bound vacuoles (78). Bacteria with P- and type 1 fimbriae also adhere to the mucosal surface of human foreskins (79).

Bacteremia
P-fimbriated *E. coli* are frequently isolated from women with community-acquired, acute pyelonephritis and bacteremia. In one study, P-fimbriated strains were present in 100% of women with uncomplicated pyelonephritis and bacteremia compared to 71% with pyelonephritis alone (80). Non-P-fimbriated strains were found only in patients with complicated pyelonephritis and bacteremia. In a similar study, P-fimbria were found in 67% of women with acute pyelonephritis (23). There was no significant difference in the frequency of P-fimbria in patients with or without bac-

teremia, but the bacteremic patients were older and more often had complicated infections.

Complicated and Recurrent Infections

P-fimbriated strains are isolated less often in men (26), in nosocomial urinary tract infection (81), in complicated infections (82,83), and in children with vesico-ureteral reflux (84) and with renal scarring (85). The presence of P-fimbriated *E. coli* does not reliably predict the occurrence of parenchymal inflammation on DMSA scans in children (86). Several investigators have even suggested that when P-fimbriated strains are absent, underlying structural lesions should be considered. The presence of P-fimbria and other virulence factors does not reliably predict that a female is more likely to develop recurrent episodes of urinary tract infections (41,87). These observations reinforce the concept stressed throughout this book that more virulent strains are required to produce uncomplicated pyelonephritis and less virulent strains produce complicated infection. They also have important implications for the potential development of a pyelonephritis vaccine.

Animal Studies

In a brilliantly conceived and conducted study, O'Hanley, Lark, Falko, and Schoolnik (74) developed four strains of *E. coli*, each of which had different adhesion characteristics. One strain was encoded for both type I and P-fimbria, one possessed type I fimbria only, one possessed P-fimbria only, and one was a non-piliated strain. Mice were infected intravesically with each of these strains, and invasion of the kidneys was correlated with the presence or absence and type of fimbria. The strain containing both types of fimbria produced renal colonization and invasion. The strain with P-fimbria colonized the kidney but did not invade, whereas the type I fimbria strain did not colonize renal epithelium nor invade the kidney unless acute reflux was induced. Immunization with P-fimbria was protective against colonization and renal invasion by the fimbriated strains. Using immunohistologic methods, they demonstrated that the binding sites in the mouse kidney for types I and P-fimbria were located in the collecting tubular and convoluted distal tubular epithelial cells, but not in the glomerulus. Type I fimbria binding substance, which they confirmed to be Tamm-Horsfall glycoprotein, was also located in the loop of Henle.

Roberts, working with Winberg and his group (75), demonstrated that P-fimbriated *E. coli* bind to urothelial cells of rhesus monkeys and baboons in a manner similar to that in man. In experimentally induced infection, a P-fimbriated strain produced ureteral malfunction and pyelonephritis. Animals infected with P-fimbriated strains had more prolonged bacteriuria compared to those that received non-fimbriated organisms. Based on this work, they proposed that renal infection is augmented by the turbulent flow and mild reflux produced by P-fimbriated strains.

> **Key Points About P-Fimbria**
>
> • P-fimbriated *E. coli* are acquired from the bowel, colonize the urethra, grow in bladder urine, induce the release of interleukins IL-6 and IL-8 from urothelial cells, and recruit PMNs.
> • They are mannose-resistant and do not bind to Tamm-Horsfall proteins or PMNs.
> • The tip binds to urothelial cells by means of Gal-Gal receptors of the P blood group.
> • Receptors are present in the glomerulus, renal tubules, and the bladder.
> • They play a key role in producing acute, uncomplicated pyelonephritis and bacteremia in children and adult women.
> • They have a less important role in producing complicated, nosocomial, or recurrent urinary tract infections.
> • Their expression is inhibited by salicylate, Mar mutation, and osmotic stress mediated through OmpF and other outer membrane proteins.

S-Fimbria

S-fimbriated *E. coli* are characteristically associated with meningitis and bacteremia in the newborn. *E. coli* O18:K1:H7 is the most commonly isolated clone (22). Both the S-fimbria and K polysaccharide are important in producing experimental meningitis in animals (88). The S-fimbriae are mannose-resistant and bind to terminal sialyl-galactoside residues and the receptors are present in renal glomeruli, tubules, and bladder mucosal cells (89). S-fimbriated strains infrequently cause urinary tract infections, but the *sfaS* gene is more widespread. We recovered over twenty strains of nicotinamide-requiring *E. coli* O18:K1:H7 from young women with acute cystitis. Only a few of the strains expressed S-fimbria, but most of the remainder contained the *sfaS* gene (90). Detection of these strains in the stools or urine of pregnant women by their requirement for nicotinamide may be a means to prevent neonatal meningitis.

Dr, X, M, and G Adhesins

Many strains of *E. coli* express mannose-resistant hemagglutination in the absence of fimbria. They are referred to as nonfimbrial adhesins (NFA). The Dr (blood group antigen) family is associated with cystitis and diarrhea (27) and binds to a phosphatidylinositol-linked membrane glycoprotein in the regulation of the complement cascade. Other NFAs include X and M (M blood group). G adhesins are located on fimbria.

> **Key Points About S- and G-Fimbria and Dr, X, and M Adhesins**
>
> • They are mannose-resistant and can be mistaken for P-fimbriated strains.
> • Gal-Gal-coated latex particles are useful to differentiate them from P-fimbria.
> • They are associated with cystitis.
> • The S-fimbriated clone O18:K1:H7 is an important cause of neonatal bacteremia and meningitis. Early detection in stool and urine may help prevent these infections.

Is Bacterial Adhesion Necessary for Persistence of Urinary Tract Infections?

Bacterial adhesion to the urothelium is considered to be the first step in establishing infection in the bladder. Svanborg and her group (92) deliberately colonized women with a strain of *E. coli* that lacked adherence factors. Colonization with the avirulent strain protected against superinfection with the same strain transformed to express type 1 and P-fimbriae. The findings could not be explained by differences in growth rates of the strains. They wondered whether adherence might be disadvantageous because P-fimbria induces an inflammatory response that facilitates bacterial clearance. These observations are of great interest, but are open to interpretation. First of all, the natural route of infection was bypassed by instilling the strains with a catheter; second, it is possible that the avirulent strain had become adapted to grow in the bladder urine; and third, they could not, for ethical reasons, determine whether prior instillation of the virulent strain would prevent superinfection with the nonvirulent strain. The key point is that it is difficult to produce superinfection against an established strain. This point may explain why uncomplicated urinary tract infections are almost invariably caused by a single strain. This study supports the concept that asymptomatic bacteriuria provides a microbiologic barrier against acquisition of more virulent strains. This concept is an important rationale for not treating asymptomatic bacteriuria in children (93) or the elderly. Another advantage of nontreatment of asymptomatic bacteriuria is that the strains tend to lose O antigenicity and become more sensitive to the bactericidal effect of serum and less virulent over time (94).

Serum Resistance (O and K Antigens)

Many strains of gram-negative bacteria are killed by fresh human serum. Killing depends on activation of complement either through the classic or alternative pathways. Complement renders the organisms more sensitive to muramidase (lysozyme) which splits the cell wall peptidoglycan structure. Antibody is not essential for these reactions, but antibody-antigen complexes may trigger the classic complement cascade. Strains of gram-negative bacteria that are not killed by fresh serum are found more commonly in patients with gram-negative bacteremia and pyelonephritis than in the urine or feces (Table 10.4). Bacteremia caused by serum-resistant *E. coli* strains is more likely to be associated with shock and death (95). Smooth, O-typeable *E. coli* are more resistant to killing by serum than are rough, nontypeable strains. Serum resistance is related to the length of the carbohydrate side chains of the lipopolysaccharide the strains contain (96). There is also evidence that OmpA contributes to increased serum resistance (97).

Capsular Polysaccharides (K Antigens)

Capsular polysaccharides coat the surface of encapsulated *E. coli*. They interfere with detection of the O antigens, protect the bacteria from phagocytosis, and block complement fixation to the surface of the PMNs (98,99). Strains bearing K antigens are more frequent in patients with pyelonephritis than cystitis or the feces (Table 10.4). Five K antigens (1, 2, 3, 12 and 13) account for 70% of isolates from patients with acute pyelonephritis (100). Pyelonephritic strains contain larger amounts of capsular polysaccharide and are less susceptible to the bactericidal action of serum (101,102). The K1 capsule is of special interest because it is associated more frequently with pyelonephritis (Table 10.4), with uropathogenic clones (Table 10.1), and with neonatal bacteremia and meningitis. K1 is structurally similar to the capsular polysaccharide of *Neisseria meningitidis* group B. Several of the *E. coli* K antigens cross react with some Klebsiella and pneumococcal polysaccharides (103). K antigens are poor immunogens and only low levels of antibody are detectable. Immunization of experimental animals with homotypic protein conjugate vaccine protects against pyelonephritis (104).

Aerobactin and Iron Siderophores

The ability of microorganisms to acquire iron is a critical determinant of the host-parasite relationship and is linked to virulence (105). *E. coli* and other bacteria produce at least two iron chelating siderophores—enterochelin and aerobactin. These siderophores extract iron from host iron-binding proteins. Aerobactin is more important than enterochelin in pathogenesis of infection (106). It is a small molecule formed by the condensation of two lysine molecules and one citrate. *E. coli* that produce aerobactin are more common in patients with bacteremia and pyelonephritis than in asymptomatic bacteriuria or the feces (Table 10.4).

Hemolysin

E. coli expressing alpha hemolysins are found more often in patients with bacteremia and pyelonephritis than in feces or asymptomatic bacteriuria (Table 10.4) and are more virulent in experimental infections. Hemolysin lysis erythrocytes, is cytotoxic, and impairs chemotaxis and phagocytosis by PMNs (27). It provides the organism with more available iron. Hemolysin production often is associated with other virulence factors in uropathogenic *E. coli*.

Other Virulence Factors

OmpT is a protease associated with the outer membrane of *E. coli*. Few clinical isolates express this factor, but most carry the *ompT* gene (107). A soluble virulence, a factor that appears to be a quaternary amine resembling protamine, allows bacteria to adhere to the surface of the bladder mucosa of rabbits (108). Temperature-sensitive auxotrophs are not more virulent (109) and salt-tolerance does not differ among strains isolated from stool, blood, or urine (110).

Immune Response to Infection

An antibody response to surface components of the invading microorganism occurs within about 1 to 2 weeks after the onset of pyelonephritis and persists for many weeks depending on the antigen, the sensitivity of the assay system, and therapy. IgA, IgM, and IgG antibodies are synthesized by the kidney (111,112). Antibody-secreting lymphocytes to the urinary pathogen can be detected in the peripheral blood (113). Cystitis evokes a more muted or nondetectable response. Antibody coats the bacterial surface at the site of infection. The antibody-coated bacteria (ACB) are detected in the urine by immunofluorescence microscopy using anti-human IgG or IgM. The ACB test is purported to differentiate "upper" from "lower" urinary tract infections. This differentiation assumes that coating occurs only in the kidney, but it also can occur in the prostate and probably the bladder as well. I consider the test as reflecting tissue invasion in some part of the urinary tract.

The antibody response to the O antigen is type specific and is characterized by production of IgM and, to a lesser extent, by IgG classes. A fourfold rise is required for diagnostic purposes because low levels of antibody to virtually all of the O antigens are present in human serum. The O antibodies are acquired early in life in response to colonization of the gut by a variety of strains of *E. coli*. Human colostrum contains high concentrations of antibodies to *E. coli* O antigens, but antibody is not detectable in the serum of nursing human infants (114). A variety of methods is available to measure O antibodies, including agglutination, precipitation, hemagglutination of antigen-coated human erythrocytes, ELISA, and immunofluorescence.

Antibodies to fimbria, flagella proteins, outer membrane proteins, endotoxin, and ECA are also generated in response to pyelonephritis and bacteremia. The antibody response to K antigens is muted in natural infection (115). Antibody response can be measured for screening purposes by using a panel of the most frequent O antigens or preparations of common antigenic determinants such as ECA, core lipopolysaccharides (116), or outer membrane proteins (117,118). The most direct method is to use the microorganism recovered from the urine as the source of antigens.

Protective Immunity in Experimental Infections and Humans

Type-specific protection can be demonstrated in experimental animals immunized with O, K antigens or P-fimbria (74,75) and by maternal immunization with P-fimbriated, hemolysin-producing strains (119). Patients with gram-negative bacteremia have high titers of O or ECA antibody in acute serum specimens but are not protected against the development of shock or death (116). In contrast, high titers antibody against Re mutants (exposed core lipopolysaccharide) are protective. Antibodies to outer membrane proteins are also found in acute sera of patients with bacteremia (117) but do not appear to have a protective role. Thus, antibodies found in the early phase of infection probably reflect persistent infection rather than protective immunity.

   Some years ago Sanford and his associates performed a series of animal experiments that I believe provide important insights into protective immunity and the development of a vaccine to prevent pyelonephritis (120,121). Ascending and hematogenous infections were produced in rats with *E. coli, Klebsiella pneumoniae,* and *Proteus mirabilis.* The course of infection with *E. coli* was acute but self-limited and was associated with development of circulating agglutinins. After healing, the infected animals acquired type-specific resistance to the infecting strain. This finding corresponds to the course of acute, uncomplicated pyelonephritis in humans. *Klebsiella pneumonia* infections were chronic but did not elicit circulating agglutinins against encapsulated strains. This finding corresponds to the poor immune response noted with *E. coli* K antigens. Pyelonephritis due to *Proteus mirabilis* was associated with circulating agglutinins and resistance to reinfection, but the course was also chronic and associated with obstructive uropathy caused by deposition of calculi. This finding corresponds to complicated infection in humans. Thus, type specific immunity to surface antigens is protective in acute infections but not in chronic, obstructive uropathy.

Local Immune Response

The mucosal surface is the first point of contact between the microbe and the host. Local production of IgA is thought to have an important role in preventing acquisition of infection by interfering with bacterial attachment (122). Small amounts of serum-derived IgG, IgA, and immunoglobulin light chains may be found in the urine of healthy subjects. IgA is produced in response to bladder infection in rodents (123,124), in cynomolgus monkeys (125), and in patients with asymptomatic bacteriuria and symptomatic urinary tract infections (126). IgA isolated from the urine of patients with acute pyelonephritis can block the adherence of *E. coli* to human urinary tract epithelial cells (127), but proteases that cleave IgA are reported in patients with urinary tract infections (128).

   It has been difficult to demonstrate a protective role of IgA in humans because of the need to use indirect evidence. Stamey and his associates (129) and others (130, 131) have provided evidence that cervicovaginal immunoglobulins and local IgA prevent colonization of the vaginal introitus and periurethral zone with enteric bacteria. Other investigators were unable to find differences in IgA and IgG levels in cervicovaginal washings obtained from adult females with recurrent infection than controls (132) or urine (133). Furthermore, children with acute urinary tract infections mount a urinary IgA response (134) and elderly women with asymptomatic bacteriuria have elevated urinary IgA compared with controls (135). Factors other than cervicovaginal antibody appear to mediate adherence and may be responsible for why some women are more susceptible to introital colonization. The role of blood group antigens and susceptibility to infection is discussed in Chapter 11.

Antibody in Prostatic Secretions

Antigen-specific immunoglobulins of the IgA and IgG classes are present in the expressed prostatic secretions (EPS) of men with chronic *E. coli* prostatitis (136). The antibody response tends to persist after eradication of infection. The antibody response of the prostate appears to be independent of the response in serum. This supports the notion that they are synthesized locally. Antibody-coated bacteria (ACB) often are found in the urine of patients with bacterial prostatitis (137).

Cell-Mediated Immunity

Antibody-mediated immunity considers only one limb of the immunologic response to infection. Cell-mediated immunity in experimental pyelonephritis has been examined in detail by Miller and his associates in New Zealand (138). They found that ablation of cell-mediated immunity and macrophage blockade did not affect host defenses, but that cyclosporin A provoked an increase in lesion size and bacterial numbers. A leukocyte migration test was utilized by Bailey and co-workers (139) to assess the cell-mediated immunity of women with urinary tract infections. They found that increased migration occurred in six of seven patients with upper tract infection. They interpret these results to suggest defective cell-mediated immune responses to *E. coli* in patients with pyelonephritis.

Prospects for a Pyelonephritis Vaccine

It would seem reasonable to try to develop a vaccine that might prevent pyelonephritis and recurrent urinary tract infections. It is clear from the preceding sections that there are a large variety of antigens to choose among. The O antigens provide type specific protection in animal models, but they are numerous and difficult to separate from endotoxin. In addition, cystitis often is caused by rough strains that do not possess O antigens. The K antigens are fewer in number and more protective in animals, but they are poor immunogens unless linked to a protein carrier. Other potential antigens are P-fimbriae, alpha hemolysin, and outer membrane proteins. These have been shown to be protective in animals. Uehling and his group have focused their attention on developing a multi-strain vaccine made up of killed uropathogenic bacteria that can be administered by the vaginal route (140). Several vaccines composed of mixed antigens (SolcoUrovac and Uro-Vaxom) are available in Europe but are not licensed in the United States. They have not as yet been shown to be safe and effective for humans (141). The key features of an effective vaccine are listed as follows:

Key Features of Safe and Effective Vaccines

- Infection is acquired from an exogenous source.
- The host has minimal innate immunity to the microbial antigens.
- Natural infection is protective against reinfection.
- The immunogen is highly specific.
- Antibody provides a barrier to infection or neutralizes toxins.
- The rate of infection is sufficiently high to be cost-effective.
- Infection produces considerable morbidity or is life-threatening for an identifiable population.
- Immunization is superior to chemoprophylaxis.

Most of these conditions are not met in urinary tract infections. The difficulties in developing an effective vaccine are summarized as follows:

Difficulties in Developing an Effective Vaccine Against Urinary Tract Infections

Acute, uncomplicated pyelonephritis
- The condition is too sporadic and infrequent to warrant development of a vaccine.
- Renal damage is rare after an acute episode.
- Antimicrobial therapy is highly effective.

Complicated urinary tract infections and bacteremia
- Infection persists or may get worse despite the presence of large amounts of antibodies to the components of the invading microorganisms.
- Mechanical factors are paramount and need to be corrected whenever possible.
- Microbial virulence factors are much less important than in uncomplicated infections.
- They are often caused by microorganisms other than *E. coli*. A vaccine would need to protect against a wide variety of gram positive and gram negative bacteria and yeasts.

Recurrent cystitis
- Patients with recurrent urinary tract infection do not acquire natural protection against the microorganism that caused the preceding infection.
- Antimicrobial prophylaxis is highly effective in individuals with closely spaced infections.
- *E. coli* vaccines would not be expected to protect against *Staphylococcus saprophyticus*.

Uncomplicated Asymptomatic Bacteriuria
- This condition is not associated with renal damage or increased mortality in children or adults. The only indication for treatment is to prevent pyelonephritis of pregnancy.
- Asymptomatic bacteriuria protects against infection with a more virulent strain.

Clinical Trials
- The vaccine must be proven to be safe and effective for the indicated use.

In view of these numerous difficulties, it is doubtful that a safe and effective vaccine against urinary tract infections will be developed in the near future.

Nosocomial *E. Coli* Infections

E. coli is not only the most common cause of community-acquired urinary tract infections, but also the leading cause of nosocomial urinary tract infections, although to a lesser extent (143) (Table 10.5). *E. coli* are also over-represented in bacteremic nosocomial urinary tract infections. In a study conducted among chronically hospitalized men, many of whom were managed with indwelling urinary catheters, *E. coli* was present in the urine in 29% of the cases but was responsible for 46% of bacteremic urinary tract infections (144). The prevalence of virulence factors in nosocomial *E. coli* urinary tract infections is reported to be low, but many of the strains express P-fimbria and hemolysin (81). These strains may have special epidemic virulence.

Other Enterobacteriaceae

The other *Enterobacteriaceae* are for the most part opportunistic secondary invaders. Special attention will be given to Klebsiella and the genera Proteus, Morganella, and Providencia because of their special urovirulence properties and production of urease. Much less is known about the invasive properties of *Enterobacter aerogenes* and *Enterobacter cloacae*, *Citrobacter freundii* and *Serratia marcescens*. Low numbers of these bacteria are present in feces, but they appear to be held in check by the dominant fecal flora (colonization resistance). They do not appear to be able to colonize even heavily exposed

Table 10.5. Frequency of Major Microorganisms in Nosocomial Urinary Tract Infections

Pathogen	Number	Percent (%)
E. coli	11,135	26
Enterococci	6,720	16
P. aeruginosa	5,127	12
C. albicans	2,978	7
Enterobacter spp.	2,339	6
K. pneumoniae	2,664	6
P. mirabilis	2,312	5
Staphylococcus, coagulase negative	1,634	4
S. aureus	823	2
Citrobacter spp.	812	2
Candida spp.	853	2
S. marscescens	367	1
Streptococcus spp.	207	<1

Some of the patients with urinary catheters were infected with four or more species simultaneously. Data are from the National Nosocomial Infections Surveillance System 1986–1989 (142).

healthy hosts. For example, these microbes were no more frequent in the stools of nurses working in a medical intensive care unit, where there is intense use of antibiotics, than in coronary care nurses or college women (145).

Klebsiella

Klebsiella are non-motile, encapsulated gram negative rods. The principle pathologic species are *Klebsiella pneumoniae* and *Kl. oxytoca*. Klebsiella are part of the normal fecal flora, but they rarely cause uncomplicated cystitis and pyelonephritis. Primary invasive *Klebsiella pneumoniae* infection is well recognized among countries in the Pacific Rim, particularly in Taiwan (146). Sporadic cases are also reported in the United States (147,148). The disease is characterized by bacteremia, liver abscess, osteomyelitis, pyelonephritis, meningitis, and endophthalmitis. Diabetics are particularly vulnerable. The reservoir is unknown, but bacteremia is often preceded by Klebsiella urinary tract infections. The primary invasive strains are usually susceptible to first generation cephalosporins. In contrast, nosocomial Klebsiella are frequently resistant to multiple antibiotics. They are spread by contaminated urine, feces, and body secretions and are common in patients on long-term urinary catheter drainage. They are important causes of nosocomial pneumonia, hepato-biliary infections, and bacteremia. Individual strains can be characterized by over 70 different capsular (K-antigen) serotypes and by type-1 (mannose-sensitive) and type-3 fimbria. Virulence factors include surface adhesins and fimbria, capsules, O antigen-associated lipopolysaccharides, iron-scavenging systems, and urease production (149).

Proteus, Providencia, and Morganella

These are motile, urease-producing gram negative rods. They are considered together because of their similar taxonomy and invasive properties. The pathogenicity of these microorganisms is closely linked to the production of urease. Urease catalyses the hydrolysis of urea to yield ammonia and carbamate. Carbamate decomposes to form another molecule of ammonia and carbonic acid. This reaction results in an increase in urine pH and precipitation of coffin-shaped struvite crystals ($MgNH_4PO_4 \cdot 6H_2O$). The crystals aggregate in urine and produce infection stones. These stones are deposited in the renal pelvis, ureters, bladder, and around the surface of urinary catheters (see Figure 8.7). The concretions obstruct urine flow and can produce severe renal damage. There is also evidence that ammonia may directly damage the kidney and urothelium (150, 151). Hyperammonemia with encephalopathy may occur in patients with Proteus infections, in the absence of liver disease, when the urinary stream is diverted into the bowel, or when there is marked stasis such as in a ureterocele or hypotonic bladder (152–154).

The clinically important species include *Proteus mirabilis, Proteus vulgaris, Morganella morganii, Providencia stuartii,* and *Providencia rettgeri. Proteus mirabilis* is responsible for about 80% to 90% of urinary infections caused by this group. It is reported to be common in uncircumcised boys in Europe (155) but not in the United States (156). *Proteus mirabilis* accounts for only a small proportion of community-acquired urinary tract infections, but it has a special predilection to ascend to the kidneys and produce pyelonephritis. For this reason, it should be eradicated whenever possible even in the asymptomatic patient. *Proteus mirabilis* is usually susceptible to beta lactam antibiotics and aminoglycosides, but it may be exceedingly difficult to clear once the microorganisms are established within urinary calculi. Lithotripsy or pyelolithotomy can be used to extract the larger stones, but small calculi imbedded in the renal parenchyma are usually impossible to remove. The other species are important causes of nosocomial and urinary catheter-associated infections.

Proteus mirabilis virulence factors include urease production, capsule polymers that enhance formation of calculi (157), cytotoxic hemolysin, mannose resistant fimbriae, PMF (fimbriae), flagella, siderophores, and an IgA-degrading metalloprotease. Mobley (151) proposes that urinary tract infection with *Proteus mirabilis* is initiated by attachment of the microorganism to the bladder via PMF (fimbriae). Highly flagellated swarmer cells ascend the ureters to the kidney and bind specifically to the renal epithelium. A renal microenvironment is formed consisting of a biofilm of microbes and struvite matrix. Renal tissues are damaged by ammonia and hemolysin and the bacteria are internalized by renal tubular epithelial cells. Novel methods, in addition to antimicrobial therapy, are needed to block this complex series of events. Acetohydroxamic acid is a urease inhibitor that blocks ammonia production in experimental animals (158). We found that salicylates block expression of flagella in *E. coli, Proteus mirabilis,* and *Providencia stuartii* (159).

Key Points About Urease-Producing Microorganisms

- Urease splits urea into ammonia and carbonic acid.
- Ammonia produces an alkaline urine resulting in precipitation of struvite crystals.
- The crystals aggregate with the microorganism and urine matrix to produce infection stones and encrustations on catheters and cause urinary obstruction.
- The major microorganisms that produce urease include: Proteus, Providencia, Morganella, *Klebsiella pneumoniae, Staphylococcus saprophyticus, Corynebacterium urealyticum,* and *Mycoplasma urealyticum.*
- Once the stones form, they are exceedingly difficult to remove completely and may be a nidus for persistent infection.

Shigella

These bacteria are closely related to *E. coli* as shown by DNA-DNA hybridization. It is therefore not surprising to find that they produce urinary tract infections. We isolated a strain of *Shigella sonnei in* 1 of 122 school girls with asymptomatic bacteriuria (42). Sporadic cases caused by *Shigella sonnei* and *Shigella flexneri* continue to be reported in the literature (161–163). The patients may have asymptomatic bacteriuria, cystitis, and uncomplicated pyelonephritis without dysentery. Strains isolated from new cases should be saved to determine whether they possess *E. coli* virulence factors.

Salmonella

The Salmonella include *S. typhi,* the causative agent of typhoid fever, the invasive serotypes *S. choleraesuis, S. paratyphi* A and *S. typhimurium,* and well over 1,000 other serologic types associated with gastroenteritis. *S. typhi* can be transiently isolated from the urine in patients with typhoid fever and the chronic carrier state. Invasive urinary tract infections are usually associated with structural abnormalities or bilharzia (164, 165). Gastroenteritis-causing serotypes can produce prostatitis, epididymo-orchitis, pyelonephritis, renal and perinephric abscesses, and bacteremia. Severe infections have been noted after prostatectomy (164), renal transplantation (166–168) obstructive uropathy and nephrolithiasis (169–171), in diabetics (172), homosexuals (173, 174), and patients with systemic lupus erythematosus (175). Alterations in both immune and structural defenses of the urinary tract most likely increase susceptibility to Salmonella, but the exact nature of the pathogenesis of these infections is unknown. The key point is that an underlying structural lesion should be suspected in patients with Salmonella urinary tract infections.

Other Gram Negative Bacteria

Pseudomonas

Pseudomonas spp. are opportunistic, environmental microorganisms found in soil, water, and food. Most pseudomonads are motile and possess one or more polar flagella. They are usually colored by a greenish-blue pigment, pyocyanin. Unlike Proteus, they do not produce urease. Their occurrence in human disease is closely related to the selective pressure of antimicrobial drugs in structurally compromised and leukopenic patients. *Pseudomonas aeruginosa* is the predominant species and is isolated more often than *P. fluorescens* and *P. putida* from patients with respiratory problems, urinary tract infections, and burns. *Pseudomonas aeruginosa* grows well in urine and is a common cause of catheter-associated infections (176). It is the third most common bacterial species in nosocomial urinary tract infections (Table 10.5). *Pseudomonas* bacteriuria and tissue infections tend to persist even after urinary drainage devices are removed. Suppurative infections may extend to the kidney and involve adjacent structures such as the urethral glands, prostate, and epididymis. There may be bacteremia and metastatic infection. Vertebral osteomyelitis is an important complication.

Pseudomonas aeruginosa can be traced for epidemiologic studies by pyocyanin, phage, serologic types, and modern molecular methods (Table 10.2). A variety of virulence factors have been identified (177). These include adhesins and fimbriae, protease, hemolysin, phospholipase C, and several exotoxins. Pyoverdin is an iron siderophore that appears to be essential for virulence (178). It is not clear which of these virulence factors are most important in urinary tract infections.

Outbreaks of *Pseudomonas* urinary tract infections on urologic services have been traced to contaminated irrigation solutions and instruments. The organism grows well in solutions of hexachlorophene or benzalkonium chloride. Corrective measures include use of alkalinized glutaraldehyde or iodophor solutions or gas sterilization. One outbreak, caused by Pseudomonas EO-1, was traced to contaminated commercially packaged urinary catheter kits. Cross infection with a particular epidemic strain of *Pseudomonas* is common among paraplegic patients and patients in long-term care facilities. The reservoirs are contaminated urine found in condom catheters, catheter drainage bottles, and bedpans. Serotypes 1,6, and 11 are particularly common nosocomial strains. Spread appears to occur both by the hands of patients and health care personnel and by fluids and inanimate objects. Meticulous bathing with bar soap will not eliminate colonization.

Ciprofloxacin and other quinolones are promoted heavily for treatment of *Pseudomonas* infections. Resistant strains rapidly emerge, as expected, because host factors that favor these infections have not changed. The frequency of antibiotic-resistant bacteria on a urologic ward can be reduced by decreasing antibiotic consumption. Several cases of acute cystitis caused by *Pseudomonas aeruginosa* have been traced to hot whirlpool tubs (see "Environmental Factors" in Chapter 4).

Acinetobacter

Acinetobacter spp. are opportunistic enteric gram negative bacteria. They are generally rod shaped, but can appear coccoid and be mistaken for Neisseria. They are important causes of hospital-associated infections in wounds, drainage sites, and long-term urinary catheters. Their reservoir is feces, skin, food, and water.

Hemophilus

Haemophilus influenzae and *H. parainfluenzae* are usually considered to be respiratory pathogens, but are also known to cause prostatitis, epididymo-orchitis, cystitis, and pyelonephritis in both children and adults (179–193). Hemophilus also causes female genital infections, including intrauterine device-associated endometritis, salpingitis, cervicovaginitis, and Bartholin's gland abscess. They may be sexually transmitted (192), particularly in homosexual men (193). Some of the strains are encapsulated type b, but nonencapsulated strains biotype 4 are more frequent (192). Non-typeable *Hemophilus influenzae* bind to respiratory mucins (194). Cervico-vaginal and bladder mucous may play a role in genital and urinary tract infections. Hemophilus do not grow well in standard urine culture media. For this reason, *gram stain of the urine should be performed in all patients with sterile pyuria.*

Gardnerella

Gardnerella vaginalis is an important cause of nonspecific vaginitis, but it is much more difficult to delineate its role in urinary tract infections. *Gardnerella vaginalis* requires anaerobic incubation in enriched medium and survives poorly in urine at 37°C (195). It is commonly found in the male urethra and in sperm and appears to be sexually transmitted. It can cause balanoposthitis and urethritis in men and has been occasionally isolated from patients with prostatitis and pyelonephritis (196–200). Fairley and his associates have provided evidence that it causes cystitis and pyelonephritis, especially in pregnant women (201, 202). It is usually a vaginal contaminant and an uncommon urinary tract pathogen (203).

Key Points About *Gardnerella vaginalis*

- It may be present in large numbers in the vagina and readily contaminate the urine.
- Pus cells may originate in the vagina and be confused with pyuria.
- It does not grow well in urine.
- The quantitative count of this microorganism in voided urine is unreliable and needs to be confirmed by catheterization.
- Small numbers found on suprapubic aspiration may represent reflux of microorganisms from the urethra.
- It can cause urethritis, balanoposthitis and prostatitis in males.
- Well documented cases of urinary tract infection and pyelonephritis are rare.

Vibrio, Campylobacter, and Other Unusual Gram Negative Bacteria

Isolated cases of urinary tract infections have been described with unusual bacteria. These cases include *Vibrio cholerae* in a woman who had been swimming in the Chesapeake Bay (204); *Campylobacter jejuni* urinary tract infection in a young girl without diarrhea (205) and an elderly man with prostatitis (206); and with *Escherichia vulneres* (207), *Oligella urethralis* (208) and *Rahnella aquatilis* (209). It is expected that urinary tract infections with unusual microorganisms will continue to be reported in immunosuppressed patients, patients with AIDS, and renal transplant recipients.

Gram Positive Bacteria

Gram positive bacteria are almost as important as gram negative bacteria as causal agents of urinary tract infections. *Staphylococcus saprophyticus* is the second most common cause of uncomplicated cystitis and pyelonephritis in females. Enterococci are the second most common cause of nosocomial urinary tract infections. Together with the staphylococci they account for about 23% of hospital-acquired urinary tract infections (Table 10.5). *Staphylococcus aureus* is a major cause of hematogenous pyelonephritis. The relatively newly recognized species *Corynebacterium urealyticum* is an important cause of infection stones. The important role of gram positive bacteria justifies culturing urine routinely on blood agar plates or other media that support the growth of these microorganisms. It also renders the term "bacilluria" obsolete because most of the gram positive urinary pathogens are cocci. The more general term "bacteriuria" is preferable and is used throughout this book.

Staphylococci

Staphylococci pathogenic for humans are divided into coagulase positive *Staphylococcus aureus* and a large number of species of coagulase-negative staphylococci. The coagulase-negative staphylococci are differentiated on the basis of phenotypic characteristics and DNA homology. *Staphylococcus aureus* is most often associated with blood-stream invasion, *Staphylococcus epidermidis* with nosocomial infections, and *Staphylococcus saprophyticus* with uncomplicated acute cystitis and pyelonephritis in young adult females. Staphylococci account for about 6% of nosocomial urinary tract infections (Table 10.5).

Staphylococcus aureus

Staphylococcus aureus is a highly virulent organism. It can produce generalized infection and bacteremia after invasion of the skin, subcutaneous tissue, wounds, bone, and lung. Staphylococcal bacteremia, in turn, can cause endocarditis and multifocal abscesses in bone, soft tissues, and the kidney. Important sources of nosocomial infection are indwelling vascular and urinary catheters. In one large study of patients with *Staphylococcus aureus* bacteremia, the microorganism was isolated from the urine in pure culture at counts >10^5 cfu/ml in 27% of patients (210). In another study, the rate of secondary bacteremia among hospitalized patients with *Staphylococcus aureus* bacteriuria was 5.5% (211). Diabetics are particularly susceptible to pyelonephritis with this microorganism (see Fig. 8.5).

In the preantibiotic era, *Staphylococcus aureus* was the leading cause of hematogenous infection of the kidney (212). It continues to be an important cause of prostatic, renal, and perinephric abscesses. The classic signs and symptoms of sepsis and urinary infection may be absent. Their absence may delay diagnosis until the appearance of unexplained bacteremia, renal and perinephric masses, paraspinous abscesses, or osteomyelitis. Bacteriuria appears when the abscesses penetrate the renal tubules. Gram stain of the urine provides an important clue to the diagnosis as illustrated by the following case. A discussion of the virulence factors of *Staphylococcus aureus* is beyond the scope of this book.

An Illustrative Case
The patient was a 45-year-old intravenous drug addict. About a year before admission he underwent a spinal fusion for a ruptured intervertebral disc.

The site became infected with *Staphylococcus aureus* and he was treated with β lactam antibiotics for 6 weeks. About 3 months before admission he developed pain in his left hip. He was seen on multiple occasions in emergency rooms, but he was not admitted because he remained afebrile and did not have leukocytosis. The sedimentation rate was 50 mm on one occasion. Radiographs and CT scan of his left hip were interpreted as old osteoarthritis. He was finally admitted because of persistent hip pain. He was afebrile and had no other complaints. The examination was unremarkable except for thrombosed veins and skin pop marks and pain on movement of the left hip and the adjacent soft tissues. There were no heart murmurs. There was no swelling, tenderness, or erythema in the left thigh. There were >50 WBCs and WBC casts on urinalysis. Gram stain of the urine revealed numerous gram positive cocci in clusters. *Staphylococcus aureus* was isolated from the urine and blood. An MRI scan showed extensive destruction of the left acetabulum, femoral head, and surrounding soft tissue. The kidneys were diffusely enlarged by renal ultrasound without definite evidence of abscesses.

This case illustrates the sometime insidious nature of disseminated *Staphylococcus aureus* infections and the key role of the sedimentation rate, microscopic examination of the urine, and the MRI scan to help make the diagnosis.

Coagulase-negative Staphylococci

The most clinically significant species include *Staphylococcus epidermidis, S. saprophyticus, S. haemolyticus, S. lugdunensis, S. cohni, S. warnii, S. schlieferi, S. intermedius,* and *S. hyicus.* For epidemiologic studies, individual strains can be characterized by susceptibility to antibiotics, phage typing, and molecular markers (Table 10.2). *Staphylococcus saprophyticus* is identified presumptively by resistance to novobiocin, but other less common species share this property. Characteristics such as phosphatase production, fermentation of sugars, and colonial morphology are used for more specific identification.

Coagulase-negative staphylococci are part of the normal urethral flora. They commonly colonize the fossa navicularis of the male urethra and may contaminate the ejaculate and expressed prostatic secretions obtained from patients suspected of having chronic prostatitis. The principle importance of the coagulase negative staphylococci, other than *S. saprophyticus,* is as secondary invaders in patients with complicated urinary tract infections and indwelling urinary catheters. They account for about 4% of nosocomial urinary tract infections (Table 10.5). *Staphylococcus epidermidis* is the most common species, isolated from urine in about 70% of cases, and is frequently resistant to many antimicrobial drugs. We examined the distribution of staphylococci adherent to urinary catheters at the time they were removed (213). *Staphylococcus epidermidis* accounted for 70.2%

of coagulase-negative staphylococci followed by *S. hominis* (16.9%), *S. haemolyticus* (10.8%), and a few isolates of *S. cohni* and *S. warnii*. *S. saprophyticus* was not found even though most of the patients were young women.

Coagulase-negative staphylococci do not grow as rapidly as *E. coli or S. aureus* in urine or routine culture media (213,214). Quantitative bacterial counts should be considered significant, even though present at $<10^5$ cfu/ml, when the organism is recovered repeatedly or obtained from a catheter or suprapubic aspirate.

Staphylococcus saprophyticus

This species has received a great deal of attention because of its remarkable prevalence among young women with acute urinary tract infections. Torres Pereira is credited with identifying the first cases in 1962 (215). He described 40 patients, mostly women, with urinary tract infection caused by coagulase-negative staphylococcus 51. His work was preceded by an earlier report by Hellström in 1938 (216) who described renal and ureteral stones caused by *Staphylococcus albus*. He noted that "the staphylococci had the capacity to split urea, although to a varying degree." Urease production is one of the important characteristics of *Staphylococcus saprophyticus.*

Staphylococcus saprophyticus is the second most common cause of urinary tract infections in young adult women, accounting for about 6% to 30% or more of cases depending on the clinical setting and time of year (217–220). The clinical presentation and findings in the urine are indistinguishable from acute cystitis and pyelonephritis caused by *E. coli*. When tested, many of the patients will have defects in urinary concentrating ability and antibody-coated bacteria (ACB) suggestive of tissue invasion (219,221). Infection with this microorganism almost always occurs in outpatients and is a rare cause of nosocomial infection (220). It can cause nephrolithiasis (216–222), prostatitis, bacteremia and sepsis (223–225), and endocarditis (226).

The reservoir of infection is not established. In one study (227), 6.9% of women were found to be colonized. The rectum was the most frequent site, followed by the urethra, urine, and cervix. None of the women developed urinary tract infections over the next 6 months. *Staphylococcus saprophyticus* has been isolated from carcasses of slaughtered pigs, cattle, or goats and may be acquired by eating contaminated meat (220). Both colonization and clinical infections are more frequent in the summer and fall. It does not appear to be a sexually transmitted disease, but infection has been described in males. The virulence factors include adherence to urothelial cells by means of a surface-associated protein, lipoteichoic acid, a hemagglutinin that binds to fibronectin, a hemolysin, and extracellular slime (220).

Key Points About Staphylococcus Infections

Staphylococcus aureus
- *Staphylococcus aureus* remains a major cause of hematogenous pyelonephritis, perinephric, and prostatic abscesses.
- Bacteriuria occurs in about a quarter of cases of bacteremia and provides an important clue to the diagnosis.
- Secondary bacteremia from the urinary tract is less common—5.5% in one series.

Coagulase-negative Staphylococci*
- They commonly colonize the urethra in both males and females.
- They cause about 4% of nosocomial urinary tract infections.
- *Staphylococcus epidermidis* accounts for about 70% of the isolates.
- They often are resistant to multiple antibiotics.
- They should not be treated in patients with urinary catheters unless there is evidence of systemic infection.

*Other than *Staphylococcus saprophyticus*

Staphylococcus saprophyticus
- It is the second most common cause of acute cystitis and pyelonephritis in young women.
- Signs and symptoms of infection are indistinguishable from those of *E. coli* infections.
- Recurrent urinary tract infections should be anticipated.
- They occur all during the year round with peaks in the summer and fall.
- Reservoir is the large bowel; contaminated meat is a possible source.
- They rarely cause nosocomial infections and are uncommon in males.
- Urease production predisposes to urinary calculi.
- Presumptive diagnosis is based on novobiocin-resistance, but is not unique to this species.
- They are susceptible to most antimicrobial drugs used to treat urinary tract infections.

Streptococci

The two important streptococci that cause urinary tract infections are *Streptococcus agalactiae* (group B) and the genus *Enterococcus*. The group B streptococcus is commonly found in the periurethral area and is usually considered to be a contaminant unless present in large numbers in the urine. It is an important cause of neonatal sepsis and can produce bacteremia and pyelonephritis in infants, and in adults with diabetes and with urinary obstruction (228–230). Pneumococcuria is described in adults with urinary symptoms and bacteremia but appears to be transient and does not appear to require specific therapy other than for the underlying disease (231).

Enterococci

Enterococci are part of the normal fecal flora. The two most common species in humans are *Enterococcus faecalis* and *Enterococcus faecium*. They are the second most common cause of nosocomial urinary tract infections (Table 10.5).

Most urinary infections with these microbes are catheter-related. *Enterococcus faecalis* is by far the more common species. Enterococci may be uropathogenic because of salt tolerance and ability to grow in urine. Other virulence factors are aggregation substance that enhances adherence to matrix proteins and a hemolytic cytolysin (220). The increasing frequency of nosocomial enterococcal infections is caused by the selective pressure of cephalosporins and other antibiotics (232). *Enterococcus faecalis* is often susceptible to ampicillin and nitrofurantoin, but ampicillin, gentamicin, and vancomycin-resistant strains pose major therapeutic problems (233–236). This is of critical concern because the enterococci can cause subacute bacterial endocarditis, particularly in males with prostatic obstruction. Catheterized patients should not be treated unless there is evidence of systemic infection.

Corynebacteria urealyticum

Corynebacteria urealyticum is a gram positive, aerobic, non-spore-forming, slow-growing, urea-splitting, multi-antibiotic-resistant bacterium. It was first reported in 1985 as Corynebacterium group D2 by Soriano and his associates in Spain (237,238). Since then it has been reported in several other countries, including the United States (239–241). The remarkable features of this microorganism are its ability to produce urease and cause encrusted cystitis, struvite calculi, and even urethral encrustation (240). The microorganism colonizes the skin (242) and may produce cutaneous infections at sites of intravenous catheters (243), bacteremia in association with Hickman catheters (244), and pneumonia in immunocompromised hosts. It is susceptible to ofloxacin, doxycycline, rifampin, vancomycin, and teicoplanin, but resistant to most other antimicrobial drugs (245). Treatment of encrusted cystitis requires surgery, prolonged antimicrobial therapy, and the urease inhibitor, acetohydroxamic acid (246). Fortunately, infections with the microorganism are thus far rare in the United States (241).

Key Points About Gram Positive Urinary Tract Infections

- They account for about a quarter of all cases of nosocomial urinary tract infections.
- The gram stain provides rapid presumptive identification and must be interpreted within the clinical context:
    Acute uncomplicated infections—*Staphylococcus saprophyticus*
    Systemic infections—*Staphylococcus aureus*
    Urinary calculi—*Staphylococcus saprophyticus* and *Corynebacterium urealyticum*
    Nosocomial infections—Enterococci, coagulase-negative staphylococci and *Staphylococcus aureus*
    Unusual infections—Group B streptococci, *Streptococcus pneumoniae*
- *Corynebacterium urealyticum* grows slowly and may be missed on routine culture.

Anaerobes

Strict (obligate) anaerobic bacteria do not grow or survive in the presence of atmospheric oxygen. For clinical purposes, they can be divided into anaerobic gram negative bacilli (Bacteroides and Fusobacteria), anaerobic gram negative cocci (Veillonella), anaerobic gram-positive cocci (Peptostreptococcus), gram-positive spore-forming rods (Clostridia), and gram-positive non-spore forming bacilli (Propionibacterium and Eubacterium). They are commensal microorganisms of the gut, vagina, and periurethral flora. They rarely produce urinary tract infections unless there is tissue necrosis or foreign bodies. They can produce periurethral abscesses, cowperitis, Bartholin cystitis, emphysematous cystitis, epididymo-orchitis, prostatitis, pyelonephritis, and perinephric abscess (247,248). Transient bacteremia may occur with urinary instrumentation. Anaerobic infections usually consist of a mixture of several species of anaerobic and aerobic microorganisms. Anaerobes grow poorly in urine presumably because urine contains oxygen at concentrations slightly lower than venous blood (249,250).

Suprapubic punctures may be needed to make a definitive diagnosis of anaerobic urinary tract infections because of ready contamination from the periurethral zone (251). At times the diagnosis may be made by gram stain of voided urine. This may reveal large numbers of Clostridia in patients with emphysematous cystitis (252) or on occasion sulfur granules, denoting the presence of Actinomycosis (253).

Urinary infections due to anaerobes should be suspected in patients with pyuria in whom routine urine cultures are negative and have suppurative complications of long-standing infection. *This is another reason why the Gram stain is an extremely useful diagnostic test and should be done routinely in patients with unexplained pyuria.*

L-forms and Protoplasts

Bacteria may exist in forms other than the classic coccus or bacillus whose shape is limited by a rigid, relatively osmotically resistant cell wall. Morphologic variants termed "L-forms," "phase variants," or "protoplasts" may be formed when the cell-wall structure is weakened by β lactam antibiotics and enzymes, such as lysozyme or lysostaphin, that attack the wall. These forms usually assume bizarre shapes and are osmotically fragile. They retain the ability to grow and multiply in hypertonic media. L-forms or protoplasts are induced during the course of treatment of urinary tract infections with drugs that interfere with cell-wall synthesis. The high osmolality of urine within the kidney and collecting system protects them from destruction (254,255).

L-forms or protoplasts have been shown to be responsible for some human cases of recurrent urinary tract infection, particularly with Proteus

(256). In vivo conversion of classic bacteria to L-forms occurs in chronic enterococcal pyelonephritis in rats (257). The microorganisms can be eradicated by erythromycin (257) or water diuresis (258).

The clinical significance of L-forms and protoplast formation is not entirely clear. The phenomenon is real and may account for some episodes of relapse in patients treated with β lactam antibiotics. The most reasonable maneuver is to treat the relapse with a non-β lactam antibiotic. This treatment is much simpler and probably more effective than water diuresis.

It is important to keep an open mind about the possibility that hitherto unknown microorganisms can produce urinary tract infections. Cryptic bacterial forms and dormant microbes have been described in renal immunologic diseases and interstitial cystitis (259,260). More work needs to done in this field.

Mycoplasma

Mycoplasma urealyticum

Mycoplasmas are small pleomorphic microorganisms with a cell membrane, but without a cell wall. The major two species that colonize the urogenital tract are *Mycoplasma hominis* and *Ureaplasma urealyticum*. These microorganisms are common in the vagina of healthy women and have been implicated in intrauterine and pelvic infections. *Ureaplasma urealyticum*, as its name implies, splits urea, alkalinizes the urine, and produces struvite calculi. It has been recovered from patients with infection stones (261), prostatitis (262,263), and urinary tract infections (264,265). It has been localized to the upper urinary tract in patients with sterile pyuria, reflux nephropathy, pregnancy, and renal allograft recipients (266). Large inocula instilled into the bladder of rats can produce ascending pyelonephritis. Viable organisms can be isolated from the kidney, and the infection exhibits a humoral response (267). Experimental infection can also be produced in dogs (268).

Mycobacteria

Infection of the kidney due to *M. tuberculosis* should be considered in patients with unexplained persistent hematuria and pyuria, particularly in those with healed or active tuberculosis at another site or with AIDS. Atypical mycobacteria (*M. kansasii, M. avium-intracellulare*) usually produce more generalized infections in immunocompromised hosts, but may invade or obstruct the kidney (269,270). The cardinal signs of genitourinary tuberculosis are distortion of the renal collecting system, renal calcification, and ureteral strictures (271,272). The tuberculin test may be negative in patients with miliary tuberculosis, AIDS, and the elderly. Tuberculosis can involve the prostate, epididymis, ureters, testes, bladder, and seminal vesicles (273,274).

BCG therapy for bladder cancer can result in disseminated infection and osteomyelitis (275,276).

The diagnosis is based on clinical suspicion and confirmed by culture of the urine. Three clean morning urine specimens should be submitted for culture. The highest yield is obtained with the first specimen and falls off rapidly thereafter. Nephrectomy need not be done even for the nonfunctioning kidney unless there is intractable pain, major urinary hemorrhage, suspicion of renal malignancy, or when the disease is refractory to, or the patient is intolerant of, chemotherapy. Ureteral stenosis is an important complication of renal tuberculosis and may occur during the course of therapy. It is recommended that intravenous urography or renal ultrasound examinations be obtained periodically during follow-up.

Antimicrobial chemotherapy is highly effective provided that the microbe is susceptible. Three drugs were customarily given for 2 years in the past, but shorter periods have been reported to be effective (277). The combinations include isoniazid, ethambutol, pyrazinamide, streptomycin, and rifampin, depending on the susceptibility of the invading microorganism.

Yeasts and Fungi

Urinary tract infections with these microorganisms can be divided for clinical purposes into those caused by Candida and related yeasts (candidiasis), opportunistic fungi (mucormycosis, aspergillosis), and systemic fungi (histoplasmosis, blastomycosis, coccidioidomycosis, cryptococcosis). They cause urinary tract infections in special clinical settings (278–280) (Table 10.6).

Candida

The genus Candida includes more than 80 species. The important members that cause urinary tract infections include *Candida albicans, C. glabrata (Torulopsis glabrata), C. tropicalis* and *C. parapsilosis, C. quilliermondii,* and *C. krusei. Candida albicans* accounts for over half of urinary tract infections. *C. glabrata* is responsible for another quarter to a third. *Candida* spp. are the fourth most common cause of nosocomial urinary tract infections (Table 10.5). The diagnosis is readily made by finding gram positive, budding yeasts in the urine. Identification of individual members of the genus is accomplished by the germ tube test and biochemical reactions. *Candida albicans* produces pseudohyphae and true hyphae when invading tissue. Torulopsis does not produce pseudohyphae. In experimental *Candida* infection in mice, pseudohyphae grow within the renal tubule and can reinvade the parenchyma at a distant site (281,282). Candida may also form large mycelial clumps or "fungus balls" (283–286). These may obstruct the renal pelvis, ureters, and bladder, particularly in diabetics and neonates. *Candida* can produce gas, ethanol, and can cause pneumaturia (287).

Table 10.6. Risk Factors for Yeast and Fungal Infections of the Urinary Tract*

Type of Infection	Risk Factors
CANDIDIASIS—*Candida albicans, Candida glabrata and other Candida* spp.	
Ascending infections of the bladder and kidneys; obstructing fungus balls in the ureter and bladder.	Urinary catheters and drainage tubes, obstructive uropathy, diabetes, females, antibacterial therapy, extremes of age and renal transplantation.
Metastatic infection to the kidney	Neutropenia, intravascular catheters, intravenous drug use, burns, recent abdominal or thoracic surgery and systemic infection.
MUCORMYCOSIS—*Rhizopus, Rhizomucor, Absidia*	
Invasive renal and genital mucormycosis	Diabetes with ketoacidosis, corticosteroids, and alcoholism.
ASPERGILLOSIS—*Aspergillus fumigatis, Aspergillus flavus, Aspergillus niger*	
Renal aspergilloma, obstructing fungus balls, invasive infection of the kidney.	Diabetes, AIDS, cancer chemotherapy, corticosteroids and obstructive uropathy.
SYSTEMIC MYCOSES—*Histoplasma capsulatum, Blastomyces dermatitidis, Coccidioides immitis, Cryptococcus neoformans*	
Penile infection, prostatitis, epididymitis, orchitis and pyelonephritis.	Disseminated infections in apparently healthy hosts, AIDS, immunosuppression, and corticosteroids.

*Based on recent reviews (278–280).

Candida spp. are part of the normal flora of the gastrointestinal tract and are commonly found in the vagina and skin. They are widespread in nature and can be recovered from soil and plants. Invasive infection rarely occurs unless the normal microbial flora is altered by antimicrobial drugs or host resistance is decreased by diabetes, granulocytopenia, glucocorticosteroids, and immunosuppressive agents, or the skin and mucous membranes are bypassed by intravascular or urinary devices (Table 10.6).

Ascending infection is the most common route, particularly in patients with indwelling urinary catheters. The infection is usually limited to the bladder, but may progress to ulceration and the bladder, ureter and renal pelvis, and, in rare instances, to formation of fungus balls that can obstruct the urinary tract. Asymptomatic infection need not be treated. Eradication of *Candida* may result in superinfection with more virulent gram negative enteric bacteria when the catheter remains in place. The catheter should be removed whenever possible. Treatment should be reserved for patients with symptomatic infection.

Candiduria may be the first clue to disseminated *hematogenous infection* in a febrile patient with prolonged leukopenia or an intravascular line. Parenteral hyperalimentation is responsible for major outbreaks of *Candida* sepsis. The kidneys are involved frequently in systemic candidiasis. Usually there are multiple renal abscesses with intense leukocytic reaction and mycelia in the renal tubules. Systemic candidiasis is a life threatening infection. It requires early diagnosis, removal of the lines, and prompt therapy.

Blood cultures may be negative in about half of the patients with disseminated Candida infection. A search for surrogate markers such as arabinitol and other metabolites, antigens, and humoral antibodies is promising but often unsuccessful (288–291). Mannan, the major capsular material, can be detected by ELISA or gas-liquid chromatography. Antibodies to the organism are measured by immunoprecipitant, counter immunoelectrophoresis, ELISA, and other serologic methods. The major problems are the lack of a standardized antigen and the presence of low levels of antibody in uninfected subjects.

The diagnosis of *Candida* urinary tract infection is based on recovery of the organism from the urine. The differentiation between hematogenous and ascending infection usually is determined by the clinical setting and presence of Candidemia (Table 10.6). Localization of infection using the antibody-coated method is not satisfactory because *Candida* bind immunoglobulins nonspecifically.

The quantitative count is helpful in differentiating between contaminants (from the vagina or perineum) and significant candiduria. *Candida* grows well in urine and is expected to reach counts of $> 10^5$ cfu/ml. Some authors have proposed that counts of $<10^5$ cfu/ml should be considered significant (279). It is reasonable to make a presumptive diagnosis of candiduria with counts of $<10^5$ cfu/ml provided that the organism is isolated repeatedly from clean-catch specimens or obtained by urethral or suprapubic catheters. Any number of *Candida* in the urine should be considered significant in patients at high risk of hematogenous infection.

Opportunistic Fungus Infections

Aspergillus spp. most often invade the lung in immunocompromised, diabetic, and granulocytopenic patients. The infection may extend to the brain, liver, and kidneys. Renal involvement includes formation of aspergillomas, urinary tract fungus balls, and invasive infection similar to disseminated candidiasis (292–296). Mucormycosis is associated with penile necrosis and invasive renal infection, particularly in patients with poorly controlled diabetes mellitus and in alcoholics (297–300). Sporotrichosis has been described in a renal transplant recipient (301). Nocardia is not a fungus, but can produce invasive infections of the kidney (302).

Systemic Mycoses

Blastomycosis may involve the prostate and epididymis in otherwise normal hosts (303, 304). The kidney is rarely involved. The organism may be isolated directly from the urine or prostatic secretions or cultured from biopsy specimens. The presenting findings are dysuria and difficulty in urination with "sterile" pyuria.

Coccidioidomycosis usually is localized to epididymis and prostate but can cause renal abscesses (305–309). The initial presentation may be painful scrotal swelling with a draining perineal draining sinus. Small numbers of the organism can be recovered from the urinary sediment of infected patients.

Histoplasmosis also causes infections of the penis, epididymitis, and prostatitis and can involve the kidney as part of disseminated disease in compromised hosts and in patients with AIDS (310, 311).

Cryptococcosis can produce extensive involvement of the kidneys in patients treated with corticosteroids, with lymphoma, and in renal transplant recipients (312–314). An important feature in some cases is papillary necrosis associated with budding yeasts in the collecting ducts.

Schistosomiasis

Schistosomiasis (bilharziasis) is a chronic infection caused by a group of trematode worms, *Schistosoma mansoni, S. japonicum,* and *S. haematobium.* Of these, only *S. haematobium* invades the urinary tract. The disease is endemic in Africa and the Middle East. The chronic disease in man is caused by persistent infestation and granulomatous reaction to the eggs lodged in the wall of the bladder and ureter. These eggs are laid by female worms living in the vesical and ureteral veins. The eggs may extrude into the urinary cavity and be passed in the urine. Long standing infection leads to formation of granulomas, fibrosis, and calcification of the ureter and bladder and may produce obstruction and hydronephrosis. The disease may be asymptomatic or characterized by dysuria, hematuria, colic, or urinary incontinence. The major radiologic findings are (1) bladder calcification, (2) ureteric deformity, (3) hydronephrosis, (4) nonfunctioning kidney, and (5) urinary calculus. These lesions are more common in males. Death may be caused by renal failure from obstruction and secondary bacterial infection with *Salmonella typhi* and *S. paratyphi* (163,315–317). Massive proteinuria and nephrotic syndrome have been described in males with chronic salmonellosis superimposed on bilharzia (317). Praziquantel is the drug of choice for treatment of bilharzia (318).

References

1. Kunin CM, Beard MV, Halmagyi NE. Evidence for a common hapten associated with endotoxin fractions of *E. coli* and other *Enterobacteriaceae.* Proc Soc Exp Biol Med 1962;111: 160–166.
2. Young LS. Gram-negative rod bacteremia: Microbiologic, immunologic, and therapeutic considerations. Ann Intern Med 1977;86:456–471.
3. Westphal O, Jann K, Himmelspach K. Chemistry and immunochemistry of bacterial lipopolysaccharides as cell wall antigens and endotoxins. In: Hanson LA, Kallos P, Westphal O, eds. Progress in allergy 33. New York: Karger, 1983:9–39.
4. McCabe WR. Endotoxin tolerance. II. Its occurrence in patients with pyelonephritis. J Clin Invest 1963;42:618–625.

5. Wenzel RP. Anti-endotoxin monoclonal antibodies—a second look. N Engl J Med 1992;326: 1151–1153.
6. Boyarsky S, Labay P. Ureteral motility. Annu Rev Med 1969;20:383–394.
7. Roberts JA. Vesicoureteral reflux and pyelonephritis in the monkey: a review. J Urol 1992;148:1721–1725.
8. Linder H, Engberg I, Mattsby-Baltzer I, et al. Natural resistance to urinary tract infection determined by endotoxin-induced inflammation. FEMS Microbiol Lett 1988;49:219–222.
9. Aronson M, Medalia O, Amichay D, et al. Endotoxin-induced shedding of viable uroepithelial cells is an antimicrobial defense mechanism. Infect Immun 1988; 56:1615–1617.
10. Linder H, Engberg I, Baltzer IM, et al. Induction of inflammation by E. coli on the mucosal level: requirement for adherence and endotoxin. Infect Immun 1988;56:1309–1313.
11. Hedges S, Anderson P, Lidin-Janson G, et al. Interleukin-6 response to deliberate colonization of the human urinary tract with gram-negative bacteria. Infect Immun 1991;59: 421–427.
12. Ko YC, Mukaida N, Ishiyama S, et al. Elevated interleukin-8 levels in the urine of patients with urinary tract infections. Infect Immun 1993;61:1307–1314.
13. Agace W, Connell H, Svanborg C. Host resistance to urinary tract infection. In: Mobley HLT, Warren JW, eds. Urinary tract infections: molecular pathogenesis and clinical management. Washington DC: ASM Press, 1986:221–243.
14. Acker G, Kammerer C. Localization of enterobacterial common antigen immunoreactivity in the ribosomal cytoplasm of E. coli cells cryosubstituted and embedded at low temperature. J Bacteriol 1990;172:1106–1113.
15. Mäkelä PH, Mayer H. Enterobacterial common antigen. Bact Rev 1976;40:591–632.
16. Frentz G, Domingue G. Effects of immunization with ethanol-soluble enterobacterial common antigen in vivo bacterial clearance and hematogenous pyelonephritis. Proc Soc Exp Biol Med 1973;142:246–252.
17. McCabe WR, Greely A. Common enterobacterial antigen. II. Effect of immunization on challenge with heterologous bacilli. Infect Immun 1973;7:386–392.
18. McCabe WR, Johns M, DiGenio T. Common enterobacterial antigen. III. Initial titers and antibody response in bacteremia caused by gram-negative bacilli. Infect Immun 1973; 7:393–397.
19. Lagercrantz R, Hammarstrom S, Perlmann P, et al. Immunological studies in ulcerative colitis IV. Origin of autoantibodies. J Exp Med 1968;128:1339–1352.
20. Holmgren J, Hammarstrom S, Hom SE, et al. An antigenic relationship between human kidney, colon and common antigens of Enterobacteriaceae. Int Arch Allergy Immunol 1972;43:89–97.
21. Ørskov F, Ørskov I. Clonal structures of Escherichia coli populations. In: Kass EH, Svanborg-Edén C, eds. Host-parasite interactions in urinary tract infections. Chicago: University of Chicago Press, 1989:81–85.
22. Korhonen TK, Valtonen MV, Parkkinen J, et al. Serotypes, hemolysin production, and receptor recognition of Escherichia coli associated with neonatal sepsis and meningitis. Infect Immun 1985;48:486–491.
23. Ikäheimo R, Siitonen A, Kärkkäinen, et al. Community-acquired pyelonephritis in adults: Characteristics of E. coli isolates in bacteremic and non-bacteremic patients. Scand J Infect Dis 1994;26:289–296.
24. Ikäheimo R, Siitonen A, Kärkkäinen U, et al. Characteristics of Escherichia coli in acute community-acquired cystitis of adult women. Scand J Infect Dis 1993;25:705–712.
25. Sandberg T, Kaijser B, Lidin-Janson G, et al. Virulence of E. coli in relation to host factors in women with symptomatic urinary tract infection. J Clin Microbiol 1988;26:1471–1476.
26. Ulleryd P, Lincoln K, Scheutz F, et al. Virulence characteristics of Escherichia coli in relation to host response in men with symptomatic urinary tract infection. Clin Infect Dis 1994;18:579–584.
27. Johnson JR. Virulence factors in Escherichia coli urinary tract infection. Clin Microbiol Rev 1991;4:80–128.
28. Su C, Brandt LJ. Escherichia coli O145:H7 infection in humans. Ann Intern Med 1995;123: 698–714.
29. Gaillard JL, Cheron G, Mougenot JF, et al. Pyelonephritic Escherichia coli strains as intestinal pathogens in two newborn infants. Lancet 1989;1:327–328.
30. Wetter LA, Hamadeh RM, Griffiss JM, et al. Differences in outer membrane characteristics between gall-stone associated bacteria and normal bacterial flora. Lancet 1994;343: 444–448.

31. Vosti KL, Monto AS, Rantz LA. The importance of sample size in studies based upon the serologic classification of *Escherichia coli*. Proc Soc Exp Biol Med 1962;111:201–204.
32. Miller TE, Creaghe E. Bacterial interference as a factor in renal infection. J Lab Clin Med 1976;87:792–803.
33. Ryan FJ. Natural selection in bacterial populations. Atti Del VI Congr Internat Di Microbiol 1953;1:649.
34. Stamey TA, Timothy M, Miller M, et al. Recurrent urinary infections in adult women. Calif Med 1971;115:1–19.
35. Bollgren J, Winberg J. The periurethral aerobic flora in girls highly susceptible to urinary infections. Acta Paediatr Scand 1976;65:81–87.
36. Kunin CM, Polyak F, Postel E. Periurethral bacterial flora in women. JAMA 1980;243:134–139.
37. Brauner A, Jacobson SH, Kuhn I. Urinary *Escherichia coli* causing recurrent infections—a prospective follow-up of biochemical phenotypes. Clin Nephrol 1992;38:318–323.
38. Schlager TA, Hendley JO, Lohr JA, et al. Effect of periurethral colonization on the risk of urinary tract infection in healthy girls after their first urinary tract infection. Pediatr Infect Dis J 1993;12:988–993.
39. Foxman B, Zhang L, Tallman P, et al. Virulence characteristics of *Escherichia coli* causing first urinary tract infection predict risk of second infection. J Infect Dis 1995;172:1536–1541.
40. Russo TA, Stapleton A, Wenderoth S, et al. Chromosomal restriction fragment length polymorphism analysis of *Escherichia coli* strains causing recurrent urinary tract infection in young women. J Infect Dis 1995;172:440–445.
41. Ikäheimo R, Siitonen A, Heiskanen T, et al. Recurrence of urinary tract infection in a primary care setting: Analysis of a 1-year follow-up of 179 women. Clin Infect Dis 1996;22:91–99.
42. Kunin CM, Deutscher R, Paquin AJ. Urinary tract infection in school children: epidemiologic, clinical and laboratory study. Medicine 1964;43:91–130.
43. Bergström T, Lincoln K, Ørskov F, et al. Studies of urinary tract infections in infancy and childhood VIII. Reinfection vs. relapse in recurrent urinary tract infections. Evaluation by means of identification of infecting organisms. J Pediatr 1967;71:13–20.
44. McGeachie J. Recurrent infection of the urinary tract: reinfection or recrudescence? Br Med J 1966;1:952–954.
45. Kunin CM. A ten-year study of bacteriuria in school girls: final report of bacteriologic, urologic and epidemiologic findings. J Infect Dis 1970;122:382–393.
46. Donnenberg MS, Welch RA. Virulence determinants of uropathogenic *Escherichia coli*. In: Mobley HLT, Warren JW, eds. Urinary tract infections: molecular pathogenesis and clinical management. Washington DC: ASM Press,1986:135–174.
47. Duguid JP, Clegg S, Wilson MI. The fimbrial and non-fimbrial hemagglutinins of *Escherichia coli*. J Med Microbiol 1979;12:213–227.
48. Beachey EH. Bacterial Adherence: adhesin-receptor interactions mediating the attachment of bacteria to mucosal surfaces. J Infect Dis 1981;143:325–345.
49. Silverblatt FJ, Dreyer JS, Schauer S. Effect of pili on susceptibility of *Escherichia coli* to phagocytosis. Infect Immun 1979;24:218–223.
50. Blumenstock E, Jann K. Adhesion of piliated *Escherichia coli* strains to phagocytes: Differences between bacteria with mannose-sensitive pili and those with mannose-resistant pili. Infect Immun 1982;35:264–269.
51. Bjorksten B, Wadstrom T. Interaction of *Escherichia coli* with different fimbriae and polymorphonuclear leukocytes. Infect Immun 1982;38:298–305.
52. Mangan DF, Snyder IS. Mannose-sensitive interaction of *Escherichia coli* with human peripheral leukocytes in vitro. Infect Immun 1979;26:520–527.
53. Ørskov I, Ferencz A, Ørskov F. Tamm-Horsfall protein or uromucoid is the normal urinary slime that traps Type 1 fimbriated *Escherichia coli*. Lancet 1980;2:887.
54. Kuriyama SM, Silverblatt FJ. Effect of Tamm-Horsfall urinary glycoprotein on phagocytosis and killing of type I-Fimbriated *Escherichia coli*. Infect Immun 1986;51:193–198.
55. Chick S, Harber MJ, Mackenzie R, et al. Modified method for studying bacterial adhesion to isolated uroepithelial cells and uromucoid. Infect Immun 1981;34:256–261.
56. Reinhart H, Obedeanu N, Merzbach D, et al. Effect of Tamm-Horsfall protein on chemoluminescence response of polymorphonuclear leukocytes to uropathogenic *Escherichia coli*. J Infect Dis 1991;164:404–406.

57. Duncan JL. Differential effects of Tamm-Horsfall protein on adherence of *Escherichia coli* to transitional epithelial cells. J Infect Dis 1988;158:1379–1382.

58. Venegas MF, Navas EL, Gaffney RA, et al. Binding of type 1-piliated *Escherichia coli* to vaginal mucus. Infect Immun 1995;63:416–422.

59. Ofek I, Goldman J, Zafriri D, et al. Anti-*E. coli* adhesion activity of cranberry and blueberry juices. N Engl J Med 1991;324:1599.

60. Schmidt DR, Sobota AE. An examination of the anti-adherence activity of cranberry juice on urinary and nonurinary bacterial isolates. Microbios 1988;55:173–181.

61. Eisenstein BI. Phase variation of type 1 fimbria in *Escherichia coli* is under transcriptional control. Science 1981;214:337–339.

62. Pere A, Nowicki B, Saxen H, et al. Expression of P, Type-1, and Type-1C of *Escherichia coli* in the urine of patients with acute urinary tract infection. J Infect Dis 1987;156:567–574.

63. Ofek I, Mosek A, Sharon N. Mannose-specific adherence of *Escherichia coli* freshly excreted in the urine of patients with urinary tract infections, and of isolates subcultured from the infected urine. Infect Immun 1981;34:708–711.

64. Ofek I, Hadar S, Heiber R, et al. Effect of urea and urine dialysate on the growth of type-1 fimbriated and nonfimbriated phenotypes of isolates of *Escherichia coli*. In: Kass EH, Svanborg-Edén C, eds. Host-parasite interactions in urinary tract infections. Chicago: University of Chicago Press, 1989:122–126.

65. Kunin CM, Tong HH, Guerrant RI, Bakaletz LO. Effect of salicylate, bismuth, osmolytes, and tetracycline resistance on expression of fimbriae by *Escherichia coli*. Infect Immun 1994;62:2178–2186.

66. Aronson M, Medalia O, Schori L, et al. Prevention of colonization of the urinary tract of mice with *Escherichia coli* by blocking of bacterial adherence with methyl-D-mannopyranoside. J Infect Dis 1979;139:329–332.

67. Abraham SN, Babu JP, Giampapa CS, et al. Protection against *Escherichia coli*-induced urinary tract infections with hybridoma antibodies directed against type 1 fimbriae or complementary D-mannose receptors. Infect Immun 1985;48:625–628.

68. Svenson SB, Kallenius G, Mollby R, et al. Rapid identification of P-fimbriated *Escherichia coli* by a receptor-specific particle agglutination test. Infection 1982;10:209–214.

69. Johnson JR, Ross AE. P1-antigen-containing avian egg whites as inhibitors of P adhesins among wild-type *Escherichia coli* strains from patients with urosepsis. Infect Immun 1993;61:4902–4905.

70. Jones CH, Dodson K, Hultgren SJ. Structure, function, and assembly of adhesive P pili. In: Mobley HLT, Warren JW eds. Urinary tract infections: molecular pathogenesis and clinical management. Washington DC: ASM Press, 1986:175–219.

71. Svanborg-Edén C, Eriksson B, Hanson LA. Adhesion of *Escherichia coli* to human uroepithelial cells in vitro. Infect Immun 1977;18:767–774.

72. Leffler H, Svanborg-Edén C. Chemical identification of a glycosphingolipid receptor for *Escherichia coli* attaching to human urinary tract epithelial cells and agglutinating human erythrocytes. FEMS Microbiol Lett 1980;8:127–134.

73. Kallenius G, Mollby R, Svenson SB, et al. The Pk antigen as receptor for the hemagglutinin of pyelonephritis *Escherichia coli* in urinary tract infections. Lancet 1981;2:1369–1372.

74. O'Hanley P, Low D, Romero I, et al. Gal-Gal Binding and Hemolysin Phenotypes and genotypes associated with uropathogenic *Escherichia coli*. N Engl J Med 1985;313:414–420.

75. Roberts JA, Hardaway K, Kaack B, et al. Prevention of pyelonephritis by immunization with P-fimbriae. J Urol 1984;131:602–607.

76. Korhonen TK, Virkola R, Holthofer H. Localization of binding sites for purified *Escherichia coli* P Fimbriae in the Human Kidney. Infect Immun 1986; 54:328–332.

77. Smith J. Microbial and host factors that influence adherence of *Escherichia coli* to kidney epithelium. Amer J Kid Dis 1986;7:368–374.

78. Donnenberg MS, Newman B, Utsalo SJ, et al. Internalization of *Escherichia coli* into human kidney epithelial cells: comparison of fecal and pyelonephritis-associated strains. J Infect Dis 1994;169:831–838.

79. Fussell EN, Kaack MB, Cherry R, et al. Adherence of bacteria to human foreskins. J Urol 1988;140:997–1001.

80. Otto G, Sandberg T, Marklund BI, et al. Virulence factors and pap genotype in *Escherichia coli* isolates from women with acute pyelonephritis, with or without bacteremia. Clin Infect Dis 1993;17:448–456.

81. Ikäheimo R, Siitonen A, Kärkkäinen U, et al. Virulence characteristics of *Escherichia coli* in nosocomial urinary tract infection. Clin Infect Dis 1993;16:785–791.

82. Domingue GJ, Roberts JA, Laucirica R, et al. Pathogenic significance of P-fimbriated *Escherichia coli* in urinary tract infections. J Urol 1985;133:983–989.

83. Johnson JR, Ørskov I, Ørskov F, et al. O, K, and H antigens predict virulence factors, carboxylesterase B pattern, antimicrobial resistance, and host compromise among *Escherichia coli* strains causing urosepsis. J Infect Dis 1994;169:119–126.

84. Lomberg H, Hellström M, Jodal U, et al. Virulence-associated traits in *Escherichia coli* causing first and recurrent episodes of urinary tract infection in children with or without vesicoureteral reflux. J Infect Dis 1984;150:561–569.

85. Plos K, Lomberg H, Hull S, et al. *Escherichia coli* in patients with renal scarring: genotype and phenotype of galα1–4galβ Forssman- and mannose-specific adhesins. Pediatr Infect Dis 1991;10:15–19.

86. Rushton HG, Majd M. Dimercaptosuccinic acid renal scintigraphy for the evaluation of pyelonephritis and scarring: a review of experimental and clinical studies. J Urol 1992;148: 1726–1732.

87. Schlager TA, Whittam TS, Hendley JO, et al. Comparison of expression of virulence factors by *Escherichia coli* causing cystitis and *E. coli* colonizing the periurethra of healthy girls. J Infect Dis 1995;172;772–777.

88. Korhonen TK, Parkkinen J, Hacker J, et al. Binding of *Escherichia coli* S Fimbriae to human kidney epithelium. Infect Immun 1986;54:322–327.

89. Parkkinen J, Korhonen TK, Pere A, et al. Binding sites in the rat brain for *Escherichia coli* S Fimbriae associated with neonatal meningitis. J Clin Invest 1988;81:860–865.

90. Kunin CM, Tong HH, Krishnan C, et al. Isolation of a nicotinamide-requiring clone of *Escherichia coli* O18:K1:H7 from women with acute cystitis: resemblance to strains found in neonatal meningitis. Clin Infect Dis 1993;16:412–416.

91. Johnson JR, Skubitz KM, Nowicki BJ, et al. Nonlethal adherence to human neutrophils mediated by Dr antigen-specific adhesins of *Escherichia coli*. Infect Immun 1995;63: 309–316.

92. Andersson P, Engberg I, Lidin-Janson G, et al. Persistence of *Escherichia coli* bacteriuria is not determined by bacterial adherence. Infect Immun 1991;59:2915–2921.

93. Hansson S, Jodal U, Noren L, et al. Untreated bacteriuria in asymptomatic girls with renal scarring. Pediatrics 1989;84:964–968.

94. Lindberg U, Hanson LÅ, Lidin-Janson G, et al. Studies of *Escherichia coli* strains in asymptomatic bacteriuria of schoolgirls. In: Kass EH, Brumfitt W, eds. Infections of the urinary tract. Chicago: University of Chicago Press, 1978:44–48.

95. McCabe WR, Kaijser B, Olling S, et al. *Escherichia coli* in bacteremia: K and O antigens and serum sensitivity of strains from adults and neonates. J Infect Dis 1978;138:33–41.

96. Porat R, Johns MA, McCabe WR. Selective pressures and lipopolysaccharide subunits as determinants of resistance of clinical isolates of gram-negative bacilli to human serum. Infect Immun 1987;55:320–328.

97. Weiser JN, Gotschlich EC. Outer membrane protein A (OmpA) contributes to serum resistance and pathogenicity of *Escherichia coli* K-1. Infect Immun 1991;59:2252–2258.

98. Horwitz MA, Silverstein SC. Influence of the *Escherichia coli* capsule on complement fixation and on phagocytosis and killing by human phagocytes. J Clin Invest 1980;65:82–94.

99. Stevens P, Chu CL, Young LS. K-1 antigen content and the presence of an additional sialic acid-containing antigen among bacteremic K-1 *Escherichia coli*: correlation with susceptibility to opsonophagocytosis. Infect Immun 1980;29:1055–1061.

100. Kaijser B. Immunology of *Escherichia coli*: K antigen and its relation to urinary-tract infections. J Infect Dis 1973;127:670–677.

101. McCabe WR, Carling PC, Bruins S, et al. The relation of K-antigen to virulence of *Escherichia coli*. J Infect Dis 1975;131:6–10.

102. Glynn AA, Brumfitt W, Howard CK. Antigens of *Escherichia coli* and renal involvement in urinary tract infections. Lancet 1971;1:514–516.

103. Jann K, Jann B. The K antigens of *Escherichia coli*. In: Hanson LA, Kallos P, Westphal O, eds. Progress in allergy 33. New York: Karger, 1983:53–79.

104. Kaijser B, Larsson P, Olling S, et al. Protection against acute, ascending pyelonephritis caused by *Escherichia coli* in rats, using isolated antigen conjugated to bovine serum albumin. Infect Immun 1983;39:142–146.

105. Finkelstein RA, Scirotino CV, McIntosh MA. Role of iron in microbe-host interactions. Rev Infect Dis 1983;5:S759–S777.
106. Montgomerie JZ, Bindereif A, Neilands JB, et al. Association of hydroxamate siderophore (aerobactin) with *Escherichia coli* isolated from patients with bacteremia. Infect Immun 1984;46:835–838.
107. Lundrigan MD, Webb RM. Prevalence of OmpT among *Escherichia coli* isolates of human origin. FEMS Microbiol Lett 1992;97:51–56.
108. Mostafavi M, Stein PC, Parsons L. Production of soluble virulence factor by *Escherichia coli*. J Urol 1995;153:1441–1443.
109. Kunin CM, Tong HH, Krishnan C, White LV. Do temperature-sensitive auxotrophs of *Escherichia coli* have special virulence? J Clin Microbiol 1993;31:47–49.
110. Kunin CM, Tong HH, White LV, et al. Growth of *Escherichia coli* in human urine: role of salt tolerance and accumulation of glycine betaine. J Infect Dis 1992;166:1311–1315.
111. Hand WL, Smith JW, Miller TE, et al. Immunoglobulin synthesis in lower urinary tract infection. J Lab Clin Med 1970;75:19–29.
112. Lehman JD, Smith JW, Miller TE, et al. Local immune response in experimental pyelonephritis. J Clin Invest 1968;47:2541–2550.
113. Kantele A, Papunen R, Virtanen E, et al. Antibody-secreting cells in acute urinary tract infection as indicators of local immune response. J Infect Dis 1994;169:1023–1028.
114. Kunin CM. Distribution of antibodies against various nonenteropathic *E. coli* groups: relation to age, sex and breast feeding. Arch Intern Med 1962;110:676–686.
115. Hanson LA, Ahlastedt S, Fasth A, et al. Antigens of *Escherichia coli*, human immune response and the pathogenesis of urinary tract infections. J Infect Dis 1977;136:114–150.
116. McCabe WR, Kreger BE, Johns M. Type-specific and cross-reactive antibodies in gram-negative bacteremia. N Engl J Med 1972;287:261–267.
117. Henriksen AZ, Maeland JA. Serum antibodies to outer membrane proteins of *Escherichia coli* in healthy persons and patients with bacteremia. J Clin Microbiol 1987;25:2181–2188.
118. Nicolle LE, Brunka J, Ujack E, et al. Antibodies to major outer membrane proteins of *Escherichia coli* in urinary infection in the elderly. J Infect Dis 1989;160:627–633.
119. Kaak MB, Roberts JA, Baskin G, et al. Maternal immunization with P fimbriae for the prevention of neonatal pyelonephritis. Infect Immun 1988;56:1–6.
120. Sanford JP, Hunter BW, Souda LL. The role of immunity in the pathogenesis of experimental hematogenous pyelonephritis. J Exper Med 1962;115:383–410.
121. Hunter BW, Akins LL, Sanford JP. The role of immunity in the pathogenesis of experimental retrograde pyelonephritis. J Exper Med 1964;119:869–879.
122. Tomasi TB. Mechanisms of immune regulation at mucosal surfaces. Rev Infect Dis 1983;5:S784–S792.
123. Hjelm EM. Local cellular immune response in ascending urinary tract infection: occurrence of T-cells, immunoglobulin-producing cells, and Ia-expressing cells in rat urinary tract tissue. Infect Immun 1984;44:627–632.
124. Hand WL, Smith JW, Miller TE, et al. Immunoglobulin synthesis in lower urinary tract infection. J Lab Clin Med 1970;75:19–29.
125. Hopkins WJ, Uehling DT, Balish E. Local and systemic antibody responses accompany spontaneous resolution of experimental cystitis in cynomolgus monkeys. Infect Immun 1987;55:1951–1956.
126. Jodal U, Ahlstedt S, Carlsson B, et al. Local antibodies in childhood urinary tract infection. Int Arch Allergy 1974;47:537–546.
127. Svanborg Edén C, Svennerholm AM. Secretory immunoglobulin A and G antibodies prevent adhesion of *Escherichia coli* to human urinary tract epithelial cells. Infect Immun 1978;22:790–797.
128. Milazzo FH, Delisle GJ. Immunoglobulin A proteases in gram-negative bacteria isolated from human urinary tract infections. Infect Immun 1984;3:11–13.
129. Stamey TA, Howell JJ. Studies of introital colonization in women with recurrent urinary infections. IV. The role of local vaginal antibodies. J Urol 1976;115:413–415.
130. Tuttle JP Jr, Sarvas H, Koistinen J. The role of vaginal immunoglobulin A in girls with recurrent urinary tract infections. J Urol 1978;120:742–744.
131. Riedasch G, Heck P, Rauterberg E, et al. Does low urinary sIgA predispose to urinary tract infection? Kidney Int 1983;23:759–763.

132. Kurdydyk LM, Kelly K, Harding GKM, et al. Role of cervicovaginal antibody in the pathogenesis of recurrent urinary tract infection in women. Infect Immun 1980;29:76–82.
133. Floege J, Boddeker M, Stolte H, et al. Urinary IgA, secretory component in women with recurrent urinary tract infections. Nephron 1990;56:50–55.
134. Uehling DT, Steihm RE. Elevated urinary secretory IgA in children with urinary tract infection. Pediatrics 1971;7:40–46.
135. Nicolle LE, Brunka J. Urinary IgG and IgA antibodies in elderly individuals with bacteriuria. Gerontol 1990;36:345–355.
136. Fowler JE, Mariano M. Immunologic response of the prostrate to bacteriuria and bacterial prostatitis. J Urol 1982;128:165–170.
137. Riedasch G, Ritz E, Mohring K, et al. Antibody-coated bacteria in the ejaculate: a possible test for prostatitis. J Urol 1977;118:787–788.
138. Miller T, Findon G. Cellular basis of host defenses in acute pyelonephritis. In: Kass EH, Svanborg-Edén C, eds. Host-parasite interactions in urinary tract infections. Chicago: University of Chicago Press, 1989:380–385.
139. Bailey RR, Roberts AP, Rowe B, et al. The leukocyte migration test in urinary tract infection. N Z Med J 1974;81:10–15.
140. Uehling DT, Hopkins WF, Dahmer LA, et al. Phase I clinical trial of vaginal mucosal immunization for recurrent urinary tract infection. J Urol 1994;152:2308–2311.
141. O'Hanley P. Prospects for urinary tract infection vaccines. In: Mobley HLT, Warren JW, eds. Urinary tract infections: molecular pathogenesis and clinical management. Washington DC: ASM Press,1986:405–425.
142. Schaberg DR, Culver DH, Gaynes RP. Major trends in the microbial etiology of nosocomial infection. Am J Med 1991;91(Suppl 3B):72s–75s.
143. Muder RR, Brennen C, Wagener MM, et al. Bacteremia in a long-term-care facility: a five-year prospective study of 163 consecutive episodes. Clin Infect Dis 1992, 14:647–654.
144. Senay H, Goetz MB. Epidemiology of bacteremic urinary tract infections in chronically hospitalized elderly men. J Urol 1991;145:1201–1204.
145. Chambers ST, Steele C, Kunin CM. Enteric colonization with antibiotic resistant bacteria in nurses working in intensive care units. J Antimicrob Chemother 1987;19:685–693.
146. Cheng D-L, Liu Y-C, Yen M-Y, et al. Septic metastatic lesions of pyogenic liver abscesses. Their association with *Klebsiella pneumoniae* bacteremia in diabetic patients. Arch Intern Med 1991;151:1557–1559.
147. Goldman JM, Kowalec JC. Hepatic abscess and osteomyelitis from *Klebsiella pneumoniae.* JAMA 1978;240:2660.
148. Margo CE, Mames RN, Guy JR. Endogenous *Klebsiella* endophthalmitis. Ophthalmology 1994;101:1298–1301.
149. Collins CM, D'Orazio SEF. Virulence determinants of uropathogenic *Klebsiella pneumoniae.* In: Mobley HLT, Warren JW, eds. Urinary tract infections: molecular pathogenesis and clinical management. Washington DC: ASM Press,1986:299–312.
150. Braude AI, Siemienski J. Role of bacterial urease in experimental pyelonephritis: a histological and biochemical study. J Bacteriol 1960;80:171–179.
151. Mobley HLT. Virulence of Proteus mirabilis. In: Mobley HLT, Warren JW, eds. Urinary tract infections: Molecular pathogenesis and clinical management. Washington DC: ASM Press,1986:245–269.
152. Sinha B, Gonzalez R. Hyperammonemia in a boy with obstructive ureterocele and Proteus infection. J Urol 1984,131:330–331.
153. Drayna CJ, Titcomb CT, Varma RR, et al. Hyperammonemic encephalopathy caused by infection in a neurogenic bladder. N Engl J Med 1981;304:766.
154. Samtoy B, DeBeaukelaer MM. Ammonia encephalopathy secondary to urinary tract infection with Proteus mirabilis. Pediatrics 1980;65:294.
155. Saxena DR, Bassett DC. Sex-related incidence in Proteus infection of the urinary tract in childhood. Arch Dis Child 1975,50:899–901.
156. Wiswell TE, Smith FR, Bass JW. Decreased incidence of urinary tract infections in circumcised male infants. Pediatrics 1985;75:901–903.
157. Dumanski AJ, Hedelin H, Edin-Liljegren A, et al. Unique ability of the *Proteus mirabilis* capsule to enhance mineral growth in infectious urinary calculi. Infect Immun 1994;62: 2998–3003.

158. Griffith DP, Musher DM. Acetohydroxamic acid. Potential use in urinary infection caused by urea-splitting bacteria. Urology 1975;5:299–302.
159. Kunin CM, Tong HH, Bakaletz LO. Effect of salicylate on expression of flagella by *Escherichia coli* and *Proteus, Providencia* and *Pseudomonas* spp. Infect Immun 1995;63: 1796–1799.
160. Jao RL, Jackson GG. Asymptomatic urinary tract infection with *Shigella sonnei* in a chronic fecal carrier. N Engl J Med 1963;268:1165–1168.
161. Ekwall E, Ljungh A, Selander B. Asymptomatic urinary tract infection caused by *Shigella sonnei*. Scand J Infect Dis 1984;16:121–122.
162. Papasian CJ, Enna-Kifer S, Garrison B. Symptomatic *Shigella sonnei* urinary tract infection. J Clin Microbiol 1995;33:2222–2223.
163. Neva FA. Urinary enteric carriers in Egypt: incidence in 76 cases and observations on the urinary carrier state. Am J Trop Med 1949;29:909–919.
164. Mathai E, John TJ, Rani M, et al. Significance of *Salmonella typhi* bacteriuria. J Clin Microbiol 1995;33:1791–1792.
165. Scott MB, Cosgrove MD. Salmonella infection and the genitourinary system. J Urol 1977;118:64–68.
166. Dupuis F, Vereerstraeten P, Van Geertryden J, et al. *Salmonella typhimurium* urinary infections after kidney transplantation. Report of 7 cases. Clin Nephrol 1974;2:131–135.
167. Berk MR, Meyers AM, Cassal W, et al. Nontyphoid salmonella infections after renal transplantation. A serious clinical problem. Nephron 1984;37:186.
168. Hasham AI, Uehling DT. Salmonella lithiasis. J Urol 1976;115:110–111.
169. Hagood PG, Steinhardt GF. Salmonella urinary tract infection associated with ureteropelvic junction obstruction. J Urol 1988;140:351–352.
170. Ross SA, Townes PL, Hopkins TB. *Salmonella enteritidis*. A rare cause of pyelonephritis in children. Clin Pediatr 1986;25:325–326.
171. Mitchell RG, Oxon BM. Urinary-tract infections caused by salmonellae. Lancet 1965;1: 1092–1093.
172. Foster RS, Rink RC, Mulcahy JJ. Focal *Salmonella enteritidis* infection of urinary tract. J Urol 1987;29:646–647.
173. Green JB, Adler M, Holzman RS. *Salmonella enteritidis* genitourinary tract infection in a homosexual man. J Urol 1982;128:1046.
174. Eng RHK, Smith SM, Kloser P. Nontyphoid salmonella urinary tract infections. Diagn Microbiol Infect Dis 1987;6:223–228.
175. Frayha RA, Jizi I, Saadeh G. *Salmonella typhimurium* bacteriuria: an increased infection rate in systemic lupus erythematosus. Arch Intern Med 1985;145:645–647.
176. Kunin CM. Infections of the urinary tract due to *Pseudomonas aeruginosa*. In: Baltch A, Smith RP, eds. *Pseudomonas aeruginosa* infections and treatment. New York: Dekker, 1994:237–256.
177. Woods DE, Vasil ML. Pathogenesis of *Pseudomonas aeruginosa* infections. In: Baltch A, Smith RP, eds. *Pseudomonas aeruginosa* infections and treatment. New York: Dekker, 1994:21–50.
178. Meyer J-M, Neely A, Stintzi A, et al. Pyoverdin is essential for virulence of Pseudomonas aeruginosa. Infect Immun 1996;64:518–523.
179. Wright JD. An observation on the occurrence of the bacillus of influenza (*Bacterium influenzae*) in pyelonephrosis. Boston Med Surg J 1905;152:496.
180. Davis DJ. A hemophilus bacillus found in urinary infections. J Infect Dis 1910;7:599–608.
181. Albright F, Dienes L, Sulkowitch HW. Pyelonephritis with nephrocalcinosis caused by *Haemophilus influenzae* and alleviated by sulfanilamide: report of two cases. JAMA 1938;110:357–360.
182. Burkland CE, Leadbetter WF. Pyelitis cystica associated with a *Haemophilus influenzae* infection in the urine. J Urol 1939;42:14–20.
183. Granoff DM, Roskes S. Urinary tract infection due to *H. influenzae* type b -report of two cases. J Pediatr 1974;84:414–416.
184. Farrand RJ. *Haemophilus influenzae* infections of the genital tract. J Med Microbiol 1971;4:357–358.
185. Albritton WL, Brunton JL, Meier M, et al. *H. influenzae:* comparison of respiratory tract isolates with genitourinary tract isolates. J Clin Microbiol 1982;16:826–831.
186. Blaylock BL, Baber S. Urinary tract infection caused by *Haemophilus parainfluenzae*. Am J Clin Pathol 1980;73:285–287.

187. Chesney PJ. Acute epididymo-orchitis due to *Hemophilus influenzae* type b. J Pediatr 1977;91:685.
188. Waldman RJ, Kosloske AM, Parsons DW. Acute epididymo-orchitis as the presenting manifestation of *Haemophilus influenzae* septicemia. J Pediatr 1977;90:87–89
189. Schuit KE. Isolation of Haemophilus in urine cultures from children. J Pediatr 1979;95: 565–566.
190. Thomas D, Simpson K, Ostojic H, et al. Bacteremic epididymo-orchitis due to *Hemophilus influenzae* type B. J Urol 1981;126:832–833.
191. Goetz MB, Craig WA. *Haemophilus influenzae* prostatitis. JAMA 1982;247:3118.
192. Quentin R, Musser JM, Mellouet M, et al. Typing of urogenital, maternal, and neonatal isolates of *H. influenzae* and *H. parainfluenzae* in correlation with clinical source of isolation and evidence for a genital specificity of *H. influenzae* biotype IV. J Clin Microb 1989;27:2286–2294.
193. Cross J, Davidson K, Bradsher R. *Haemophilus influenzae* epididymo-orchitis and bacteremia in a man infected with the human immunodeficiency virus. Clin Infect Dis 1994;19:768–769.
194. Davies J, Carlstedt I, Nilsson A-K, et al. Binding of *Haemophilus influenzae* to purified mucins from the human respiratory tract. Infect Immun 1995;63:2485–2492.
195. Lam M, Birch DF. Survival of *Gardnerella vaginalis* in human urine. Am J Clin Pathol 1991;95:234–239.
196. Burdge DR, Bowie WR, Chow AW. *Gardnerella vaginalis*-associated balanoposthitis. Sex Trans Dis 1986;14:159–162.
197. Catlin BW. *Gardnerella vaginalis:* characteristics, clinical considerations, and controversies. Clin Microbiol Rev 1992;5:213–237.
198. Denoyel GA, Drouet EB, DeMontclos HP, et al. *Gardnerella vaginalis* bacteremia in a man with prostatic adenoma. J Infect Dis 1990;161:367–368.
199. Finkelhor RS, Wolinsky E, Kim CH, et al. *Gardnerella vaginalis* perinephric abscess in a transplanted kidney. N Engl J Med 1981;304:846.
200. Patrick S, Garnett PA. *Corynebacterium vaginale* bacteraemia in a man. Lancet 1978;1:987.
201. Fairley K, Birch D. Unconventional bacteria in urinary tract disease: *Gardnerella vaginalis.* Kidney Int 1983;23:862–65.
202. Lam MH, Birch DF, Birch DF, et al. Prevalence of *Gardnerella vaginalis* in the urinary tract. J Clin Microbiol 1988;26:1130–1133.
203. Woolfrey BF, Ireland GK, Lally RT. Significance of *Gardnerella vaginalis* in urine cultures. Am J Clin Pathol 1986;86:324–329.
204. Dumler JS, Osterhout GJ, Spangler JG, et al. *Vibrio cholerae* Non-Serogroup 01 cystitis. J Clin Microbiol 1989;27:1898–1899.
205. Davies JS, Penfold JB. Campylobacter urinary infection. Lancet 1979;1:1091–1092.
206. Feder HM Jr, Rasoulpour M, Rodriguez AJ. Campylobacter urinary tract infection. Value of the urine gram's stain. JAMA 1986;256:2389.
207. McElroy Jr EA, Marks GL. A case report of *Escherichia vulneres* urosepsis. Rev Infect Dis 1991;13:1247–1248.
208. Pugliese A, Pacris B, Schoch PE, et al. *Oligella urethralis* urosepsis. Clin Infect Dis 1993;17:1069–1070.
209. Alballaa SR, Qadri SMH, Al-Furayh O, et al. Urinary tract infection due to *Rahnella aquatilis* in a renal transplant patient. J Clin Microbiol 1992;30:2948–2950.
210. Lee BK, Crossley K, Gerding DN. The association between *Staphylococcus aureus* bacteremia and bacteriuria. Am J Med 1978;65:303–306.
211. Demuth PJ, Gerding DN, Crosley K. *Staphylococcus aureus* bacteremia. Arch Intern Med 1979;139:78–80.
212. Nesbit RM, Dick VS. Acute staphylococcal infections of the kidney. J Urol 1940;43: 623–636.
213. Kunin CM, Steele C. Culture of the surface of urinary catheters to sample the urethral flora and study the effect of antimicrobial therapy. J Clin Microbiol 1985;21:902–908.
214. Almeida RJ, Jorgensen JH. Comparison of adherence and urine growth rate properties of *Staphylococcus saprophyticus* and *Staphylococcus epidermidis.* Eur J Clin Microbiol 1984;3: 542–545.
215. Torres Pereira A. Coagulase-negative strains of staphylococcus possessing antigen 51 as agents of urinary infection. J Clin Pathol 1962;15:252–253.

216. Hellström J. The significance of Staphylococci in the development and treatment of renal and ureteral stones. Br J Urol 1938;10:348–372.
217. Mitchell R. Urinary tract infections due to coagulase-negative staphylococci. J Clin Pathol 1964;17:105–106.
218. Wallmark G, Arremark I, Telander B. Staphylococcus saprophyticus: a frequent cause of acute urinary tract infection among female outpatients. J Infect Dis 1978;138:791–797.
219. Hovelius B, Mardh P-A. Staphylococcus saprophyticus as a common cause of urinary tract infections. Rev Infect Dis 1984;6:328–337.
220. Gatermann SG. Virulence factors of Staphylococcus saprophyticus, Staphylococcus epidermidis, and enterococci. In: Mobley HLT, Warren JW, eds. Urinary tract infections: molecular pathogenesis and clinical management. Washington DC: ASM Press,1986:313–340.
221. Latham RH, Running K, Stamm WE. Urinary tract infections in young adult women caused by Staphylococcus saprophyticus. JAMA 1983,250:3063–3066.
222. Fowler Jr JE. Staphylococcus saprophyticus as the cause of infected urinary calculus. Ann Intern Med 1985;102:342–343.
223. Carson CC, McGraw VD, Zwadyk P. Bacterial prostatitis caused by Staphylococcus saprophyticus. Urol 1982;19:576–578.
224. Golledge LC. Staphylococcus saprophyticus bacteremia. J Infect Dis 1988;157:215.
225. Lee W, Carpenter RJ, Phillips LE, et al. Pyelonephritis and sepsis due to Staphylococcus saprophyticus. J Infect Dis 1987;155:1079–1080.
226. Singh VR, Raad I. Fatal Staphylococcus saprophyticus native valve endocarditis in an intravenous drug addict. J Infect Dis 1990;162:783–784.
227. Rupp ME, Soper DE, Archer GL. Colonization of the female genital tract with Staphylococcus saprophyticus. J Clin Microbiol 1992;30:2975–2979.
228. Bayer As, Chow AW, Anthony BF, et al. Serious infections in adults due to group B streptococci. Am J Med 1976;61:498–503.
229. Shehab Z, Lohr JA. Group B streptococcal urinary infection in an infant. JAMA 1979;124:1327–1328.
230. Munoz P, Coque T, Rodriguez Creixems M, et al. Group B streptococcus: a cause of urinary tract infection in nonpregnant adults. Clin Infect Dis 1992;14:492–496.
231. Nguyen VQ, Penn RL. Pneumococcuria in adults. J Clin Microbiol 1988;26:1085–1087.
232. Pallares R, Pujol M, Pena C, et al. Cephalosporins as risk factor for nosocomial Enterococcus faecalis bacteremia. Arch Inter Med 1993;153:1581–1586.
233. Nachamkin I, Axelrod P, Talbot G, et al. Multiply high-level-aminoglycoside-resistant enterococci isolated from patients in a university hospital. J Clin Microbiol 1988;26:1287–1291.
234. Chirurgi VA, Oster SE, Goldberg AA, McCabe RE. Nosocomial acquisition of β-Lactamase-negative, ampicillin-resistant Enterococcus. Arch Intern Med 1992; 152:1457–1461.
235. Chow JW, Kuritza A, Shlaes DM, et al. Clonal spread of vancomycin-resistant Enterococcus faecium between patients in three hospitals in two states. J Clin Microbiol 1993;31:1609–1611.
236. Handwerger S, Raucher B, Altarac D, et al. Nosocomial outbreak due to Enterococcus faecium highly resistant to vancomycin, penicillin, and gentamicin. Clin Infect Dis 1993;16:750–755.
237. Soriano F, Ponte C, Santamaria M, et al. Corynebacterium group D2 as a cause of alkaline-encrusted cystitis: report of four cases and characterization of the organisms. J Clin Microbiol 1985;21:788–792.
238. Soriano F, Aguado JM, Ponte C, et al. Urinary tract infection caused by Corynebacterium group D2: report of 82 cases and review. Rev Infect Dis 1990;12:1019–1034.
239. Ronci-Koenig TJ, Tan JS, File TM, et al. Infections due to Corynebacterium group D2. Report of a case. Arch Intern Med 1990;150:1965–1966.
240. Park JM, Faerber GJ. Corynebacterium induced urethral encrustation. J Urol 1994;151:1636–1637.
241. Ryan M, Murray PR. Prevalence of Corynebacterium urealyticum in urine specimens collected at a university-affiliated medical center. J Clin Microbiol 1994;32:1395–1396.
242. Soriano F, Rodrigues-Tudela JL, Fernandez-Roblas R, et al. Skin colonization by Corynebacterium groups D2 and JK in hospitalized patients. J Clin Microbiol 1988;26:1878–1880.

243. Lipsky BA, Goldberger AC, Tompkins LS, et al. Infections caused by nondiphtheria corynebacteria. Rev Infect Dis 1982;4:1220–1225.
244. Wood C. Bacteremia in a patient with non-urinary-tract infection due to *Corynebacterium urealyticum*. Clin Infect Dis 1994; 19:367–368.
245. García-Rodriguez JA, García-Sanchez E, Muñoz-Bellido JL, et al. In vitro activity of 79 antimicrobial agents against Corynebacterium group D2. Antimicrob Agents Chemother 1991;35:2140–2143.
246. Soriano F, Rodriguez-Tudela JL, Castilla C, et al. Treatment of encrusted cystitis caused by Corynebacterium group D2 with norfloxacin, ciprofloxacin, and teicoplanin in an experimental model in rats. Antimicrob Agents Chemother 1991;35:2587–2590.
247. Feingold SM. Anaerobic bacteria in human disease. New York: Academic Press, 1977.
248. Brook I. Anaerobic bacteria in suppurative genitourinary infections. J Urol 1989;141: 889–893.
249. Rennie DW, Reeves RB, Pappenheimer JR. Oxygen pressure in urine and its relation to intrarenal blood flow. Am J Physiol 1958;195:120–132.
250. Leonhardt KO, Landes RR. Oxygen tension of the urine and renal structures. N Engl J Med 1963;269:115–121.
251. Segura JW, Kelalis PO, Martin WJ, et al. Anaerobic bacteria in the urinary tract. Mayo Clin Proc 1972;47:30–33.
252. West TE, Holley HP, Lauer AD. Emphysematous cystitis due to *Clostridium perfringens*. JAMA 1981;246:363–364.
253. Wajszczuk C, Logan T, Pasculle AW, et al. Intra-abdominal actinomycosis presenting with sulfur granules in the urine. Am J Med 1984;77:1126–1128.
254. Braude AI, Siemienski J, Jacobs I. Protoplast formation in human urine. Trans Assoc Am Physicians 1961;74:234–245.
255. Kalmanson GM, Guze LB. Role of protoplasts in pathogenesis of pyelonephritis. JAMA 1964;190:1107–1109.
256. Gutman LT, Schaller J, Wedgwood RJ. Bacterial L-forms in relapsing urinary-tract infection. Lancet 1967;1:464–466.
257. Guze LB, Kalmanson GM. Action of erythromycin on "protoplasts" in vivo. Science 1964;146:1299–1300.
258. Eastridge RR, Farrar WE. L-form infection of the rat kidney: effect of water diuresis. Proc Soc Exp Biol Med 1968;128:1193–1196.
259. Domingue GJ. Filterable cell-associated cryptic bacterial forms in immunologic renal diseases. Urol Survey l980;30:1–4.
260. Domingue GJ, Ghoniem GM, Bost KL, et al. Dormant microbes in interstitial cystitis. J Urol 1995;153:1321–1326.
261. Grenabo L, Hedlin H, Pettersson S. Urinary infection stones caused by *Ureaplasma urealyticum*: a review. Scand J Infect Dis l988;S53:46–49.
262. Brunner H, Weidner W, Schiefer H. Studies on the role of *Ureaplasma urealyticum* and *Mycoplasma hominis* in prostatitis. J Infect Dis 1983;147:807–812.
263. Meseguer MA, Martinez-Ferrer M, DeRafael L, et al. Differential counts of *Ureaplasma urealyticum* in male urologic patients. J Infect Dis 1984;149:657.
264. McDonald MI, Lam DF, Birch DF, et al. *Ureaplasma urealyticum* in patients with acute symptoms of urinary tract infection. J Urol 1982;128:517–519.
265. McDowall DRM, Buchanan JD, Fairley KF, et al. Anaerobic and other fastidious microorganisms in asymptomatic bacteriuria in pregnant women. J Infect Dis 1981;144: 114–122.
266. Birch DF, D'Apice AJF, Fairley KF. *Ureaplasma urealyticum* in the upper urinary tracts of renal allograft recipients. J Infect Dis 1981;144:123–127.
267. Pickering WJ, Birch DF. Bacteriologic and serologic findings in experimental pyelonephritis caused by *Ureaplasma urealyticum*. Infect Immun 1989;57:1235–1239.
268. Krieger JN, Boatman ES, Kenny GE. *Ureaplasma urealyticum* upper urinary tract infection: persistence and pathogenicity in a canine model. J Urol 1989;141:1437–1443.
269. Pergament M, Gonzalez R, Fraley EE. Atypical mycobacteriosis of the urinary tract. A case report of extensive disease caused by the Battey bacillus. JAMA 1974;229:816–817.
270. Grange JM, Yates MD. Survey of mycobacteria isolated from urine and the genitourinary tract in south-east England from 1980 to 1989. Brit J Urol 1992;69:640–646.

271. Teklu B, Ostrow JH. Urinary tuberculosis: a review of 44 cases treated since 1963. J Urol 1976;115:507–509.

272. Christensen WI. Genitourinary tuberculosis: review of 102 cases. Medicine 1974;53: 377–390.

273. Gorse GJ, Belshe RB. Male genital tuberculosis: a review of the literature with instructive case reports. Rev Infect Dis 1985;7:511–523.

274. Gorostarzu JF, Avisrror MU. Genitourinary tuberculosis in Spain: review of 81 cases. Clin Infect Dis 1994;18:557–561.

275. Deresiewicz RL, Stone RM, Aster JC. Fatal disseminated mycobacterial infection following intravesical bacillus Calmette-Guerin. J Urol 1990;144:1331–1334.

276. Kristjansson M, Green P, Manning HL, et al. Molecular confirmation of bacillus Calmette-Guerin as the cause of pulmonary infection following urinary tract instillation. Clin Infect Dis 1993;17:228–230.

277. Wong SH, Lau WY, Poon ST, et al. The treatment of urinary tuberculosis. J Urol 1984;131:297–301.

278. Fisher JF, Newman CL, Sobel JD. Yeast in the urine: solutions for a budding problem. Clin Infect Dis 1995;20:183–189.

279. Wise GJ, Silver DA. Fungal infections of the genitourinary system. J Urol 1993;149: 1377–1388.

280. Sobel JD, Vazquez JA. Urinary tract infections due to Candida species. In: Mobley HLT, Warren JW, eds. Urinary tract infections: molecular pathogenesis and clinical management. Washington DC: ASM Press, 1986:119–131.

281. Louria DB, Stiff DP, Bennett B. Disseminated moniliasis in the adult. Medicine 1962;41: 307–337.

282. Louria DB, Brayton RG, Finkel G. Studies on the pathogenesis of experimental *Candida albicans* urinary tract infection in mice. Sabouraudia 1963;2:217–283.

283. Chisholm ER, Hutch JA. Fungus ball (*Candida albicans*) formation in the bladder. J Urol 1961;86:559–562.

284. Shelp WD, Wen SF, Weinstein AB. Ureteropelvic obstruction caused by Candida pyelitis in a homotransplanted kidney. Arch Intern Med 1966;117:401–404.

285. Khan MY. Anuria from Candida pyelonephritis and obstructing fungal balls. Urology 1983;21:421–423.

286. Baetz-Greenwalt B, Debaz B, Kumar ML. Bladder fungus ball: a reversible cause of neonatal obstructive uropathy. Pediatrics 1988;81:826–829.

287. Ball W, Lichtenwalner M. Ethanol production in infected urine. N Engl J Med 1979;301: 614.

288. Greenfield RA, Bussey MJ, Stephens JL, et al. Serial enzyme-linked immunosorbent assays for antibody to Candida antigens during induction chemotherapy for acute leukemia. J Infect Dis 1983;148:275–283.

289. Strockbine NA, Largen MT, Zweibel SM, et al. Identification and molecular weight characterization of antigens from *Candida albicans* that are recognized by human sera. Infect Immun 1984;43:715–721.

290. Van Deventer AJM, Van Vliet HJA, Voogd L, et al. Increased specificity of antibody detection in surgical patients with invasive candidiasis with cytoplasmic antigens depleted of mannan residues. J Clin Microbiol 1993;31:994–997.

291. Wells CL, Sirany MS, Blazevic DJ. Evaluation of serum arabinitol as a diagnostic test for candidiasis. J Clin Microbiol 1983;18:353–357.

292. Comings DE, Turbow BA, Callahan DH, et al. Obstructing aspergillus cast of the renal pelvis: report of a case in a patient having diabetes mellitus and Addison's disease. Arch Intern Med 1962;110:255–261.

293. Warshawsky AB, Keiller D, Gittes RF. Bilateral renal aspergillosis. J Urol 1975;113:8.

294. Salgia P, Mani MK. Renal aspergillosis-case report. Nephron 1985;40:376–378.

295. Bibler MR, Gianis JT. Acute ureteral colic from an obstructing renal Aspergilloma. Rev Infect Dis 1987;9:790–794.

296. Halpern M, Szabo S, Hochberg E, et al. Renal aspergillosis: an unusual cause of infection in a patient with acquired immunodeficiency syndrome. Am J Med 1992;437–440.

297. Prout GR Jr, Goddard R. Renal mucormycosis: survival after nephrectomy and amphotericin B therapy. N Engl J Med 1960;263:1246–1248.

298. Davila RM, Moser SA, Grosso LE. Renal mucormycosis: a case report and review of the literature. J Urol 1991;145:1242–1244.
299. Scully RE, Mark EJ, McNeely WF, et al. Case 36–1988. N Engl J Med 1988;319:629–640.
300. Sherwood JA, Dansky AS. Paecilomyces pyelonephritis complicating nephrolithiasis and review of paecilomyces infections. J Urol 1983;130:525–528.
301. Agarwal SK, Tiwari SC, Dash SC, et al. Urinary sporotrichosis in a renal allograft recipient. Nephron 1994;66:485.
302. Salahuddin F, Purnendu S, Chechko S. Urinary tract infection with an unusual pathogen (Nocardia asteroides). J Urol 1996;155:654–655.
303. Eickenberg HU, Amin M, Lich R. Blastomycosis of the genitourinary tract. J Urol 1975;113:650–652.
304. Inoshita T, Youngberg GA, Boelen LJ, et al. Blastomycosis presenting with prostatic involvement: Report of 2 cases and review of the literature. J Urol 1983;130:160–162.
305. Goldman MJ, Movitt E. Disseminated coccidioidomycosis: isolation of the causative organism from the urine. Calif Med 1948;69: 456–458.
306. Rohn JG, Davila JC, Gibbon TE. Urogenital aspects of coccidioidomycosis: review of the literature and report of two cases. J Urol 1951;65:660–667.
307. Conner WR, Drach GW, Bucher WC Jr. Genitourinary aspects of disseminated coccidioidomycosis. J Urol 1975;113:82–88.
308. Petersen EA, Friedman BA, Crowder ED, et al. Coccidioiduria: clinical significance. Ann Intern Med 1976;85:34–38.
309. Chen KT. Coccidioidomycosis of the epididymis. J Urol 1983;130:978–979.
310. Redy P, Gorelick DF, Brasher CA, et al. Progressive disseminated histoplasmosis as seen in adults. Am J Med 1970;48:629–636.
311. Marans HY, Mandell W, Kislak JW, et al. Prostatic abscess due to *Histoplasma capsulatum* in the acquired immunodeficiency syndrome. J Urol 1991;145:1275–1276.
312. Randall RE, Stacy WK, Toone EC, et al. Cryptococcal pyelonephritis. N Engl J Med 1968;279:60–65.
313. Salyer WR, Salyer DC. Involvement of the kidney and prostate in cryptococcosis. J Urol 1973;109:695.
314. Hellman RN, Hinrichs J, Sicard G, et al. Cryptococcal pyelonephritis and disseminated cryptococcosis in a renal transplant recipient. Arch Intern Med 1981;141:128–130.
315. Hathout SE, El-Gaffar YA, Awny AY, et al. Relation between urinary schistosomiasis and chronic enteric urinary carrier state among Egyptians. Am J Trop Med 1966;15:156–161.
316. Lehman JS Jr, Farid Z, Bassily S. Salmonellosis and schistosomiasis of urinary tract. N Engl J Med 1970;283:1291.
317. Farid Z, Higashi GI, Bassily S, et al. Chronic salmonellosis, urinary schistosomiasis and massive proteinuria. Am J Trop Med Hyg 1972;21:578–581.
318. Doehring E, Reider F. Reduction of pathological findings in urine and bladder lesions in infection with *Schistosoma haematobium* after treatment with praziquantel. J Infect Dis 1985;152:807–810.

11

Pathogenesis of Infection—The Host Defenses

Overview

The urinary tract possesses powerful defense mechanisms against microbial invasion. The most important of these are the hydrodynamic properties of the collecting system. The healthy bladder empties almost completely, leaving only a small volume of residual urine. Any condition that alters the wash-out effect of the urinary stream favors colonization with microorganisms that grow in urine. This concept provides a rather straight forward explanation for the ability of relatively avirulent microorganisms to produce complicated infections. The kidneys are remarkably resistant to infection unless the nephrons are damaged structurally or mobilization of leukocytes is delayed (1). More virulent P-fimbriated strains of *E. coli* are needed to invade the normal kidney and produce uncomplicated pyelonephritis and bacteremia (see Table 10.4).

The pathogenesis of uncomplicated infections in females is more difficult to explain. Most females never acquire urinary tract infections, some have unpredictable, sporadic episodes, and a small proportion are remarkably susceptible to recurrent infection. The short female urethra and its complex ductal structure are obvious explanations for differences in the rates of urinary infections in males and females. Nevertheless it is not entirely clear why some females are more susceptible than others to recurrent urinary tract infections. The uropathogenic properties of the invading microorganisms must have an important role, as was described in the preceding chapter. There are no epidemics of uncomplicated urinary tract infections except for occasional nursery outbreaks. This finding suggests that special host factors are involved. The key determinants appear to be the ecology and uropathogenicity of the invading microorganisms, interactions between the microbes and urothelial cells, and the host cellular response.

The sequential steps in ascending infections in females are listed in Table 11.1. The invading microorganisms must be able to grow in bladder urine

Table 11.1. Sequential Steps in Ascending, Uncomplicated Urinary Tract Infections in Females

Colonization of the colon with *Enterobacteriaceae* and *Staphylococcus saprophyticus*
Migration of uropathogenic microorganisms to the periurethral region
Colonization of the vaginal vestibule and distal urethra
Migration to the bladder and attachment to mucosal cells
Resistance to bladder wash-out, shedding of cells, and local killing
Growth in bladder urine
Ascent to kidney against the urinary stream
Colonization and invasion of the renal medulla
Growth and inflammation within renal tubular segments
Bacteremia
Metastatic infection back to the kidney

Table 11.2. Determinants of Host Susceptibility and Resistance in Ascending, Uncomplicated Urinary Tract Infections in Females

Fecal Flora	Complex ecological competition and the selective effects of antimicrobial therapy,
Vagina	Resistance to colonization with enteric microorganisms by acid-producing Lactobacilli, under the influence of estrogens,
Urothelial surfaces	Short urethra, relative abundance of receptors to microbial adhesins, local production of IgA antibodies,
Bladder mucosa	Resistance of mucous layer, local killing, shedding of urothelial cells and mobilization of leukocytes in response to P-fimbriae and endotoxin,
Urine Defenses	Binding of Type-1 fimbriae by Tamm-Horsfall protein and oligosaccharides,
Growth in Urine	pH, organic acids, osmolality and osmoprotective mechanisms,
Urinary Hydrodynamics	Rate of flow, voiding and volume of residual urine,
Renal Defense	Mobilization of leukocytes, production of antibodies to capsules, O antigens and P-fimbriae, cellular immune response,
Bacteremia	Resistance to complement, opsonization and clearance by the reticuloendothelial system.

and evade the bladder mucosal defense mechanisms. The determinants of host susceptibility and resistance to infection are summarized in Table 11.2.

Several pathogenetic mechanisms have received considerable attention in recent years. These include:

- Attachment of uropathogenic *E. coli* to urothelial cells by fimbrial adhesins
- Phase variation to elude host recognition by Tamm-Horsfall protein and leukocytes
- Polymorphonuclear leukocyte response to P-fimbriae and endotoxin mediated by a urothelial cytokine network

Paradoxically, less invasive strains that lack P-fimbriae have a special advantage in colonizing the bladder. They are found much more commonly in patients with asymptomatic bacteriuria and cystitis (see Table 10.4), and can prevent superinfection by more virulent strains (see "Is Adhesion Necessary?" in Chapter 10).

This chapter will consider the nonimmune host mechanisms that appear to protect or enhance microbial invasion of the urinary tract. The key topics include:

- The mucosal defense mechanism
- The osmoprotective activity of urine for bacteria
- The urokinetic defense mechanism and its impact on antimicrobial therapy
- P and Lewis blood group antigens as surrogate markers for host cell receptors

The humoral and cellular immune responses to infection and the potential for a pyelonephritis vaccine are considered elsewhere (see "Immune Response to Infection" in Chapter 10). Toward the end of the chapter we will consider several theories that might explain why some females appear to be susceptible to urinary tract infections. Males usually acquire urinary tract infections from instrumentation, but some episodes appear "out of the blue." The prostate produces an antibacterial substance and can synthesize IgA locally.

Ascending Infection

Colonization of the Colon and Skin

The bowel skin and vagina possess unique resident flora. Anaerobic bacteria are the most abundant organisms in the bowel, exceeding *E. coli* and other *Enterobacteriaceae by* 100 to 1000 fold. In addition, the bacterial population is constantly turning over, as evidenced by transient colonization with specific serologic types. In certain environments, such as hospitals, endemic bowel flora are selected by antibiotic pressure and cross-colonize among patients and health care workers. The situation is confounded by genetic exchange among the bacteria in the bowel through plasmid-mediated-DNA encoded resistance. Extensive use of antimicrobial agents selects resistant strains in the gut. Resistant microorganisms are often responsible for subsequent infections.

The Vaginal Flora and Estrogens

The normal resident flora of the human vagina includes over 50 species of aerobic, facultative anaerobic and obligate anaerobic bacteria. Lactobacilli are the most abundant species in adult women and are usually present in concentrations of 10^7 to 10^9 cfu/ml. Vaginal estrogen increases the glycogen content of the vaginal epithelial cells and favors the growth of Lactobacilli. Lactobacilli generate lactic acid and hydrogen peroxide (2), lower the vaginal pH, and interfere with the growth of other microorganisms (3).

In prepubertal girls, the vaginal pH is about 7.0 (4). With menarche, the pH falls to about 4.9 (range 3.7 to 7.5) and rises in postmenopausal women who are not on estrogen replacement (5). The vaginal introitus harbors *E. coli, Proteus mirabilis,* and Enterococci more often in women whose vaginal pH is ≥ 4.4 than in those with a pH of ≤ 4.4 (5). Uropathogens are rare when the vaginal pH is < 4.0. The vaginal pH can be reduced slightly (4.9 to 4.6) with intravaginal buffer cream (pH 3.0), but this has no significant effect on colonization of the vaginal introitus by uropathogens (6).

The evidence that Lactobacilli and estrogens protect against urinary tract infections is conflicting. Lack of estrogen does not appear to explain why rates of urinary tract infections are lower in premenarchal girls than in adult women. Furthermore, the common resident organisms of the vagina do not differ quantitatively in premenopausal women with or without recurrent urinary tract infections (7). Experimental animals develop hydronephrosis and are more susceptible to hematogenous and ascending urinary tract infections during pregnancy (8) and after administration of estradiol (9). Female contraceptive hormones also enhance the adhesion of *E. coli* to urothelial cells in estrogenized rats (10) and to women given oral contraceptives (11). However, use of oral contraceptives does not appear to increase susceptibility to infection (see Table 6.1) and the rate of asymptomatic bacteriuria increases only slightly during pregnancy.

Estrogens are presumed to exert a protective force against recurrent urinary tract infections in postmenopausal women because they enhance the growth of Lactobacilli and decrease vaginal pH (12–14). Even this notion has been challenged by a report of increased risk of urinary tract infections associated with estrogen use in older women (15). The key point is that gram-negative enteric bacteria do not ordinarily colonize the vagina in postmenopausal women unless these women are prone to recurrent urinary tract infection (16).

Migration to the Periurethral Region

The periurethral zone is colonized with staphylococci, diphtheroids, streptococci, and anaerobic bacteria (17). Small numbers of enteric gram-negative bacteria may be present in the vaginal vestibule and the distal one-third of the urethra of otherwise healthy females without causing urinary tract infections (see Figs. 10.4 and 10.5). The role of personal hygiene and sexual intercourse on acquisition of urinary tract infections in females is discussed in Chapter 6 (see Table 6.1). The key point is that women prone to recurrent infections tend to be persistently colonized by a single strain for prolonged periods of time. An attractive hypothesis is that surface adhesins of *E. coli,* other enteric bacteria, and *Staphylococcus saprophyticus* enable them to adhere to the urothelium and colonize the urethra of susceptible females. There is considerable evidence that type-1 fimbriae play an important role in the genesis of asymptomatic bacteriuria and cystitis (see Table 10.4). The mechanism by which bacteria enter the bladder is not known. Possibilities include migration along the urethral mucosa or reflux into the bladder with the turbulent urinary stream or during the termination of voiding. Colonization of the vaginal introitus and perineum with uropathogens is increased in women with recurrent infections and controls by more frequent micturition, suggesting transfer of microorganisms from the feces by the urinary stream (18).

Growth in Urine

Urine is a variable, but generally good, culture medium (19). The rate and extent of microbial growth depend on the pH, tonicity, and chemical constituents. The composition of urine reflects the diet, use of drugs, and fluid intake. Most of the aerobic bacteria that colonize the urinary tract grow well at neutral or slightly alkaline pH and can resist moderate changes in tonicity. Lactobacilli, streptococci, and Corynebacteria and other commensal microorganisms grow poorly, if at all, in human urine (20). Strict (obligate) anaerobes barely survive or are killed, presumably because small amounts of oxygen are dissolved in urine. Gonococci readily infect the urethra and genital tract but do not multiply and are often killed rapidly in urine. Growth of gonococci is inhibited by low pH and high concentrations of urea and NaCl (21).

Unfavorable growth conditions in urine are extremes of pH (below 5.5 and above 7.5), high tonicity and dietary-derived weak organic acids. Glucose content in urine is not a limiting factor for growth of enteric bacteria. The small amounts of glucose present in urine are used by E. coli. Addition of larger amounts does not alter the generation time, but prolongs the logarithmic growth phase (22). High concentrations of glucose (1 g/L) do not augment growth further. As the bacteria metabolize glucose, the pH tends to be lowered and becomes inhibitory. Glycosuria does not account for the increased susceptibility of diabetics to urinary tract infections.

pH, Osmolality, and Urea
The pH of the urine is determined by the diet and limited by the buffering capacity of phosphates and bicarbonate in urine. Claude Bernard demonstrated over 100 years ago that a meat diet or protein catabolism from starvation lowers the pH of urine in animals (23). Methionine and cysteine are the principal sulfur-containing amino acids in meat. These amino acids are metabolized to inorganic sulfate and excreted along with hydrogen ions to produce an acid urine (24,25). Large populations of the world whose diet is deficient in meat-derived protein tend to have an alkaline urine (see Fig. 3.3) but do not appear to be at increased risk of urinary tract infections.

Growth of E. coli in urine is inhibited by a combination of extremes of pH and high osmolality (26). The rate of multiplication is markedly reduced at pH 5.0 in combination with an osmolality of > 600 mOsm/kg. In contrast, at pH 7.0, multiplication occurs at osmolalities of up to 1600 mOsm/kg. Urea is the principal antibacterial osmolyte in urine (27,28). The antibacterial effect of urea is modulated by pH and concentrations of electrolytes (28). Growth of E. coli is less rapid in concentrated overnight urine than in dilute daytime urine (29). This growth is compensated by prolonged incubation time during the night.

Ascorbic Acid and Cranberry Juice
Ascorbic acid and cranberry juice are not effective urinary acidifying agents unless taken in large amounts (30–34). The antibacterial effect of cranberry juice is derived from hippuric acid. Quinic acid present in cranberry juice is aromatized to benzoic acid by bacteria in the gut. Benzoic acid is absorbed and conjugated with glycine in the liver to form hippuric acid (33). Hippuric acid is a weak antimicrobial compound that is most active at acid pH. Large volumes of cranberry juice must be taken to inhibit bacterial growth in

urine. Cranberry and blueberry juice contain lectins that bind type-1 fimbriae, but the clinical significance is unknown. The purported therapeutic effect of cranberry juice may be a result of water diuresis.

Natural Inhibitors of Microbial Adhesins
Urine contains substances that bind type-1 and S, but not P-fimbriae. The major inhibitor is Tamm-Horsfall protein (THP). There are also low molecular weight α mannosides in urine that bind type 1-fimbria and other adhesins (35). Human milk fat globulin membranes and mucins and a protein isolated from bovine colostrum bind S-fimbriae, suggesting that they may inhibit bacterial adhesion to intestinal cells (36,37). Oligosaccharides that bind mannose-resistant *E. coli* have also been described in human breast milk during the first month after delivery (38). This finding supports the notion that breast feeding may be beneficial in preventing colonization with enteropathic and uropathic *E. coli*.

Several investigators have attempted to determine whether susceptibility to urinary tract infections might be related to the presence of THP in the urine. The excretion of THP in infants with urinary tract infections is lower than in controls, but the authors conclude that the role of THP, if any, remains unresolved (39). Urinary excretion of THP is not significantly different among women with recurrent urinary tract infections and controls (40). Urinary disaggregated THP is decreased in elderly women, and aggregated THP is decreased in elderly women and children with active urinary tract infections. These findings are difficult to interpret, but they may indicate that THP is consumed by bacteria during active urinary tract infection (41).

Osmoprotective Activity of Urine
Bacteria are partially protected from the osmotic forces of the medium by their cell wall. This wall is relatively elastic in gram negative enteric bacteria. The cytoplasmic membrane shrinks or expands in response to external osmotic forces (42). The turgor pressure of *E. coli* is maintained at approximately 303 kPa over a broad range of osmolality of the external medium (43). *E. coli* respond to hypertonic environments by several osmoprotective mechanisms. These mechanisms include uptake of potassium, synthesis of glycine betaine from choline, and intracellular transport of glycine betaine, proline, glutamine, and trehalose (44). These small molecules are said to be compatible solutes. They accumulate intracellularly when the microorganisms are exposed to high concentrations of solute and protect the cells from dehydration. Glycine betaine is the most important compatible solute. Under conditions of osmotic stress, it is taken up from the medium and concentrated 100,000-fold intracellularly. *E. coli* are also able to alter their permeability to water and solutes by changing the expression of their outer membrane proteins in response to osmotic stress (45,46) and in hypertonic urine (47). *E. coli* mutants that cannot synthesize glycine betaine do not grow well in urine (48).

Staphylococci (*Staphylococcus aureus, Staphylococcus saprophyticus,* and co-agulase-negative staphylococci) possess a much more rigid, spherical cell wall. The cytoplasm is often hyperosmolar to the medium and resists plasmolysis. The internal turgor pressures are maintained at 2020 to 3030 kPa (49). Staphylococci are considerably more salt tolerant than *Enterobacteriaceae* and can grow in up to 20% NaCl. They contain large constitutive concentrations of glycine betaine and potassium regardless of the osmolality of the external medium (50). Enterococci are also relatively salt tolerant and respond to osmotic stress principally by increasing intracellular concentrations of potassium (50).

Enterobacteriaceae do not grow well in synthetic urine unless small amounts of broth, serum, or urine are added (28,51). The ability of *E. coli* to grow in hypertonic urine is associated with the presence of glycine and proline betaines (52,53). Proline betaine is derived from the diet. Glycine betaine is synthesized from choline by the inner medulla of the kidney. It is accumulated by renal tubular cells to counteract the osmotic forces of the urine (54,55) (Fig. 11.1). Human urine is even more osmoprotective for *Enterobacteriaceae* than for glycine betaine (Fig. 11.2), suggesting the presence of additional osmoprotectants. All human urine tested has osmoprotective

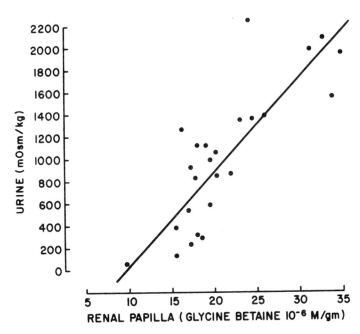

Figure 11.1. Correlation between urinary osmolality and concentration of glycine betaine in the renal inner medulla of rabbits given various osmotic loads. Reproduced with permission from Chambers and Kunin (54).

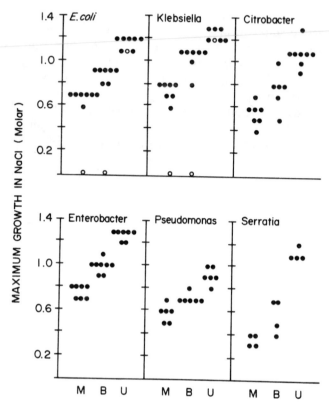

Figure 11.2. Highest molar concentrations of NaCl in which enteric organisms grew in minimal media (M), minimal medium containing 1 x 10⁻⁴M glycine betaine (B), and a 1:10 dilution of human urine in minimal medium (U). Reproduced with permission from Chambers and Kunin (52).

activity (Fig. 11.3). *E. coli* obtained from the stool, urine, or blood do not differ in their salt-sensitivity (48). It is doubtful that a defect in synthesis of glycine betaine renders some individuals more resistant to urinary tract infections or that salt-resistant *E. coli* are responsible for urinary tract infections. Glycine betaine does not protect against the osmotic effects of urea because urea can passively diffuse into the cells.

Thus, the favorable growth properties of urine for *Enterobacteriaceae* are caused by an independent renal osmoprotective mechanism that coincidentally protects the microorganisms from the osmotic forces of urine.

Effect of Diuresis on the Susceptibility of the Bladder and Kidney to Infection
The osmolality of urine in humans ranges from 38 to as high as 1400 mOsm/kg. It may exceed 3000 mOsm/kg in rodents. The osmolality of the

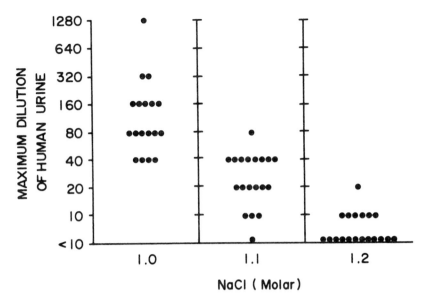

Figure 11.3. Osmoprotective activity for *E. coli* against NaCl added to the urine obtained from 19 healthy young men. In the absence of urine, growth of the organism was limited to 0.7 M NaCl. Reproduced with permission from Chambers and Kunin (52).

urine has a profound effect on the susceptibility of rodents to experimental urinary tract infection (56–59). Under conditions of intense diuresis, rats become less susceptible to the intravenously-induced infection, but more susceptible to the ascending infection. This apparent paradox is explained by differences in the defense mechanisms of the kidney and bladder. Diuresis tends to protect the kidney from infection and augments the effect of antimicrobial drugs by improving mobilization of leukocytes in the renal medulla (60) and by diluting solutes that inhibit phagocytic activity (61–69). Diuresis dilutes urea and salts in hypertonic rodent urine and provides a more suitable media for bacteria to grow in the bladder. Diuresis has also been shown to disrupt the layer of mucin coating the surface of the bladder mucosa and to interfere with its antimicrobial properties (70).

These observations are of considerable theoretical interest in experimental infections, but are probably not relevant to humans. Unlike rodents, the osmolality of human urine rarely exceeds 800 mOsm/kg and is generally much more dilute. The reason to advise patients with recurrent urinary tract infections to drink fluids is not to improve leukocyte function, but for the hydrodynamic purposes.

Urinary Hydrodynamics

The hydrodynamic properties of the urinary tract are considered to be the most important protective mechanisms. High rates of urine flow coupled with voiding dilute the invading microorganisms and eliminate all but a few that remain in the residual urine or that are attached to the urothelium. This finding is illustrated by a study of the effect of high fluid intake and frequent voiding in infected patients with small or large residual urinary volumes (71) (Fig. 11.4). Note the marked washout of bacteria by subject A who had a small residual volume, and the persistence of large numbers of bacteria in the urine of subject B who could not empty the bladder completely. The response to treatment of urinary tract infection in females is not as good when even small residual volumes of urine are left in the bladder after voiding (72). This may explain why some girls with asymptomatic bacteriuria and diabetics with urodynamic abnormalities are more susceptible to urinary tract infections (73,74).

People with urinary tract infections often are advised to drink large volumes of fluid, void frequently, and try to completely empty the bladder. Only

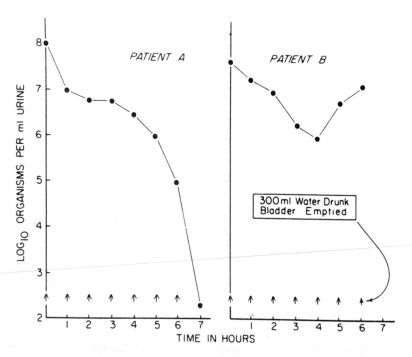

Figure 11.4. Effect of water diuresis and voiding on concentration of bacteria in the urine in a patient without residual volume (A) and one unable to completely empty the bladder (B). Reproduced with permission from O'Grady and Cattell (71).

a few clinical studies have examined the issue of whether these measures are of value in preventing recurrent infection. Eckford et al. (75) used a self-administered conductivity probe to encourage women with recurrent urinary tract infections to maintain a dilute urine. They found that women using the probe tended to have a lower urine osmolality and fewer recurrent infections, but the number of subjects was small and many dropped out because of unwillingness to use the device. It has also been shown that some women spontaneously clear their infection after undergoing a Fairley wash-out test. There are anecdotal accounts that incipient urinary tract infections can be aborted by forced diuresis. Antimicrobial drugs are much more powerful, and high water intake is not needed (see next section). Bacteriostatic drugs are effective in patients with uncomplicated infection and an intact voiding mechanism. Bactericidal drugs often are ineffective in complicated infections.

Kinetics of the Upper and Lower Urinary Tract
The theoretical foundation for the mechanisms by which the bladder and kidneys "wash-away" bacteria was developed by Cox and Hinman (76) and expanded by O'Grady, Cattell, and Greenwood and others (77–82). In vitro bladder models and kinetic equations have helped understand how antimicrobial agents and voiding work together to eradicate urinary tract infections. These concepts are summarized briefly as follows.

The urinary washout kinetics are quite different for the upper and lower tracts. According to O'Grady and Cattell (71), the "conditions in the upper tract correspond with those in continuous cultivation systems in which fresh medium (in this case urine) is constantly supplied and the culture drained off at the same rate. Conditions in the bladder are more complicated in that while they approximate cultivation in a static chamber there are important differences: the volume of culture medium is continuously increased by addition of fresh urine and the whole culture is discarded at intervals which may be varied, but are, to some extent at least, governed by the rate at which fresh medium is added."

UPPER TRACT. The factors that govern persistence of bacteria in the upper tract include:

1. The bacterial multiplication rate: The maximum doubling time for enteric bacteria in urine is about 20 minutes. This duration may be altered depending on the character of the urine (pH, osmolality, and other factors described above) and the effect of antimicrobial agents.
2. The perfusion volume ratio: The concentration of organisms will remain steady if the rate of addition of fresh urine is just fast enough to halve the concentration of bacteria at each doubling time interval. The rate of change depends on the rate of urine flow divided by the volume in the system (the perfusion volume of ratio). The volume of the upper tract of adult humans is estimated to be about 5 to 15 ml.

3. Critical perfusion/volume ratio: The value at which the concentration of organisms in the urine will remain steady. When the rate of urine flow is increased, the concentration of bacteria will fall, and when it decreases, the concentration of bacteria will rise.

O'Grady and Cattell examined the effect of different perfusion/volume ratios on the ability of bacterial populations to achieve full growth or become sterile over time. They determined the critical perfusion/volume ratio in the upper urinary tract that is required to allow a bacterial population to reach a steady state. This turns out to be at about the ordinary physiologic rates of urine flow (assuming that the average volume of the upper tract is 10 ml and urine flow is 0.35 ml per minute or about 1 liter per day). Higher rates of flow will tend to raise the ratio and gradually eliminate bacteria from the system. Lower rates of flow, as occur overnight, tend to increase the bacterial population. The kinetic analysis explains how the normal upper tract can remain sterile simply by increasing urine flow in excess of 1 liter per day at all times. It also explains why an antimicrobial drug can eradicate bacteria from the urine in the upper tract by prolonging the doubling time even without killing the microorganism if the rate of urine flow is adequate.

These calculations for the upper tract are based on the assumption that there is complete mixing of urine, that there is a steady rate of urine flow, and that bacteria do not remain adherent to cells, foreign bodies, or mucosal surfaces. A large dilated renal pelvis, a stone, unequal perfusion of nephrons, or low rate of flow (such as at night) tend to permit the bacteria to persist. Even bactericidal agents may not be effective under such conditions.

LOWER TRACT. The factors that determine the rate at which bacterial populations will change in the bladder urine depend on the size of the inoculum, rate of growth of the organisms, the residual volume, rate of urine flow, and frequency of voiding. The number of bacteria left in the bladder after voiding is equal to the concentration in the urine (C) and the residual volume (V). The larger the residual volume, the more the organisms are left in the bladder to grow. The more organisms that are left behind, the more frequent the voidings will have to be to remove them. The change in bacterial concentration is also affected by dilution with fresh urine or bladder refilling rate (r). High volumes of urine will dilute the bacteria left behind in the residual volume but will not change their absolute number. O'Grady and Cattell have developed the following formula to describe bladder kinetics. The number of bacteria that will be in the bladder at time t after it is emptied will be:

$$CV \times e^{kt}$$

(Concentration times Residual Volume times Rate of Growth at a Given Interval). Because the bladder is always being refilled with urine, this rate must be added to the equation as:

$$\frac{CV \times e^{kt}}{V + rt}$$

(rt is the increase in urine volume over a given period of time).

It can be seen from these equations that factors that favor eradication of bacteriuria are: a small residual volume, increase in doubling time (decreased rate of growth), rapid flow of urine, and a short voiding interval. Hinman (76) calculated that the residual volume in normal people is about 0.5 ml or just enough to wet the mucosal surfaces. Residual urine will be increased in patients with vesicoureteral reflux (as the ureter empties into the bladder after voiding) and any other factor that interferes with complete emptying.

O'Grady and Cattell made the following calculations to illustrate the washout mechanism of the bladder. Assuming a bacterial doubling time of 20 minutes, a bladder volume of 300 ml, and a residual volume of 3 ml, the bacterial population will achieve its previous density in about 2 hours. It can be seen from these calculations why overnight incubation of bacteria in the absence of voiding is critical for the initiation and persistence of infection. This is the rationale for use of bed-time doses of chemoprophylactic agents. The critical nature of a low residual volume explains why it is so important to empty the bladder as completely as possible when performing intermittent catheterization. The formula also explains why large amounts of fluids are effective in preventing infection by diluting the bacteria in the urine and by increasing the frequency of voiding. This voiding effect is limited by the physical constraints of taking large volumes of fluid and voiding frequently. Antimicrobial drugs are highly effective because they decrease the doubling time so that high voiding frequency becomes much less critical.

The bladder is not a simple flask in which the contents are limited to the fluid phase. This is one of the problems in extrapolating the in vitro models to man. Bacteria can adhere to the surface of the mucosa or to particulate matter on the surface. Therefore, VC (the amount of bacteria left behind after voiding) should include all bacteria in the bladder regardless of whether they are in the urine or attached to some surface. Another mode of defense of the bladder is its ability to remove adherent organisms. This mucosal defense mechanism will be discussed later.

THERAPEUTIC IMPLICATIONS. The customary method for predicting clinical efficacy of an antimicrobial agent is to determine the minimum inhibiting concentration (MIC). The tests are performed using a relatively small inoculum in artificial culture fluids at neutral pH and under static conditions. Most of the standards for assessing whether an organism is sensitive, intermediate, or resistant to a given drug are based on achievable concentrations in the blood rather than urine. Laboratory conditions are different from those in the bladder urine. The MIC does not take into account the highly variable characteristics of urine, kinetics of flow, the postantibiotic effect, or achievable concentrations of a drug in various portions of the urinary tract.

Urinary Kinetic Effects That Work in Favor of the Drug
- High concentrations are achieved in concentrated urine.
- The bacterial population is diluted as fresh urine enters the tract.
- The activity of most antimicrobial drugs is enhanced in a dilute urine.
- Large portions of the bacterial population are removed by voiding.

Urinary Kinetic Effects That Work Against the Drug
- Diuresis dilutes the drug in urine.
- Fresh nutrients are supplied as new urine is formed.
- The activity of most antimicrobial drugs is reduced in hypertonic urine.
- The drug is eliminated from the bladder with each voiding.

Although the in vitro bladder model has its limitations, it has helped predict potential efficacy of drugs to treat urinary tract infections. For example, MICs do not adequately predict synergistic effects of antimicrobial agents in the bladder model (81). The model also shows that penicillin G is more effective against gram-negative bacteria than would be predicted from MIC (79).

Bladder Mucosal Defense Mechanism

The washout of bacteria, by a combination of urinary flow and periodic voiding, is a powerful but incomplete mechanism for ridding microorganisms from the bladder. Comparative studies between humans and mechanical models strongly suggest that the intact bladder mucosa must be able to remove microorganisms left behind on the thin film of urine after voiding. In simulated bladder models, droplets of fluid containing residual bacteria provide an inoculum for sterile urine added to the system. In contrast, healthy volunteers clear all the bacteria from the bladder under virtually identical circumstances (76).

Several independent investigators have demonstrated that bladder mucosa can destroy surface bacteria (83–89). The mechanism is unknown, but a viable bladder is required. It cannot be accounted for by local antibody or phagocytosis. The bladder is able to kill bacteria adherent to the urothelium but has no effect on those suspended in the urine (88).

Mucin coats the surface of the transitional epithelial cells. It provides a permeability barrier against water and solutes, protects the urothelium from invasion, and enhances clearance of microorganisms from the bladder (90–93). Disruption of the mucous sheath by washing the bladder with solutions of acid, detergents, or pentachlorophenol increases susceptibility to infection and delays clearance of the microorganisms from the bladder. The protective activity can be restored by adding bladder mucin, heparin, or sodium pentosanpolysulfate. Estrogen-depleted animals are more susceptible to infection, possibly because of decreased production of bladder mucin (94). An anion exchange resin has been used to simulate adherence of bacteria to bladder mucosal cells. Bladder washes from patients with recurrent urinary tract infections are significantly less potent in inhibiting bacterial adherence than are extracts from controls (95). A soluble *E. coli* virulence factor, which appears to be a quaternary amine resembling protamine, is reported to enhance attachment of bacteria to the bladder mucosa of rabbits (96).

Mobilization of Bladder Leukocytes and Cell Shedding

Svanborg and her group (97) have shown that mice generate a marked cellular response to intravesical infection with P-fimbriated *E. coli* and endotoxin by means of a cytokine network. Clearance of the microorganisms from the bladder is associated with mobilization of leukocytes and shedding of urothelial cells (98). Anti-inflammatory drugs blunt the leukocyte response and increase susceptibility to infection (99). Mice genetically resistant to lipid A- (LPS or endotoxin) respond to intravesical challenge less vigorously and do not clear the bacteria as well as normal responder mice (97). It is also conceivable that bacteria may be caught up in mucin and eliminated during urination in a manner analogous to the respiratory defense mechanism.

Structure and Function of the Cells that Line the Bladder

In view of the potential importance of the bladder mucosa in resisting infection, it is instructive to briefly review the structure and function of the squamous epithelial cells that line the bladder. The following account is based on a review by Hicks (100). The function of the mammalian bladder is to retain water and solutes. Unlike that of amphibian bladders, it does not modify the composition of the urine. The transitional epithelium is made up of three layers (basal, intermediate, and superficial). The cells are connected by desmosomes. They retain the same relationship to each other when the bladder is contracted, except that they take on a more cuboidal appearance. The rate of turnover is slow. For example, the cycle time of the basal cells is estimated as 6 weeks in the guinea pig and 48 weeks in the mouse. Some epithelial cells may have a life span of more than 200 days. Humans can rapidly regenerate and close large denuded areas of the bladder within 6 weeks.

Bladder epithelial cells contain a unique structure on the luminal side. This structure consists of multiple thickened discoid plaques united to each other by thinner regions. When the bladder is full, the surface is even. On emptying, it buckles at the thin "hinge" region, producing fusiform vacuoles that extend into the cell cytoplasm, giving it a foamy appearance. The ultrastructure consists of a lattice of hexagonal subunits containing cerebrosides, which are also found in myelin. Functionally, the membrane is impermeable to water. It entraps only small amounts into the fusiform vacuoles on contraction.

Healthy bladder mucosal cells are not ordinarily phagocytic. If the epithelium is regenerating in response to damage, the rapidly dividing cells behave like phagocytes and can engulf cells and debris, including erythrocytes. Hicks states "we have not seen any uptake of foreign cells such as infecting organisms during an episode of bacterial cystitis." Other investigators have described bacteria on electron microscopy to form microcolonies in bladder mucus and to be localized in the intracellular space and intracellularly (93).

Ascent and Invasion of the Kidney

Pyelonephritis in animals can be produced by either injecting the bacteria intravenously or instilling them into the bladder. To produce hematogenous infection with enteric bacteria, large inocula are required and the kidney must be injured in some way. This can be accomplished by external massage, local trauma, obstruction, burns, hypokalemia, or acidosis. To produce ascending infections, smaller inocula can be used provided that the voiding mechanism is impaired by insertion of glass beads, sutures, or partial bladder neck obstruction. P-fimbriated strains of *E. coli* appear to ascend to the kidney by altering peristaltic function and by Brownian motion and attachment to renal cell receptors.

The renal medulla is much more susceptible than the cortex to infection by enteric gram negative bacteria and Enterococci. The striking difference in resistance to infection between the cortex and medulla has been worked out by Beeson and his co-workers (1). They demonstrated that as few as 10 *E. coli* injected into the renal medulla of rabbits are sufficient to initiate infection, whereas 100,000 are required to infect the cortex. The most likely explanation for these differences is the relatively poor blood supply of the medulla, delay in mobilization of leukocytes, and the deleterious effect of hypertonicity and low pH in the medulla on phagocytic function. *Staphylococcus aureus* is much more virulent and produces renal cortical abscesses similar to those seen in acute staphylococcal pyelonephritis in humans.

Renal damage and scar formation in acute, experimental pyelonephritis is caused by release of lysosomal enzymes from PMNs (101,102). Chronic pyelonephritis and renal damage can be prevented by antibiotic therapy administered within 3 days after initiation of infection. Thereafter, renal damage is inevitable despite eradication of the microorganisms by antimicrobial drugs and a vigorous humoral and cellular immune response. Dexamethasone prevents renal swelling but does not interfere with leukocyte infiltration, and it fails to prevent scarring (103).

The kidney also elaborates cytokines (IL-1, IL-6, G-CSF, and TNFα) in response to bacterial invasion (104). It is now known that Tamm-Horsfall protein (THP) not only binds type-1 fimbriae but is also a renal ligand for lymphokines and is identical to uromodulin. THP binds to and regulates the circulating activity of IL-1 and TNF (105). Thus, THP appears to have several roles in the defense of the urinary tract against microbial invasion.

Proteus mirabilis is much more invasive and destructive than *E. coli*. Renal invasion is associated with the production of urease. When urease activity is blocked by acetohydroxamic acid or thiourea, tissue destruction is markedly reduced (106,107). Mutants of *Proteus* that lack urease are no more virulent than *E. coli* in mouse models of pyelonephritis. Ammonia has a direct toxic effect on kidney tissue, decreases human PMN cytoskeletal actin (108), and inhibits complement (109).

Extrapolating Experiments in Animals to Humans

Animal models of urinary tract infection and pyelonephritis have improved our understanding of susceptibility to infection and the pathogenesis of pyelonephritis. However, it is not always appropriate to extrapolate animal experiments to the human condition. The experimental conditions, such as inoculum size, route of infection, and microorganisms, can be manipulated to meet the expectations of the investigator. Rodents differ from humans. They have a small bladder capacity, void frequently, reflux into the ureters, maintain a high urine osmolality, eat a laboratory diet, are genetically variable, and possess different gastrointestinal and vaginal flora and cell receptors.

Genetic Susceptibility

Some females are more susceptible to urinary tract infection than others and are at higher risk of periurethral colonization with *E. coli* and recurrent infection. Because bacterial attachment to urothelial cells appears to play an important role in the pathogenesis of infection, it is possible that their urothelial cells might possess fimbrial receptors that more avidly bind *E. coli*. This concept is supported by the work of Stamey (5) and Schaeffer and his colleagues (110). They found that *E. coli* adhered more readily to vaginal cells from women with recurrent urinary tract infections. Their work is presented in greater detail later in this chapter.

Blood Group Antigens

The important role of P-fimbriae in the pathogenesis of uncomplicated pyelonephritis (see Chapter 10) led investigators to determine whether a relationship exists between the P blood group and susceptibility to infection. There are 5 phenotypes of the P blood group system. Of these, the frequency in man is 75% for P_1 and 25% for P_2. The other phenotypes, including cells which are P negative (p), are rare. Data on the distribution of P blood groups in patients with recurrent urinary tract infections are summarized in Table 11.3 (111–113). There is a clear association between

Table 11.3. Frequency of P1 Blood Group Phenotype in Females With Recurrent Urinary Tract Infection

Authors	Cases Compared with Controls
Lomberg et al. (111)	97% P_1 versus 75% without UTI, p<0.01;
(recurrent pyelonephritis in children)	82% in children with reflux, p>0.05
Mulholland et al. (112)	85% P_2 versus 21% in general population
(recurrent UTI in adult women)	Normal distribution of ABO blood groups
Tomisawa et al. (113)	50% P_1 versus 31% in Japanese population
(recurrent UTI in children)	62% P_1 in children with febrile UTI

both P_1 and P_2 blood groups and recurrent urinary tract infections except in girls with vesicoureteral reflux (111). These data suggest that the P_1 group identifies females at higher risk of recurrent infection provided that there are no risk factors for infection. Vesico-ureteral reflux is under separate genetic control.

There is also evidence that the Lewis blood group plays an important role in susceptibility to infection (Table 11.4) (114–117). Individuals who are Le (a−b−) and Le (a+b−) do not secrete A, B, or H blood group antigens in their saliva. Increased binding to bladder squamous and transitional epithelial cells occurs in nonsecretors without regard to the P blood group (118) and in the bladder cells of the nonsecretor phenotype (119,120). Immunohistologic analysis demonstrates that various blood group antigens are expressed differentially in various cell types and domains of the urinary tract and that major differences exist in the abundance of receptors among secretors and nonsecretors (121).

Further support for the notion that nonsecretors may be more susceptible to urinary tract infection is based on a prospective study of girls with

Table 11.4. Relation Between ABO, Lewis Blood Group and NonSecretor Status, and in Females with Recurrent Urinary Tract Infections

Authors	Relative Risk of Recurrent Urinary Tract Infections (95% confidence interval)
Kinane et al. (114)	3.12 (1.49 to 6.52)
(recurrent UTI in adult women)	Blood group B and AB and nonsecretors
Sheinfeld et al. (115)	3.4 (95% confidence interval 1.5 to 7.9)
(recurrent UTI adult women)	Le (a-b-) and Le (a+b-)
	No relation to ABO blood groups
Jantausch et al. (116)	3.2 (1.3 to 7.9) for Le (a-b-) phenotype
(hospitalized children)	No relation to ABO and minor blood groups
Jacobson & Lomberg (117)	Prior UTIs-60% of nonsecretors vs.
(Adults with renal scars)	16% of secretors developed renal scars

recurrent urinary tract infection. The levels of C-reactive protein, erythrocyte sedimentation rate, and body temperature with each episode of infection was significantly higher in nonsecretors than in secretors (122). Also, nonsecretors (Lewis blood group) are more likely to be colonized with adhesive, fimbriated strains of E. coli (123).

The blood group antigens are important determinants of susceptibility to other infections. For example, there is an association of ABO blood groups with cholera (124), Lewis blood group antigens with candidal vaginitis (125), and attachment of *Helicobacter pylori* to human gastric epithelium (126). Absence of the P blood group (the rare p cell phenotype) is associated with resistance to infection with parvovirus B19 (127).

Genetically-Susceptible Animals

Strains of mice differ in susceptibility to urinary tract infections (97, 128–130). Mice with severe combined immunodeficiency are more susceptible to intravesical infection than are normal controls, but congenitally T cell deficient mice do not differ in this respect from immunocompetent heterozygous controls (130).

The "Host Susceptibility" Versus the "Chance Colonization" Theory

One of the critical issues for understanding the acquisition of urinary tract infections in females with uncomplicated infection centers around our understanding of how E. coli colonize the periurethral area. As noted above, coliform organisms are recovered only rarely from the region of the vaginal vestibule and external urethra in otherwise healthy women who have not had a recent episode of urinary tract infection. To acquire infection, at least small numbers of E. coli and other "uropathogenic" organisms must colonize the urethra and gain entry into the bladder. The issue is important because it is the key to our understanding of recurrent infections and approach to prevention and management. Any theory that is offered to explain acquisition of bacteriuria must take into account the following firm observations discussed in previous chapters.

- Most females never have urinary tract infections or only a few sporadic episodes unrelated to sexual intercourse.
- There is a smaller, but definable, group of females who are at increased risk of acquiring recurrent urinary tract infections even after prolonged prophylactic therapy. Sexual intercourse is a predisposing factor in some of these women.
- Reinfections in girls are usually caused by a new serotype of E. coli or a new bacterial species.

- After repeated short courses of therapy, most girls and adult women go into long-term remission.
- Girls found to have asymptomatic bacteriuria are at increased risk of urinary infections during marriage and pregnancy.
- About one-third to one-half of frequent, recurrent infections among adult women are caused by the same strain that produced the prior infection.
- Females with highly recurrent infection are more likely to be nonsecretors and to possess P_1 and P_2 blood group antigens.
- Infection is usually preceded by rectal and periurethral colonization with the same organism.
- Persistent colonization of the periurethral zone need not produce urinary tract infection.
- Except for use of vaginal diaphragms and spermicidal jelly, there are no clear associations between body habits and personal hygiene and urinary tract infections.

Two general theories have been proposed to explain these observations. I will call one of these "The Host Susceptibility Theory" and the other "The Chance Colonization Theory." As with most theories, their validity depends on the methods and populations studied and are subject to change as new data are developed. Furthermore, one or the other may be valid depending on the host and invading microorganism.

The Host Susceptibility Theory

This theory is based on the findings of several groups (5,76,131) that show enteric bacteria tend to colonize the vaginal vestibule and urethra of females with recurrent urinary tract infections more frequently and in higher numbers than in otherwise healthy women. Colonization with a new serotype of E. coli often is followed by recurrent urinary tract infections with the same strain. In a carefully conceived set of studies, Stamey and his group (5) presented evidence, based on quantitative consecutive cultures of the vaginal introitus, that women with recurrent infections are more likely to be colonized with Enterobacteriaceae and enterococci than women who never had urinary tract infections. They postulated that host factors rather than specific pathogenicity of the microorganisms are the prime determinants of colonization. This led them to systematically explore a variety of local factors that might favor vaginal colonization in women with recurrent infections. They found that E. coli tend to adhere more to vaginal and buccal epithelial cells obtained from women with recurrent infections than to controls (5, 110). This finding raised the possibility that some women possess more cell surface receptors for uropathogens. This notion is supported by the finding that women with recurrent urinary tract infections are more likely to be nonsecretors (Lewis blood-group nonsecretor (Le(a+b−)) and recessive

(Le(a−b−)) phenotypes) and more frequently belong to P_1 and P_2 blood groups.

This theory would explain why certain women are prone to frequent, recurrent infections. It also would explain why girls with asymptomatic bacteriuria are more prone to recurrent infection with marriage and pregnancy and would account for urinary tract infections associated with sexual intercourse in highly susceptible women.

The Chance Colonization Theory

The "Chance Theory" is based on the concept that females with a normal voiding mechanism are at constant risk of developing a first episode of urinary tract infection. The bladder defense is so powerful that infection is relatively rare. Some minor alteration in voiding permits microorganisms that originate in the gut to enter the bladder and adhere to the mucosal surface. Strains with low virulence do not elicit a vigorous host response and are able to survive in the bladder better than highly virulent microorganisms. Once established in the bladder, they prevent colonization by more virulent strains.

These chance occurrences account for the baseline frequency of asymptomatic bacteriuria and cystitis found in epidemiologic studies. At times, uropathogenic strains that possess P-fimbriae and other virulence factors are acquired from the gut. Under the appropriate conditions, they produce more invasive infections and pyelonephritis. Once established, each infection sets the stage for the next episode either by altering the bladder defense mechanism or by temporary colonization of the gut and periurethral zone. The longer the patient is free of colonization and infection, the more likely the bladder will resume its normal defense, and the frequency of recurrences will decrease.

Evidence for the "Chance Colonization Theory" is based on the "kinetics" of recurrent infection in girls (132) and adult women (133). After each effectively treated episode of infection, about 70% to 80% of the population will enter long-term remission (see Figs. 4.3, 10.6) independent of the number of previous episodes. The longer the period of remission, the less likely will infections reoccur. This theory explains why most women do not have urinary tract infections most of the time, why sexual intercourse is not a predisposing factor of urinary tract infections unless the periurethral zone is colonized with uropathogens, and why acute pyelonephritis is relatively rare.

Synthesis

Both theories are probably correct depending on the population studied. Women with recurrent urinary tract infections and pyelonephritis tend to be referred to research centers and accumulate disproportionately in the pool over time. This tends to obscure the significance of the much larger pool of women who do not acquire urinary tract infections or have only a few isolated episodes. Women with highly recurrent infections tend to fit the host susceptibility theory. However, they represent a relatively small proportion of women with urinary tract infections.

Women with isolated, intermittent infections usually are managed by primary care physicians and are not referred to research centers. These women tend to fit the chance colonization theory and are more representative of the general population. Population based studies are less likely to identify the smaller group of women at greater risk of frequent, recurrent infection. When reading the literature, the reader is cautioned to evaluate carefully how the population was selected for study. Conclusions drawn from a selected group of individuals may not be relevant to other patients.

Acquisition of Infection in Males

Males rarely develop urinary tract infection even when there is severe obstruction of the outflow tract. The most frequent cause of infection in males is urethral instrumentation. Occasional episodes of "spontaneous" infection occur in males, followed by recurrent infection from a persistent focus in the prostate. The causative microorganisms are similar to those in females, suggesting that they originate from the bowel. The potential routes of infection to the prostate include direct extension along the urethra, through lymphatic channels, and transient bacteremia (see "Urinary Tract Infections in Men" in Chapter 6).

Table 11.5. Patient Characteristics that Help Predict the Response to Therapy in Men with Urinary Tract Infections

Poor Prognosis
    Calculus disease of the upper urinary tract and prostatic calculi
    Focal renal atrophy with subjacent calyceal deformity
    Mixed infection
    Enterococcal infection
    Symptoms for 20 years or more
    Four or more previous courses of therapy for urinary tract infections
    Prostatic enlargement
    Recurrent bacteriuria with the same organism (relapse)
    Serum creatinine, 2 mg/D1 or more
Good Prognosis
    Symptoms present 12 months or less
    No previous therapy for urinary tract infection
    Normal prostate
    Normal intravenous urogram
    Pure *Escherichia coli* infection

From Freeman et al. (135)

Human prostatic secretions contain a potent antibacterial substance (134). It is a heat-stable zinc-containing cationic protein distinct from spermine and lysozyme. It is possible that some males may have diminished amounts of this substance and be more susceptible to bacterial prostatitis. This is difficult to prove because infection of the prostate is relatively rare and large populations would need to be studied prospectively to identify the small proportion at greater risk of bacterial prostatitis.

The characteristics of urinary tract infections that help predict the prognosis and response to therapy in males is summarized in Table 11.5 (135). Note the importance of prostatic and other calculi (see Figure 7.4).

Relation of the Host Defense to Antimicrobial Therapy

The host defense mechanisms of the urinary tract are complex, highly variable, and difficult to alter by diet, body habits, immunization, or changes in the vaginal flora or fluid intake. Debates on whether to protect the kidney, acidify or alkalize the urine, or limit or increase the urinary flow rate serve little purpose when effective antimicrobial drugs are used for therapy or prophylaxis. Once infection is eradicated by effective antimicrobial drugs, the task is to prevent colonization of the lower tract and not to be too concerned about factors that predispose the bladder or kidney to infection. *If infection of the bladder can be prevented, the kidney will be protected from ascending infection.* Patients with complicated infection can be helped by measures that ensure that the collecting system is emptied as completely as possible after voiding. Obstruction must be relieved whenever possible by appropriate use of the catheter, lithotripsy, or surgery. Antimicrobial therapy is usually effective when the voiding mechanism is intact and will often fail when not. Therapeutic strategies to accomplish these goals are presented in the next chapter.

References

1. Beeson PB, Rocha H, Guze LB. Experimental pyelonephritis: influence of localized injury in different parts of the kidney on susceptibility to hematogenous infection. Trans Assoc Am Physicians 1957;70:120–126.
2. Klebanoff SJ, Hillier SL, Eschenbach DA, et al. Control of the microbial flora of the vagina by H_2O_2-generating Lactobacilli. J Infect Dis 1991;164:94–100.
3. Reid G, Bruce AW, McGroarty JA, et al. Is there a role for Lactobacilli in prevention of urogenital and intestinal infections? Clin Microbiol Rev 1990;3:335–344.
4. Hooton TM, Stamm WE. The vaginal flora and urinary tract infections. In: Mobley HLT, Warren JW, eds. Urinary tract infections: molecular pathogenesis and clinical management. Washington DC: ASM Press, 1986:67–94.
5. Stamey TA, Timothy M, Miller M, et al. Recurrent urinary infections in adult women. Calif Med 1971;115:1–19.
6. Moorman CN, Fowler Jr JE. Impact of site release vaginal pH buffer cream on introital colonization by gram-negative bacilli. J Urol 1992;147:1576–1578.

7. Fowler JE Jr, Latta R, Stamey TA. Studies of introital colonization in women with recurrent urinary infections. VII. The role of bacterial interference. J Urol 1977;118:296–298.
8. Andriole VT, Cohn GL. The effect of diethylstilbestrol on the susceptibility of rats to hematogenous pyelonephritis. J Clin Invest 1964;43:1136–1145.
9. Corriere JN, Murphy JJ. The effect of estrogen upon ascending urinary tract infection in rats. Brit J Urol 1968;40:306–314.
10. Sobel JD, Kaye D. Enhancement of *E. coli* adherence to epithelial cells derived from estrogen-stimulated rats. Infect Immun 1986;53:53–56.
11. Sharma S, Madhur BS, Singh R, et al. Effect of contraceptives on the adhesion of *Escherichia coli* to uroepithelial cells. J Infect Dis 1987;156:490–494.
12. Kirkengen AL, Andersen P, Gjersøe GR, et al. Oestriol in the prophylactic treatment of recurrent urinary tract infections in postmenopausal women. Scand J Prim Health Care 1992;10:139–142.
13. Privette M, Cade R, Peterson J, et al. Prevention of recurrent urinary tract infections in postmenopausal women. Nephron 1988;50:24–27.
14. Raz R, Stamm WE. A controlled-trial of intravaginal estriol in postmenopausal women with recurrent urinary tract infections. N Engl J Med 1993;329:753–756.
15. Orlander JD, Jick SS, Dean AD, et al. Urinary tract infections and estrogen use in older women. J Amer Geriat Soc 1992;40:817–820.
16. Pfau A, Sacks T. The bacterial flora of the vaginal vestibule, urethra and vagina in the normal premenopausal woman. J Urol 1977;118:292–295.
17. Marrie TJ, Swantee CA, Hartlen M. Aerobic and anaerobic urethral flora in healthy females in various physiological age groups and of females with urinary tract infections. J Clin Microbiol 1980;11:654–659.
18. Seddon JM, Bruce AW, Chadwick P, et al. Frequency of micturition and urinary tract infection. J Urol 1980;123:524–526.
19. Pasteur ML. Examen du rôle attribue au gaz oxygène atmosphérique dans le destruction des matières animales et végétales après la mort. Comp Rend Acad Sci 1863;56:734.
20. Stamey TA, Mihara G. Observations on the growth of urethral and vaginal bacteria in sterile urine. J Urol 1980;124:461–463.
21. McCutchan JA, Wunderlich A, Braude AI. Role of urinary solutes in natural immunity to gonorrhea. Infect Immun 1977;15:149–155.
22. Weiser R, Asscher AW, Sussman M. Glycosuria and the growth of urinary pathogens. Invest Urol 1969;6:650–656.
23. Bernard C. An introduction to the study of experimental medicine. Schuman, NY: Henderson, 1927.
24. Hunt JN. The influence of dietary sulphur on the urinary output of acid in man. Clin Sci (Colch) 1956;15:119–134.
25. Lemann J Jr, Relman AS, Connors HP. The relation of sulfur metabolism to acid-base balance and electrolyte excretion: the effects of dl-methionine in normal man. J Clin Invest 1959;12:2215–2223.
26. Asscher AW, Sussman M, Waters WE, et al. Urine as a medium for bacterial growth. Lancet 1966;2:1037–1041.
27. Schlegel JU, Cuellar J, O'Dell RM. Bactericidal effect of urea. J Urol 1961;86:819–822.
28. Kaye D. Antibacterial activity of human urine. J Clin Invest 1968;47:2374–2390.
29. Cicmanec JF, Shank RA, Evans AT. Overnight concentration of urine. Urology 1985;26:157–159.
30. Murphy FJ, Zelman S, Mau W. Ascorbic acid as a urinary acidifying agent, 2: its adjunctive role in chronic urinary infections. J Urol 1965;94:300–305.
31. Nahata MC, Shimp L, Lampman T, et al. Effect of ascorbic acid on urine pH in man. Am J Hosp Pharm 1977;34:1234–1237.
32. Travis LB, Dodge WF, Mintz AA, et al. Urinary acidification with ascorbic acid. J Pediatr 1965;67:1176–1178.
33. Fellers CR, Redmon BC, Parrott EM. Effect of cranberries on urinary acidity and blood alkali reserve. J Nutr 1933;6:455–463.
34. Bodel PT, Cotran R, Kass EH. Cranberry juice and the antibacterial action of hippuric acid. J Lab Clin Med 1959;54:881–888.
35. Parkkinen J, Virkola R, Korhonen TK. Identification of factors in human urine that inhibit the binding of *Escherichia coli* adhesins. Infect Immun 1988;56:2623–2630.

36. Schroten H, Hanisch FG, Plogmann R, et al. Inhibition of adhesion of S-fimbriated *Escherichia coli* to buccal epithelial cells by human milk fat globule membrane components: a novel aspect of the protective function of mucins in the nonimmunoglobulin fraction. Infect Immun 1992;60:2893–2899.
37. Ouwehand AC, Conway PL, Salminen SJ. Inhibition of S-fimbria-mediated adhesion to human ileostomy glycoproteins by a protein isolated from bovine colostrum. Infect Immun 1995;63:4917–4920.
38. Coppa G, Gabrelli O, Giogi P, et al. Preliminary study of breast feeding and bacterial adhesion to uroepithelial cells. Lancet 1990;335:569–571.
39. Israele V, Darabi A, McCracken GH Jr. The role of bacterial virulence factors and Tamm-Horsfall protein in the pathogenesis of *Escherichia coli* urinary tract infection in infants. Am J Dis Child 1987;141:1230–1234.
40. Reinhart H, Obedeanu N, Hooton T, et al. Urinary excretion of Tamm-Horsfall protein in women with recurrent urinary tract infections. J Urol 1990;144:1185–1187.
41. Reinhart HH, Obedeanu N, Robinson R, et al. Urinary excretion of Tamm-Horsfall protein in elderly women. J Urol 1991;146:806–808.
42. Koch AL. Shrinkage of growing *Escherichia coli* cells by osmotic challenge. J Bacteriol 1984;159:919–924.
43. Ingraham J. Effect of temperature, pH, water activity, and pressure on growth. In: Neidhardt FC, ed. *Escherichia coli* and *Salmonella typhimurium*. Cellular and molecular biology. American Society for Microbiology. Washington DC, 1987:1543–1544.
44. Le Rudulier D, Strom AR, Dandekar AM, et al. Molecular biology of osmoregulation. Science 1984;224:1064–1068.
45. Lugtenberg B, Peters R, Bernheimer A, et al. Influence of cultural conditioners and mutations on the composition of the outer membrane proteins of *E. coli*. Mol Gen Genet 1976;147:251–262.
46. Van Alphen WV, Lugtenberg B. Influence of osmolarity of the growth medium on the outer membrane protein pattern of *Escherichia coli*. J Bacteriol 1977;131:623–630.
47. Robledo JA, Serrano A, Domingue GJ. Outer membrane proteins of *E. coli* in the host-pathogen interaction in urinary tract infection. J Urol 1990;143:386–391.
48. Kunin CM, Tong HH, White LVA, et al. Growth of *Escherichia coli* in human urine: role of salt tolerance and accumulation of glycine betaine. J Infect Dis 1992;166:1311–1315.
49. Mitchell PD, Moyle J. Osmotic function and structure in bacteria. Symp Soc Gen Microbiol 1956;6:150–178.
50. Kunin CM, Rudy J. Effect of NaCl-induced osmotic stress on intracellular concentrations of glycine betaine and potassium in *Escherichia coli, Enterococcus faecalis* and staphylococci. J Lab Clin Med 1991;118:217–224.
51. Jackson GG, Grieble HG. Pathogenesis of renal infection. Arch Intern Med 1957;100:692–700.
52. Chambers ST, Kunin CM. The osmoprotective properties of urine for bacteria: the protective effect of betaine and human urine against low pH and high concentrations of electrolytes, sugars and urea. J Infect Dis 1985;152:1308–1315.
53. Chambers ST, Kunin CM. Isolation of glycine betaine and proline betaine from human urine. Assessment of their role as osmoprotective agents for bacteria and the kidney. J Clin Invest 1987;79:731–737.
54. Chambers ST, Kunin CM. Osmoprotective activity for *Escherichia coli* in mammalian renal papilla and urine: correlation of glycine and proline betaines and sorbitol with response to osmotic stress. J Clin Invest 1987;80:1255–1260.
55. Bagnasco S, Balaban R, Fales HM, et al. Predominant osmotically active organic solutes in rat and rabbit renal medullas. J Biol Chem 1986;261:5872–5877.
56. Freedman LR. Experimental pyelonephritis. XIII. On the ability of water diuresis to induce susceptibility to *Esch. coli* bacteriuria in the normal rat. Yale J Biol Med 1967;39:255–266.
57. Andriole VT. Water, acidosis, and experimental pyelonephritis. J Clin Invest 1970;49:21–30.
58. D'Alessio DJ, Jackson GG, Olexy VM, et al. Effects of water and furosemide-induced diuresis on the acquisition and course of experimental pyelonephritis. J Lab Clin Med 1971;78:130–137.
59. Kaye D. The effect of water diuresis on spread of bacteria through the urinary tract. J Infect Dis 1971;124:297–305.

60. Rocha H, Fekety FR Jr. Acute inflammation in the renal cortex and medulla following thermal injury. J Exp Med 1964;119:131–138.
61. Chernew I, Braude AI. Depression of phagocytosis by solutes in concentrations found in the kidney and urine. J Clin Invest 1962;41:1945–1953.
62. Knoll BF, Johnson AJ, Pearce CW, et al. The effect of autogenous urine on leukocytic defenses in man. Invest Urol 1969;6:406–411.
63. Maeda S, Deguchi T, Kanimoto Y, et al. Studies of the phagocytic function of urinary leukocytes. J Urol 1983;129:427–429.
64. Matsumoto T, Kumazawa J, Van der Auwera P. Suppression of leukocyte function and intracellular content of ATP in hyperosmotic condition comparable to the renal medulla. J Urol 1989;142:399–402.
65. Allison F Jr, Lancaster M. Pathogenesis of acute inflammation. VI. Influence of osmolarity and certain metabolic antagonists upon phagocytosis and adhesiveness by leukocytes recovered from man. Proc Soc Exp Biol Med 1965;119:56–61.
66. Bulger RJ. Inhibition of human serum bactericidal action by a chemical environment simulating the hydropenic renal medulla. J Infect Dis 1967;117:429–432.
67. Bryant RE, Sutcliffe MC, McGee ZA. Effect of osmolalities comparable to those of the renal medulla on function of human polymorphonuclear leukocytes. J Infect Dis 1972;126:1–10.
68. Gargan RA, Hamilton-Miller JMT, Brumfitt W. Effect of pH and osmolality on in vitro phagocytosis and killing by neutrophils in urine. Infect Immun 1993;61:8–12.
69. Hampton MB, Chambers ST, Vissers MC, et al. Bacterial killing by neutrophils in hypertonic environments. J Infect Dis 1994;169:839–846.
70. Harrison G, Cornish J, Vanderwee MA, et al. Host defense mechanisms in the bladder: I. Role of mechanical factors. Br J Exp Path 1988;69:145–154.
71. O'Grady F, Cattell WR. Kinetics of urinary tract infection: II. The bladder. Br J Urol 1966;38:156–962.
72. Shand DG, Nimmon CC, O'Grady F, et al. Relation between residual urine volume and response to treatment of urinary infection. Lancet 1970;1:1305–1306.
73. Hansson S, Hjalmas K, Jodal U, et al. Lower urinary tract dysfunction in girls with untreated asymptomatic or covert bacteriuria. J Urol 1990;143:333–335.
74. Kaplan SA, Te AE, Blaivas JG. Urodynamic findings in patients with diabetic cystopathy. J Urol 1995;153:342–344.
75. Eckford SD, Keane DP, Lamond E, et al. Hydration monitoring in the prevention of recurrent idiopathic urinary tract infections in pre-menopausal women. Brit J Urol 1995;76:90–93.
76. Cox CE, Hinman R. Experiments with induced bacteriuria, vesical emptying and bacterial growth on the mechanism of bladder defense to infection. J Urol 1961;86:739–748.
77. O'Grady F, Cattell WR. Kinetics of urinary tract infection. I. Upper urinary tract. Br J Urol 1966;38:149–1555.
78. O'Grady F, Pennington JH. Bacterial growth in an "in vitro" system stimulating conditions in the urinary bladder. Br J Exp Pathol 1966;47:152–157.
79. Greenwood D, O'Grady F. An in vitro model of the urinary bladder. J Antimicrob Chemother 1978;4:113–120.
80. Boen JR, Sylvester DL. The mathematical relationship among urinary frequency, residual urine, and bacterial growth in bladder infection. Invest Urol 1965;2:468–473.
81. Anderson JD. Relevance of urinary bladder models to clinical problems and to antibiotic evaluation. J Antimicrob Chemother 1985;15:111–115.
82. Hyman ES. Computer algorithm offers a comprehensive view of quantitative bacteriuria. Nephron 1993;65:549–558.
83. Vivaldi E, Munoz J, Cotran RS, et al. Factors affecting the clearance of bacteria within the urinary tract. In: Kass EH, ed. Progress in pyelonephritis. Philadelphia: FA Davis, 1965: 531–535.
84. Paquin AJ, Perez J, Kunin CM, et al. Does the bladder possess an intrinsic antibacterial defense mechanism? J Clin Invest 1965;44:1084.
85. Cobbs GG, Kaye D. Antibacterial mechanisms in the urinary bladder. Yale J Biol 1967;40:93–108.
86. Norden CW, Green GM, Kass EH. Antibacterial mechanisms of the urinary bladder. J Clin Invest 1968;47:2689–2700.

87. Gillenwater JY, Cardozo NC, Tyrone NO, et al. Antibacterial activity of rat vesical mucosa. J Urol 1970;104:687–692.
88. Mulholland SG, Foster EA, Paquin AJ, et al. The effect of rabbit vesical mucosa on bacterial growth. Invest Urol 1969;6:593–604.
89. Hand WL, Smith JW, Sanford JP. The antibacterial effect of normal and infected urinary bladder. J Lab Clin Med 1971;77:605–615.
90. Parsons CL, Greenspan C, Mulholland SG. The primary antibacterial defense mechanism of the bladder. Invest Urol 1975;13:72–76.
91. Parsons CL, Mulholland SG, Anwar H. Antibacterial activity of bladder surface mucin duplicated by exogenous glycosaminoglycan (heparin). Infect Immun 1979;24:552–557.
92. Parsons CL, Pollen JJ, Anwar H, et al. Antibacterial activity of bladder surface mucin duplicated in the rabbit bladder by exogenous glycosaminoglycan (sodium pentosanpolysulfate). Infect Immun 1980;27:876–881.
93. Cornish J, Lecamwasam JP, Harrison G, et al. Host defense mechanisms in the bladder II: disruption of the layer of mucus. Brit J Exp Pathol 1988;69:759–770.
94. Mooreville M, Fritz RW, Mulholland SG. Enhancement of the bladder defense mechanism by an exogenous agent. J Urol 1983;130:607–609.
95. Ruggieri MR, Levin RM, Hanno PM, et al. Defective antiadherence activity of bladder extracts from patients with recurrent urinary tract infection. J Urol 1988;140:157–159.
96. Mostafavi M, Stein PC, Parsons L. Production of soluble virulence factor by *Escherichia coli*. J Urol 1995;153:1441–1443.
97. Agace W, Connell H, Svanborg C. Host resistance to urinary tract infection. In: Mobley HLT, Warren JW, eds. Urinary tract infections: molecular pathogenesis and clinical management. Washington DC: ASM Press, 1986:221–243.
98. Aronson M, Medalia O, Amichay D, et al. Endotoxin-induced shedding of viable uroepithelial cells is an antimicrobial defense mechanism. Infect Immun 1988;56:1615–1617.
99. Linder H, Engberg I, van Kooten C, et al. Effects of anti-inflammatory agents on mucosal inflammation induced by infection with gram-negative bacteria. Infect Immun 1990;58:2056–2060.
100. Hicks RM. The mammalian urinary bladder: an accommodating organ. Biol Rev 1975;50:215–246.
101. Glauser MP, Lyons JM, Braude AI. Prevention of chronic experimental pyelonephritis by suppression of acute suppuration. J Clin Invest 1978;61:403–407.
102. Bille J, Glauser MP. Protection against chronic pyelonephritis in rats by suppuration: effect of colchicine and neutropenia. J Infect Dis 1982;146:220–226.
103. Meyland PR, Glauser MP. Failure of dexamethasone to prevent polymorphonuclear leukocyte infiltration during experimental acute exudative pyelonephritis and to reduce subsequent chronic scarring. J Infect Dis 1988;157:480–485.
104. Rugo HS, O'Hanley P, Bishop AG, et al. Local cytokine production in a murine model of *Escherichia coli* pyelonephritis. J Clin Invest 1992;89:1032–1039.
105. Hession C, Decker JM, Sherblom AP, et al. Uromodulin (Tamm-Horsfall glycoprotein): a renal ligand for lymphokines. Science 1987;237:1479–1484.
106. Aaronson M, Medalia O, Griffel B. Prevention of ascending pyelonephritis in mice by urease inhibitors. Nephron 1974;12:94–104.
107. Musher DM, Griffith DP, Yawn D. Role of urease in pyelonephritis resulting from urinary tract infection with Proteus. J Infect Dis 1975;31:177–178.
108. Brunkhorst B, Niederman R. Ammonium decreases human polymorphonuclear leukocyte cytoskeletal actin. Infect Immun 1991;59:1378–1386.
109. Beeson PB, Rowley D. The anticomplementary effect of kidney tissue; its association with ammonia production. J Exp Med 1959;110:685–697.
110. Schaeffer AJ, Jones JM, Dunn JK. Association of in vitro *E. coli* adherence to vaginal and buccal epithelial cells with susceptibility of women to recurrent urinary-tract infections. N Engl J Med 1981;304:1062–1066.
111. Lomberg H, Hanson LA, Jacobsson B, et al. Correlation of P blood group, vesicoureteral reflux, and bacterial attachment in patients with recurrent pyelonephritis. N Engl J Med 1983;308:1189–1192.
112. Mulholland SG, Mooreville M, Parsons CL. Urinary tract infections and P blood group antigens. Urology 1984;24:232–235.

113. Tomisawa S, Kogure T, Kuroume T, et al. P blood group and proneness to urinary tract infection in Japanese children. Scand J Infect Dis 1989;21:403–408.

114. Kinane DF, Blackwell CC, Brettle RP, et al. ABO blood group, secretor state, and susceptibility to recurrent urinary tract infection in women. Brit Med J 1982;285:7–9.

115. Sheinfeld J, Schaeffer AJ, Cordon-Cardo C, et al. Association of the Lewis blood-group phenotype with recurrent urinary tract infections in women. N Engl J Med 1989; 320:773–777.

116. Jantausch BA, Criss VR, O'Donnell R, et al. Association of Lewis blood group phenotypes with urinary tract infection in children. J Pediatr 1994;124:863–868.

117. Jacobson SH, Lomberg H. Overrepresentation of blood group non-secretors in adults with renal scarring. Scand J Urol Nephrol 1990;24:145–150.

118. Lomberg H, Cedergren B, Leffler H, et al. Influence of blood group on the availability of receptors for attachment of uropathogenic *Escherichia coli*. Infect Immun 1986;51: 919–926.

119. Sheinfeld J, Cordon-Cardo C, Fair WR, et al. Association of type 1 blood group antigens with urinary tract infections in children with genitourinary structural abnormalities. J Urol 1990;144:469–473.

120. Stapleton A, Nudelman E, Clausen H, et al. Binding of uropathogenic *Escherichia coli* R45 to glycolipids extracted from vaginal epithelial cells is dependent on histo-blood group secretor status. J Clin Invest 1992;90:965–972.

121. Cordon-Cardo C, Lloyd K, Finsted CL, et al. Immunoanatomic distribution of blood group antigens in the human urinary tract. Lab Invest 1986;55:444–454.

122. Lomberg H, Jodal U, Leffler H, et al. Blood group non-secretors have an increased inflammatory response to urinary tract infection. Scan J Infect Dis 1992;24:77–83.

123. Stapleton A, Hooton TM, Fennell C, et al. Effect of secretor status on vaginal and rectal colonization with fimbriated *Escherichia coli* in women with and without recurrent urinary tract infection. J Infect Dis 1995;171:717–720.

124. Van Loon FPL, Clemens JD, Sack DA, et al. ABO blood groups and the risk of diarrhea due to enterotoxigenic *Escherichia coli*. J Infect Dis 1991;163:1243–1246.

125. Hilton E, Chandrasekaran V, Rindos P, et al. Association of recurrent candidal vaginitis with inheritance of Lewis blood group antigens. J Infect Dis 1995;172:1616–1619.

126. Borén T, Falk P, Roth KA, et al. Attachment of *Helicobacter pylori* to human gastric epithelium mediated by blood group antigens. Science 1993;262:1892–1895.

127. Brown KE, Anderson SM, Young NS. Erythrocyte P antigen: cellular receptor for B19 parvovirus. Science 1993;262:114–119.

128. Guze PA, Kalmanson GM, Ishida K, et al. Strain-dependent difference in susceptibility of mice to experimental ascending pyelonephritis. J Infect Dis 1987;156:523–525.

129. Miller T. Genetic factors and host resistance in experimental pyelonephritis. J Infect Dis 1983;148:336.

130. Hopkins WJ, James LJ, Balish E, et al. Congenital immunodeficiencies in mice increase susceptibility to urinary tract infection. J Urol 1993;149:922–925.

131. Bollgren J, Winberg J. The periurethral aerobic flora in girls highly susceptible to urinary infections. Acta Paediatr Scand 1976;65:81–87.

132. Kunin CM. A ten-year study of bacteriuria in school girls: final report of bacteriologic, urologic and epidemiologic findings. J Infect Dis 1970;122:382–393.

133. Kraft JK, Stamey TA. The natural history of recurrent bacteriuria in women. Medicine 1977;56:55–60.

134. Levy BJ, Fair WR. The location of antibacterial activity in the rat prostatic secretions. Invest Urol 1973;11:173–177.

135. Freeman, RB, Richardson JA, Thurm RH, et al. Long-term therapy for chronic bacteriuria in men. Ann Intern Med 1975;83:133–147.

12

Management of Urinary Tract Infections

Overview

Treatment of urinary tract infections can be one of the most gratifying experiences in clinical practice. The patient usually will have a reasonably specific complaint, definitive diagnosis can readily be made by microscopic examination of the urine and confirmed by culture, and a wide variety of effective antimicrobial agents are available for therapy. As with most infectious diseases, the efficacy of treatment or prophylaxis depends on 1) the characteristics of the host, 2) the nature of the invading microorganism, 3) the natural history of the disease, and 4) the efficacy of chemotherapy. The goal of management is to eradicate the invading organism from the entire system. Almost equally important is the necessity to anticipate, prevent, or treat recurrences. At times it is necessary to recognize failure in complicated infections and withhold antimicrobial therapy except to treat sepsis.

A general consensus has emerged during the past decade concerning the management of urinary tract infections (1–6). It is now well accepted that uncomplicated infections rarely produce renal damage. Therapeutic and prophylactic tactics are designed to reduce morbidity and prevent symptomatic recurrences. There is also a more relaxed attitude toward treatment of asymptomatic bacteriuria in females of all ages and the elderly. The only firm indications are bacteriuria during pregnancy and renal transplantation. Treatment of uncomplicated, asymptomatic bacteriuria and funguria can be counterproductive and lead to superinfection with more resistant or virulent microorganisms. Treatment of complicated infections remains difficult despite the advent of more effective antimicrobial drugs. It is more important to relieve obstruction than to eradicate microorganisms. Treatment of persistent bacteriuria in patients with indwelling urinary devices or obstruction or foreign bodies is usually ineffective. Emergence of resistant microorganisms is an increasingly important problem, particularly in regions of the world where antimicrobial drugs are available over-the-counter (7). Initiatives to make them available without prescription in the United States and Western Europe are deplored (8).

This chapter will consider strategies to prevent and treat urinary tract infection in adults. Urinary tract infections in children are discussed in Chapter 4. Many of the concepts presented in earlier chapters will be reiterated to remind the reader that successful management depends not only on the choice, dose, and duration of chemotherapy for a particular microorganism, but also on host factors and natural history.

General Principles

The general principles of management of urinary tract infections are similar to those for other infectious diseases. They include the following steps:

- Verify the diagnosis
- Distinguish uncomplicated from complicated infections
- Assess underlying medical and surgical problems
- Decide whether antimicrobial therapy might be useful
- Select the drug and dose to be used
- Determine the appropriate duration of therapy
- Confirm the diagnosis and choice of drug by culture and susceptibility tests
- Consider the need for uroradiologic studies
- Remove foreign bodies and correct underlying obstruction when indicated
- Plan follow-up
- Establish the need for long-term prophylaxis

Verify the Diagnosis

The patient will usually present with complaints referable to the urinary tract (see Chapter 7: Dysuria Syndromes). The simplest measures are to perform a dip-stick test for pyuria, nitrite, and hematuria and examine the urine microscopically for bacteriuria or funguria (see Chapter 3: Diagnostic Methods). Dip-slides and other low cost culture methods are helpful to distinguish among the various causes of the dysuria syndrome (see Fig. 7.1). A simplified, diagnostic flow diagram to help distinguish vaginitis and chlamydial and gonococcal urethritis from urinary tract infections is presented in Figure 12.1. Pyuria should not be equated with urinary tract infections.

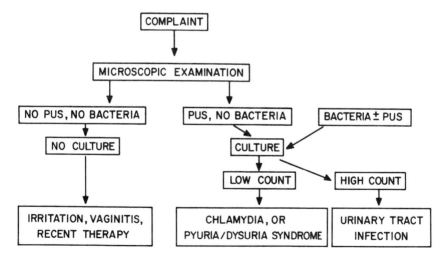

Figure 12.1. Flow diagram to help distinguish among the various causes of dysuria.

Other causes of sterile pyuria, such as vaginal contamination, need to be considered (see Table 2.3).

Distinguish Uncomplicated from Complicated Infections

The distinction between uncomplicated and complicated infections is paramount. The presence of underlying structural abnormalities determines the nature of the invading microorganisms and response to therapy. The history and microbiologic findings are more informative than localization studies in making this differentiation. Uncomplicated urinary tract infections usually are caused by *Escherichia coli* or *Staphylococcus saprophyticus* and respond well to short courses of therapy (Fig. 12.2). The major problem is recurrent infections caused by reinfection with a new microorganism or persistence of the same microorganism in periurethral and rectal reservoirs. Complicated infections often are caused by resistant microorganisms. The major problems are relapse with the same microorganism or superinfection with resistant strains. Underlying lesions need to be detected, evaluated, and corrected whenever possible. Antimicrobial therapy is an adjunct to management of complicated infections.

Assess Underlying Medical and Surgical Problems

Antimicrobial drugs are potentially toxic. It is essential to obtain baseline information on renal function, allergic reactions, recent use of antimicrobial

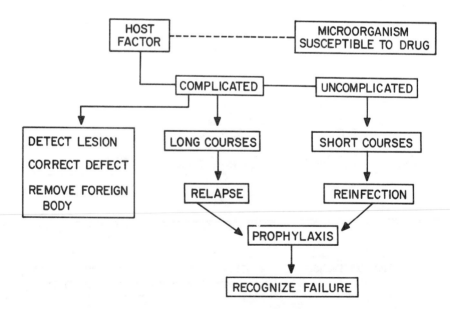

Figure 12.2. The interaction between host factors and the microorganism determines the nature of the infection and duration of therapy.

drugs, race, and underlying diseases. It is useful to know whether the patient is pregnant, has diabetes, polycystic renal disease, sickle cell anemia, or glucose-6-phosphate dehydrogenase deficiency (G-6-PD) when sulfonamides, nitrofurantoin, or quinolones may be used.

The remaining general principles will be emphasized as an integral part of the management of uncomplicated and complicated infections.

Uncomplicated Infections

Most patients with uncomplicated infections are healthy females without demonstrable structural or neurological abnormalities of the voiding mechanism. They may have asymptomatic bacteriuria, the pyuria-dysuria syndrome, bacterial cystitis, or pyelonephritis. Therapy is directed against the most common microorganisms: *Escherichia coli* and *Staphylococcus saprophyticus*. The goal is to reduce morbidity and prevent recurrent symptomatic infections. The choice of drug depends on the severity of the infection, likelihood that the organism is susceptible to a given agent, ease of administration, risk of side-effects, and relative cost. The potential outcomes of therapy are shown in Figure 12.3. The long-term prognosis for preservation of renal function is excellent.

Choice of Drug and Dose

Selection of the drug is based on probability that the invading microorganism will be susceptible, will have good oral absorption, achievable concentrations in the urine, relative cost, and toxicity (Table 12.1).

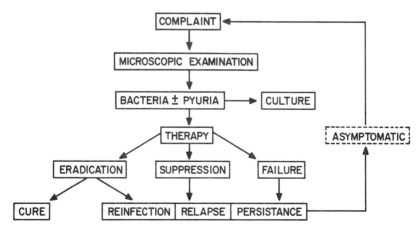

Figure 12.3. Potential outcomes for treatment of urinary tract infections.

Table 12.1. Useful Oral Drugs for Uncomplicated Urinary Tract Infections

Class of Drug	Susceptibility	Warnings	Cost	Major Toxicity
Sulfonamides[1]	Variable	Nursing mothers	Inexpensive	G-6-PD, Allergy
Trimethoprim[1]	High	Pregnancy C[9]	Inexpensive	Folate deficiency
TMP/SMZ[1]	High	Pregnancy C[9]	Inexpensive	G-6-PD, Allergy
		Nursing mothers		Folate deficiency
Older Quinolones[2]	Variable		Inexpensive	CNS effects (rare)
Fluoroquinolones[3]	High	Children	Expensive	Nausea, headache
		Pregnancy C[9]		
Nitrofurantoin[4]	High	Pulmonary	Variable	Nausea, peripheral
		reactions		neuropathy,
		Hepatitis		G-6-PD
Aminopenicillins[5]	Variable	Hypersensitivity	Inexpensive	Allergy
Amox/clavulanate[5]	Variable	Hypersensitivity	Expensive	Allergy
Cephalosporins[6]	Variable	Hypersensitivity	Expensive	Allergy
Tetracyclines[7]	Variable	Children <8 years	Inexpensive	Candida vaginitis
		(stain deciduous		Photosensitivity
		teeth)		
		Pregnancy D[9]		
Carbenicillin	Pseudomonas	Hypersensitivity	Expensive	Allergy
indanyl[8]		Pregnancy B[9]		

Customary Adult Doses (lower doses are often effective)
[1]Numerous sulfonamides available, e.g., sulfamethoxazole, 2 g followed by 1 g twice daily; trimethoprim, 100–200 mg twice daily; TMP/SMZ is trimethoprim-sulfamethoxazole, 160 plus 800 mg twice daily.
[2]Nalidixic acid, 1 g four times each day; oxalinic acid, 750 mg twice daily; cinoxacin 500 mg twice daily.
[3]Norfloxacin, 400 mg; ciprofloxacin, 250 mg; ofloxacin, 200 mg; enoxacin, 400 mg—all twice daily; lomefloxacin 400 mg daily.
[4]Macrocrystals 100 mg three or four times daily or monohydrate/macrocrystals 100 mg twice daily.
[5]Ampicillin or amoxicillin, 250 mg three times daily.
[6]Cephalexin, cephradine, cefadroxil, 250–500 mg three times daily; cefuroxime axetil, 250 mg twice daily; cefixime, 400 mg daily.
[7]Tetracycline, 250 mg three or four times daily; doxycycline, 100 mg twice daily.
[8]Each tablet contains 382 mg and is administered as one to two tablets four times daily. The higher dose is for *Pseudomonas aeruginosa*.
[9]See text for definition.

Trimethoprim

Trimethoprim (TMP) is preferred by the author to trimethoprim-sulfamethoxazole (TMP/SMZ) as the initial drug for uncomplicated urinary tract infections. The reasons are as follows:

- TMP is as effective as TMP/SMZ (9)
- Resistance to TMP is less frequent than to SMZ
- Reactions to SMZ can be severe and should be avoided
- SMZ does not delay resistance to TMP
- Synergy is not needed for urinary tract infections
- TMP, but not SMZ, is excreted in the urine in adequate concentrations in people with moderate renal impairment (10) (Fig. 12.4).

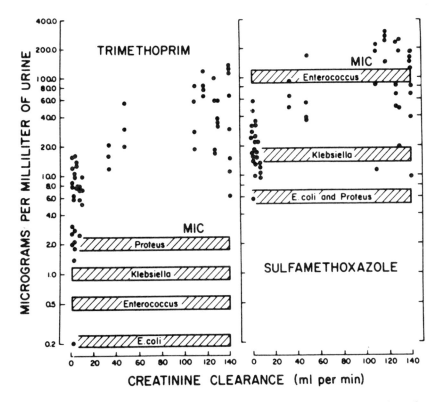

Figure 12.4. Relation between creatinine clearance and the concentration of trimethoprim and nonacetylated sulfamethoxazole after a single oral dose of the combined drugs (160 mg plus 800 mg). The shaded areas represent the minimum inhibitory concentrations for various bacteria. Reproduced with permission from Craig and Kunin (10).

Nitrofurantoin
Nitrofurantoin is an excellent drug for urinary tract infections. It is active against *E. coli, Staphylococcus aureus, Enterococcus faecalis,* but not against most strains of Proteus or Pseudomonas. Resistance to common microorganisms is minimal despite clinical use for over 35 years. It is particularly effective for recurrent infections and when susceptibility tests are not available. Nitrofurantoin exhibits a marked post-antibiotic effect (Figure 12.5). It could probably be administered twice daily, but clinical trials, using less frequent dosing, have been limited to the monohydrate/macrocrystals form. Urinary excretion is reduced as serum creatinine rises (11) (Fig. 12.6). Nitrofurantoin should not be used in patients even with moderate degrees of renal insufficiency.

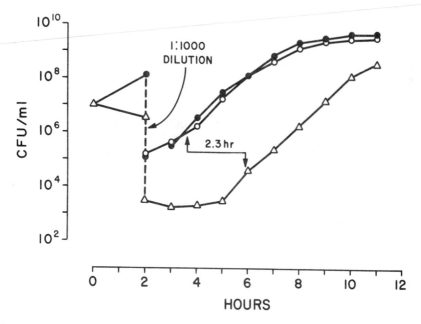

Figure 12.5. Postantibiotic effect induced by a two-hour exposure of *Escherichia coli* to five times the MIC of nitrofurantoin (Δ) followed by a 1:1000 dilution. The open circles (O) represent 0.5 times the MIC and the closed circles (●) are untreated control cultures. Unpublished data of ST Chambers.

Quinolones

The older quinolones are useful for treatment of uncomplicated urinary tract infections caused by *E. coli,* but not for *Staphylococcus saprophyticus* (12–14). The newer fluoroquinolones are much more active against *Enterobacteriaceae* and *Pseudomonas aeruginosa* and are effective in systemic infections (15). Their activity against staphylococci and *Enterococcus faecalis* and *Pseudomonas aeruginosa* is often transitory because of the emergence of resistant strains in patients with complicated infections (16–18). Some experts (19) discourage use of fluoroquinolones for *Staphylococcus saprophyticus* because of the borderline range of susceptibility. All strains tested at the Ohio State University Clinical Microbiology Laboratory were susceptible to ≤1 mcg/ml. The fluoroquinolones are expensive but are used excessively because they have a reasonably good safety profile and therapeutic efficacy. There is virtual cross resistance among the quinolones.

The lowest dosage form is more than adequate for treatment of uncomplicated urinary tract infection. Ciprofloxacin at 100 mg as a single or twice daily dose (20–22) is as effective as 250 mg; 100 mg of ofloxacin is effective for single dose therapy (23); and 250 mg of cinoxacin given twice daily (24) is as effective as 500 mg.

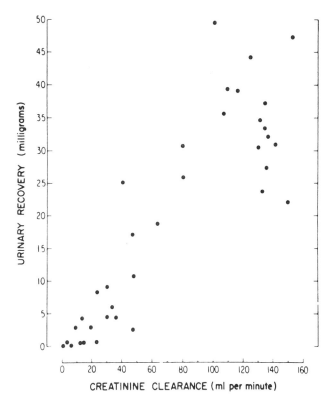

Figure 12.6. Urinary recovery of nitrofurantoin over a 10-hour period after a single oral dose according to creatinine clearance. Each dot represents an individual subject. Reproduced with permission from Sachs, Geer, Noell, and Kunin (11).

There was initial enthusiasm to use fluoroquinolones to reduce the fecal and vaginal reservoirs of coliforms. Its goal was to prevent recurrent infections without emergence of resistant strains (25–27). This concept has been tempered in recent years because of the fear that overuse will result in emergence of resistant strains. Many experts recommend that the fluoroquinolones be reserved for more difficult problems, recurrent infections, and prophylaxis (5,6,19).

Beta Lactam Antibiotics
Oral penicillin and cephalosporins are widely used for respiratory, soft tissue, and urinary tract infections. Resistance is a major problem because of exposure of fecal microorganisms to these drugs. About one-third to one-half of urinary strains of *E. coli* are resistant to ampicillin and amoxicillin in the United States, United Kingdom, and Holland (19,28,29). The rates of resistance to

amoxicillin/clavulanate and ampicillin/sulbactam are only slightly lower because susceptibility to it is often independent of β lactamase production. Ampicillin and cephalexin are excreted in adequate amounts in the urine in patients with decreased renal function provided the creatinine clearance exceeds 10 ml/min (30). The second and third generation oral cephalosporins are more active against enteric gram negative bacteria but are expensive.

Tetracyclines
The tetracyclines have been overused ever since they were introduced over 40 years ago. Their efficacy for treatment of *E. coli* urinary tract infections has progressively diminished because of selection of resistant strains in the gut. They are useful second line drugs for susceptible microorganisms.

Duration of Therapy

The current consensus is that 3 days of treatment is superior to single dose therapy and as effective as 10 to 14 days or longer (3,4,6,31). A more prolonged course of therapy (10 to 14 days) is recommended for relapses with the same microorganism.

Single dose therapy was popular until recently. It had the advantage of reduced costs, side-effects, potential for emergence of resistant strains, and compliance was more assured (32,33). Single dose therapy is most effective when given shortly after the onset of infection. It is less effective than longer courses against *Staphylococcus saprophyticus* (34,35), in inner-city than suburban patients, and when therapy may be delayed (36). Single dose therapy is not recommended for young children, diabetics, or men. It appears to be effective in adolescent girls (37) and during pregnancy (38,39).

There are occasions when an observed, single oral dose or injection of an aminoglycoside or long-acting cephalosporin can be justified. These include settings such as urgent care centers where there is potential for poor compliance and situations such as immediately after a catheter is removed from a hospitalized female. Ronald et al. (40), in their original paper published 20 years ago, used a single dose of 500 mg of kanamycin to demonstrate the efficacy of this approach to localize the site of infection. Oral therapy is equally effective.

Oral single dose therapy usually is dispensed in a larger than standard dose, i.e., TMP, 200 mg; TMP/SMZ, 320 and 1600 mg (41); cephalexin, 3 g (36); ofloxacin, 400 mg; norfloxacin, 800 mg (35,42); and cefuroxime axetil, 1 g (43).

Patients who unsuccessfully undergo single dose therapy are more likely to have tissue invasion ("upper tract infection") as evidenced by localization studies with the antibody-coated bacteria (ACB) test or Fairley wash-out studies (32,40) but a negative ACB test does not select a group of patients who are more likely to respond to single dose therapy (44), and a positive test is not an indication for uroradiologic studies.

Culture and Susceptibility Tests

Culture and susceptibility tests are not routinely needed for the management of the first few episodes of uncomplicated urinary tract infection. The decision to treat must be made before the results of these tests are available. A presumptive diagnosis can be made from the history, clinical signs, dip-stick tests, and urine microscopy. The patient should be asked to return if the symptoms do not subside within a few days. Culture and susceptibility tests are essential for the management of patients with recurrent or complicated infection. Direct susceptibility tests have the advantage of providing useful information rapidly (see "The Direct Susceptibility Test" in Chapter 3).

Therapeutic Tactics and Prophylaxis

The goal in treating urinary tract infections is to eradicate the infection and to reduce the morbidity of recurrence due to relapse or reinfection. It is not difficult to eradicate bacteria with a drug to which the organism is susceptible. The major problem is to manage recurrent infections. Each patient appears to have a unique pattern of recurrence. Some will never have another episode, others may have sporadic episodes, and others will develop multiple reinfections within a few weeks or months after treatment. The only way to determine the pattern of recurrence is to observe the patient closely over time. Most recurrences will be caused by a new strain of *E. coli* or a new bacterial species. Relapses with the same organism usually will occur within a few weeks after stopping treatment and are often the result of inadequate therapy.

Initial Approach with Intermittent Therapy

The initial approach is to treat each episode of infection with a short course of an effective antimicrobial drug. Bacteriuria should disappear from the urine (by microscopic examination or culture) within a day or two. If there is no bacteriologic response within this period, *recognize failure* and change the drug. The "in vivo susceptibility test" is more reliable than laboratory tests. Symptoms, pyuria, and hematuria may persist for several days and should not be mistaken as therapeutic failure (Fig. 12.7).

Each course of treatment will fractionally extract about 20% to 30% of patients into long-term remission (45,46). Thus, by close follow-up and repeated effective treatment of each recurrent episode, most females will eventually do well. They may have recurrent infections later in life, but these also can be managed by relatively short courses of therapy.

Anticipatory Therapy

Several different tactics can be used for management of infections in females with frequent, recurrent infection. One option is to offer patients a small supply of an effective antimicrobial drug to be taken as soon as they develop

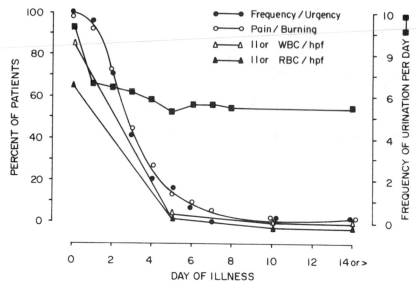

Figure 12.7. Time course of symptoms, pyuria, and hematuria among 20 young college women after treatment with an effective antimicrobial drug.

characteristic symptoms (47). I instruct the patient to pass a clean-voided specimen just before starting therapy, refrigerate the urine, and bring it to the office for examination the next day. This permits the patient to be monitored and maintain continuity of care.

In Relation to Sexual Intercourse
A second option is to prescribe a prophylactic dose just before or following sexual intercourse. It is probably not necessary to take more than one dose daily. This tactic is often highly effective and has the advantage of good compliance, minimum dosage, and patient satisfaction (42,48,49). Postcoital prophylaxis may be virtually the same as bed-time prophylaxis in women who engage in frequent intercourse. I am not aware of any controlled trials that compare dosing at the same intervals, but not synchronously with sexual activity. Coital prophylaxis should be reserved for women who believe there is a strong relationship between intercourse and infection.

Long-Term Prophylaxis for Uncomplicated Infections
A third option is to use long-term, daily, bed-time prophylaxis. This treatment is highly effective in females who have very frequent, closely spaced symptomatic episodes. There is no need to advise patients to change their life-style, sexual or hygienic practices, or fluid intake. The duration of prophylaxis in patients with recurrent infection is arbitrary, but is usually for 6 months or longer.

Prophylaxis with trimethoprim/sulfamethoxazole, trimethoprim alone, nitrofurantoin, or other drugs for as long as 5 or more years has been successful with minimal instances of development of resistance (50–52). Patients receiving long-term prophylaxis with nitrofurantoin are at risk of developing interstitial pneumonitis and hepatitis and need to be monitored closely.

Selection of Drugs for Prophylaxis
The requirements for drugs used for prophylaxis are listed in Table 12.2. Lower than therapeutic doses are effective. These doses usually are sufficient to prevent colonization with small numbers of microorganisms that may enter the bladder during the night (53). Sublethal concentrations of antimicrobial drugs that inhibit protein synthesis (trimethoprim, aminoglycosides, tetracycline, and chloramphenicol) can block the expression of type-1 and P-fimbriated strains of *E. coli* and adherence to urothelial cells (54–56). Fluoroquinolones do not exhibit this effect (57). It is possible that drugs can be developed that block expression of adhesins, capsules, and flagella without killing the microorganisms. These drugs might have the advantage of preventing infection without altering the ecosystem of the gut or periurethral zone. Salicylate is a prototype for such drugs (58) (see "P. fimbria" in Chapter 10).

Trimethoprim, trimethoprim/sulfamethoxazole, and nitrofurantoin remain excellent choices provided the organisms are susceptible. Other effective drugs include sulfonamides, cephalosporins, the older quinolones, and the fluoroquinolones (Table 12.3).

Each course of prophylaxis will extract a portion of the population into long-term remission. If the patient continues to have recurrences after completing prophylaxis, it can be resumed or short courses can be tried. Urine cultures should be obtained periodically to be certain that the drug continues to be effective.

Three outstanding studies of the efficacy of long-term prophylaxis are cited to illustrate the lessons learned about the natural history of urinary

Table 12.2. Requirements for Antimicrobial Drugs to be Used for Prophylaxis of Recurrent Urinary Tract Infections

Essential
    Can be taken orally for long periods of time
    Well tolerated with minimal toxicity or side effects
    Achieve adequate concentrations of active drug in the urine
    Active against uropathic microorganisms
    Development of resistance is rare
Desirable
    Prevent adhesion to urothelial cells
    Prevent colonization of the urethral zone
    Relative low cost

Table 12.3. Antimicrobial Drugs for Post Coital and Long-Term Bed-Time Prophylaxis*

Drug	Dose
Trimethoprim (TMP)	100 mg
TMP/SMZ	80 plus 400 mg
Nitrofurantoin	50 to 100 mg
Fluoroquinolones	Norfloxacin 200 mg, ofloxacin 100 mg, ciprofloxacin 125 mg

*Other drugs such as sulfonamides, the older quinolones, and beta lactams may be used provided that the urine is monitored for emergence of resistant bacteria.

tract infections. Stamey, Condy, and Mihara (59) found that after 6 months of prophylaxis about 60% of women still developed recurrent infections. Stansfeld (60) conducted a trial of prophylaxis in children using TMP/SMZ (see Fig. 4.4). All the children were treated for 2 weeks and then randomized to receive either no treatment or 6 months of prophylaxis. Prophylaxis was highly effective in preventing infection, but the rate of recurrent infection after stopping prophylaxis was virtually identical to that observed after 2 weeks of treatment. Stamm et al. (61) compared the efficacy of placebo, TMP/SMZ, TMP, and nitrofurantoin in a controlled trial of adult women (Fig. 12.8). All three drugs were equally effective in preventing recurrences. When prophylaxis was stopped after 6 months, 40% to 60% of the patients developed recurrent infection.

These studies show the following:

- Long-term prophylaxis does not alter the biologic behavior of recurrent infections
- Long-term prophylaxis fractionally extracts patients into long-term remission
- TMP, TMP/SMZ, and nitrofurantoin are equally effective despite different modes of action.

Methenamine Salts

Methenamine is converted to formaldehyde and ammonia in acid urine (62). It is available in combinations with mandelic acid (63) or hippuric acids (64). The urine should be acidified by a high meat diet, methionine 8 to 12 grams in daily divided doses, or acid phosphate salts. Ammonium chloride is effective as an acidifier for only a few days and is contraindicated in patients with renal failure. Cranberry juice and ascorbic acid do not acidify the urine. Methenamine salts act only in the urine and should not be used for systemic infections. Before using methenamine salts for prophylaxis bacteria should be eradicated or the count reduced with more effective drugs. Some investigators have found methenamine hippurate or methenamine mandelate to be highly effective (65–69), whereas others are less enthusi-

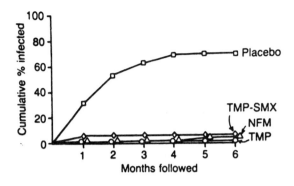

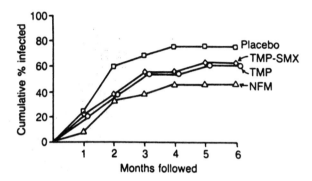

Figure 12.8. Cumulative infections during antimicrobial prophylaxis or Placebo (top panel) and in the 6 months after the study drug was discontinued (lower panel), TMP-SMX = trimethoprim-sulfamethoxazole; TMP = trimethoprim; NFM = nitrofurantoin macrocrystals. Reproduced with permission from Stamm et al. (61).

astic (53,70,71). Methenamine salts are drugs of last resort and should be used only when all other treatments have failed (Table 12.4).

Prescribing by Telephone
Physicians often are called by patients to prescribe an antibiotic for a presumed urinary tract infection. These requests are difficult to resist, particularly on a busy day or when a call is made late in the evening or on a weekend. It can be argued that treatment of a "garden-variety" urinary tract infection is harmless and the symptoms need to be addressed immediately. There should be no difficulty in complying with an urgent request from a patient whose problems are well known. It is more difficult to respond when the patient has not been seen for some time. The situation is treacherous. The patient may have vaginitis, the dysuria syndrome, a sexually transmitted disease, be receiving drugs from other physicians, or may be an antibi-

Table 12.4. Dosage of Methenamine Salts for Prophylaxis of Urinary Tract Infections*

Drug	Dose
Methenamine mandelate	1 gram four times daily
Methenamine hippurate	1 gram four times daily

*These are drugs of last resort and may only reduce the bacterial count in the urine. They should be taken after meals and are more effective at acid pH.

otic abuser. She may not return for evaluation despite sincere promises. This situation can be dealt with by providing patients with recurrent infections with a small supply of drug to be taken at the first symptoms of infection. For other patients, it is wise to question them closely about symptoms, allergic reactions, and other medications. They should be instructed to obtain a clean-voided sample of urine in a clean, but not necessarily sterile, jar, place it in an opaque bag in the refrigerator, and bring it in the next day or so. They can then be given an initial dose of a reliable antimicrobial drug and instructed to bring in their urine sample if they wish to obtain more.

Pregnancy

It is well accepted that both asymptomatic and symptomatic urinary tract infections should be treated as early as possible during pregnancy. The goal is to prevent pyelonephritis during the last trimester of pregnancy and prevent premature birth. The tactics used are the same as for uncomplicated infections. There is no need to use different doses unless there are underlying diseases that might affect the absorption or excretion of drugs.

Urine cultures should be obtained periodically during pregnancy to detect new or recurrent asymptomatic infections. Short courses of therapy are effective, including single dose (38,39). There is no advantage to use long-term prophylaxis except for highly recurrent infections (72). The patient should be treated promptly for each episode. Patients at the highest risk of prematurity are those who relapse early or have persistent infection (73). They may require more prolonged treatment.

There is no absolute contraindication to the use of any antimicrobial drug during pregnancy. Amoxicillin, cephalexin, and nitrofurantoin are preferred (74). Trimethoprim and fluoroquinolones are assigned to category C by the U.S. Food and Drug Administration. This category is defined as: "Either studies in animals reveal adverse effects on the fetus (teratogenic or embryocidal, or other), and there are no controlled studies in women or studies in women and animals are not available. Drugs should be given only if the potential benefit justifies the potential risk to the fetus." Tetracyclines are listed in Category D, which is defined as: " . . . if the drug is needed in a life-threatening situation or for a serious disease for which safer drugs cannot be used or are ineffective." Drugs listed in category X are contraindicated. The antimicrobial drugs in categories C and D and sulfonamides should not be used by nursing mothers. Acute pyelonephritis during pregnancy may be treated with a third generation cephalosporin or extended spectrum penicillin until susceptibility results are available. It is wise to avoid drugs in categories C and D whenever possible.

Key Points in the Management of Uncomplicated Urinary Tract Infection

- Verify the diagnosis by dip-stick and microscopic methods
- Select the most safe, effective and lowest cost drug
- Consider trimethoprim as the first choice for nonpregnant patients
- Consider nitrofurantoin for recurrent infections
- Reserve fluoroquinolones and new cephalosporins for more difficult problems
- Avoid aminopenicillins and combinations with beta lactamase inhibitors
- Control requests to prescribe by telephone
- Culture and susceptibility tests are helpful to manage recurrent infections
- Discuss alternate methods of management with the patient
- Three-day courses are preferred to single dose or 10 to 14-day courses
- Recurrences tend to subside with repeated short courses
- Longer courses are useful for relapses with the same microorganism
- Anticipate recurrences and provide patients at high risk with a small supply of drug
- Consider single dose prophylaxis for infections closely associated with sexual intercourse
- Consider long-term prophylaxis for highly recurrent infections
- Select the tactic that is most acceptable to the patient

Acute, Uncomplicated Pyelonephritis

Acute, uncomplicated pyelonephritis is usually caused by the same microorganisms found in other uncomplicated infections as described previously. A prompt and deliberate approach is required. The initial evaluation, in addition to the history and physical examination, should include a blood culture, gram stain of the urine by a trained observer, urine culture, and susceptibility tests, as well as white blood count and differential, serum creatinine, and electrolytes. There is no need to "cover" against both gram positive and gram negative bacteria. The gram stain of the urine will usually clearly differentiate gram positive from gram negative bacteria and suggest the presence of unusual microorganisms such as *Hemophilus influenzae*. The morphology of gram positive bacteria will usually differentiate staphylococci from streptococci. The blood culture, when positive, provides strong supportive evidence of the causative microorganism, and susceptibility tests help guide management.

Oral therapy may be used in both pregnant and nonpregnant women provided that the patient is able to eat without difficulty (75). Hospitalization is advised for people who live alone and cannot be observed, or who experience nausea, vomiting, dehydration, or possible complicating factors such as diabetes. Another option is to administer a single intravenous dose of a long-acting cephalosporin such as ceftriaxone followed by oral therapy. The recommended drugs are listed in Table 12.5. Aminopenicillins with β lactamase inhibitors are not recommended because many strains of *E. coli* are resistant to these drugs. Piperacillin/tazobactam is not recommended because piperacillin is adequate. There is no point in using an aminoglycoside with another drug because the aminoglycoside is the most active component, gram positive cocci can be excluded by gram stain, and therapy can be changed to a less toxic drug when susceptibility tests become available.

The duration of therapy need not exceed 2 weeks (76). Treatment for 5 days is often sufficient (4). Parenteral drugs should be changed to oral therapy as soon as the patient can tolerate them and the results of susceptibility tests are available. Intravenous urograms should not be done during the acute phase of illness because of poor concentration of dye. Ultrasound examination of the kidneys and bladder are recommended. CT and other scans are not needed unless a renal or perinephric abscess is suspected or *Staphylococcus aureus* is isolated from the blood.

Complicated Infections

Complicated infections are exceedingly difficult to treat even with the best antimicrobial drugs. It is essential that obstruction to urine flow, foreign bodies, and renal or perinephric abscesses be detected early and corrected

Table 12.5. Suggested Therapy for Acute, Uncomplicated Pyelonephritis

Recommended[1]	
Oral	*Parenteral*
Trimethoprim[2]	Trimethoprim/sulfamethoxazole[6]
Trimethoprim/sulfamethoxazole[3]	Fluoroquinolone[7]
Fluoroquinolone[4]	Extended spectrum cephalosporin[8]
Extended spectrum cephalosporins[5]	Extended spectrum penicillins[8]
	Aminoglycoside[9]

Not recommended
Ampicillin, amoxicillin/clavulanate, ampicillin/sulbactam, piperacillin/tazobactam Combinations of gentamicin with ampicillin or other drugs (see text for explanation)

[1]Not all of the effective drugs are included in this list
[2]200 mg every 12 hours, [3]160 mg plus 800 mg every 12 hours, [4]ciprofloxacin 500 mg, norfloxacin 400 mg, ofloxacin 200 to 400 mg every 12 hours, [5]cefuroxime axetil 250 to 500 mg, every 12 hours, cefixime 400 mg daily, [6]160 mg plus 800 mg every 12 hours, [7]ciprofloxacin or ofloxacin, 200 to 400 mg every 12 hours, [8]standard doses of ceftriaxone, ceftizoxime, piperacillin and others, [9]gentamicin or tobramycin at 5 mg per kg body weight as a single daily dose or three divided doses.

whenever possible. The causative microorganisms are often resistant to multiple drugs (see Table 1.4). Some long-standing infections are polymicrobial, particularly in patients with urinary catheters. Anaerobic organisms are found occasionally in prostatic or renal abscesses.

Aminoglycoside antibiotics are the "gold standard" against which new drugs are evaluated for treatment of enteric gram-negative bacteria. The fluoroquinolones, third generation cephalosporins, extended spectrum penicillins, imipenem/cilastatin, and aztreonam often are initially effective against susceptible microorganisms. The results are disappointing as resistant microorganisms emerge.

Cephalosporins are not effective for treatment of *Enterococcus faecalis* and *Enterococcus faecium*. The selective pressure of excessive use of these drugs in hospitals has increased the frequency of urinary tract infections caused by these bacteria. Enterococci should be treated with an aminopenicillin (ampicillin or amoxicillin), an extended spectrum penicillin, nitrofurantoin, or vancomycin depending on susceptibility tests. Synergistic effects with an aminoglycoside antibiotic is usually not necessary because of high concentrations achieved in the urine and toxic side-effects. Enterococci do not produce β lactamases and inhibitors are not needed. *Pseudomonas aeruginosa* often is initially susceptible to the fluoroquinolones, extended spectrum penicillins, ceftazidime, aminoglycosides and imipenem, but emergence of resistant strains and superinfection with enterococci and yeasts is common.

Key Points in the Management of Complicated Urinary Tract Infections

- Culture and susceptibility tests are necessary to guide therapy
- Avoid aminoglycoside antibiotics when the microorganism is susceptible to alternate drugs
- Antimicrobial drugs are adjuncts to therapy and may not be curative
- Antimicrobial drugs are ineffective in the presence of an indwelling urinary device
- Stones and foreign bodies should be removed whenever possible
- Urinary obstruction must be relieved
- Long-term prophylaxis may be useful if the microorganism remains susceptible
- Recognize failure and do not continue to use an ineffective drug

---

Management of Sepsis

Most patients with acute, uncomplicated pyelonephritis do not develop septic shock. The usual course is characterized by fever and leukocytosis accompanied by a warm and dry skin without significant change in blood pressure. These signs will gradually disappear after a few days of appropriate therapy. Some patients, particularly those who have indwelling urinary devices, may develop profound and often irreversible shock because of the liberation of endotoxin into the bloodstream. The mortality in this group of patients may exceed 50% depending on their underlying diseases, age, and the presence of preexistent antibody to core lipopolysaccharide.

There is no satisfactory treatment of endotoxin shock other than use of fluids and pressor drugs. Treatment is ineffective with corticosteroids, naloxone, nitrous oxide inhibitors, and monoclonal antibodies directed against endotoxin or tumor necrosis factor. Catheters should be removed, and antimicrobial therapy directed against the most likely invading microorganism should be instituted. Little is gained by worrying about drugs that may release endotoxin because the damage is already done. It is not known whether antimicrobial therapy is really helpful and how long it should be continued. It is common to encounter patients who recover from septic shock despite persistent infection.

Urinary Infections in Men

Urinary tract infections in males usually can be traced to prior instrumentation of the urinary tract, but they may occur without a known precipitating factor. Uncomplicated infections often are caused by *E. coli* or enterococci and often respond well to a short course (1 to 2 weeks) of chemotherapy. The infectious process may invade the prostate and persist. It is exceedingly difficult to eradicate infections in the presence of prostatic calculi, stones, obstruction, or structural abnormalities of the urinary tract (see Table 11.5). Long-term prophylaxis, as described for women, is often highly effective in preventing recurrent, symptomatic infection.

The limitations of treatment of men with long-standing, complicated infection have been examined in several well conducted trials (77,78). Rates of cure increase with duration of therapy. Single dose therapy is inadequate for most males. Six weeks of therapy is superior to 2 weeks, and 12 weeks is superior to 6 weeks. These trials included patients with diabetes or anatomic abnormalities and many had suffered from bacteremia, epididymitis, and renal abscesses in the past. Recurrent infections are common in these series and are usually caused by relapse rather than reinfection. The key point is that mortality does not differ among elderly men who are treated compared with those not treated for bacteriuria (78).

Prophylactic therapy of chronic urinary tract infection in men was evaluated in a large study that compared placebo to sulfamethizole, nitrofurantoin, or methenamine mandelate over a 2-year period (68). Continuous prophylaxis delayed recurrence of bacteriuria, reduced the clinical expression of infection, but had no effect on mortality. When treatment was discontinued most of the patients became bacteriuric. The key points are that long courses of therapy reduced morbidity, but had no effect on mortality.

Infections of the Prostate and Epididymis

Acute Bacterial Prostatitis
This is an acute septic condition characterized by perineal pain, chills, fever, and prostration. The prostatic gland, testes, and epididymis are often exquis-

itely tender. Rectal examination should be avoided whenever possible. The causative microorganism will usually be isolated from the urine, blood, or epididymal aspirates. There is no need to be concerned about penetration of drugs into the inflamed prostate. Therapy is directed against the most likely microorganisms as with acute pyelonephritis (Table 12.5). Most infections of the prostate are caused by enteric gram-negative bacteria and enterococci, but *H. influenzae* and *Staphylococcus aureus* need to be considered. The prostate specific antigen (PSA) will often be elevated and return to normal in several weeks.

Chronic Bacterial Prostatitis

This is an insidious infection that may be exceedingly difficult to eradicate. It is characterized by persistent colonization of the glandular fluid with intermittent episodes of pyuria and bacteriuria or persistent perineal tenderness and low grade fever. Bacterial prostatitis can be differentiated from prostadynia by localization tests or by evidence of recurrent urinary tract infection.

The antimicrobial drug must be able to diffuse from plasma across the prostatic epithelium to enter the noninflamed prostatic fluid. Studies in dogs indicated that nonionic diffusion plays an important role in penetration of drugs into prostatic secretions. Weak bases tend to be more ionized in the relatively acidic prostatic fluid and become trapped and concentrated. The pH of prostatic secretion in dogs is 6.4. Trimethoprim is a weak base and achieves a concentration ratio of at least 3:1 in prostatic secretions relative to plasma in dogs. Sulfamethoxazole is a weak acid and does not enter as well (79). This concept has been challenged in recent years. The pH of expressed prostatic secretions of most normal men is about 7.31 and is increased to 8.34 with prostatic infection (80–82).

The prostatic focus can be eradicated in only about one-third of patients treated with TMP/SMZ for 12 weeks (79). Lipid-soluble drugs such as minocycline, doxycycline, and fluoroquinolones diffuse into the prostate, but are rarely curative (83). Many of the reports purporting that a particular drug enters the prostate are based on measurement of concentrations of drugs in chips of prostatic tissue obtained at the time of prostatic resection. It is not known whether the drugs are in the prostatic fluid or the interstitial space of the gland. The resected prostate is usually not inflamed and does not represent conditions during infection.

Key Points in the Management of Urinary Tract Infections in Men

- Single dose therapy is usually ineffective
- Short courses (10 to 14 days) are effective when the infection is of recent onset
- Long-standing infections are exceedingly difficult to eradicate even with 12-weeks therapy
- The focus of infection is often in the prostate
- Recurrent infection is usually caused by relapse with the same microorganism from the prostate or a calculus
- Asymptomatic infections need not be treated

> • Long-term prophylaxis is effective in patients with recurrent, symptomatic infections
> • The prostate may need to be surgically removed in patients with prostatic calculi who fail prophylaxis and have recurrent episodes of sepsis

Diabetes Mellitus

Diabetics are at increased risk of complicated urinary tract infections and the most severe forms of pyelonephritis. They are a diverse group and should be managed according to their individual expression of infection and natural history. Young diabetic girls have the same rates of asymptomatic bacteriuria as age-matched girls. Pregnant diabetics are more likely to have evidence of upper tract infection and may need more prolonged therapy (84,85). Older diabetic women tend to have more recurrent infections complicated by diabetic cytopathy. It seems reasonable to treat asymptomatic bacteriuria in diabetics, but long-term efficacy is not established. More prolonged courses of therapy (2 to 6 weeks) may be needed to eradicate infection in diabetic men and women, but recurrent infection is common. Long-term prophylaxis may be useful, provided that it is effective. Progressive reduction in renal function and increased proteinuria are more closely related to diabetic nephropathy than to chronic pyelonephritis and are not, by themselves, indications for antimicrobial therapy (84). The antibody-coated bacteriuria test (ACB) is not a helpful guideline for management (84). As with other complicated infections, it may be necessary to recognize failure and withhold treatment except for septic episodes.

Should Asymptomatic Bacteriuria Be Treated?

Asymptomatic bacteriuria is meaningful only when interpreted within a clinical context as outlined in Table 1.6. Treatment is contraindicated in patients with indwelling urinary catheters because it is unsuccessful and leads to superinfection with resistant microorganisms. Treatment is optional in uncomplicated infections in females because their long-term prognosis for preservation of renal function is excellent, symptomatic episodes can be treated when they occur, and there is less likelihood of reinfection with a more virulent strain. Elderly women and men need not be treated for asymptomatic bacteriuria because therapy has no impact on mortality. Eradicating bacteriuria in nursing home residents has no short-term effect on the severity of urinary incontinence (86). Treatment of children with vesicoureteral reflux is controversial. More work needs to be done to determine how best to manage urinary tract infections in diabetic women. The situations in which treatment of asymptomatic bacteriuria may or may not be worthwhile are listed in Table 12.6.

Table 12.6. Indications for Treatment of Asymptomatic Bacteriuria

Condition
Contraindicated
With indwelling urinary catheters or other devices
Optional or Not Worthwhile
Otherwise healthy girls
Elderly men and women
With intermittent catheterization
Possibly Worthwhile
Children with vesico-ureteral reflux
Diabetic women
Worthwhile
Highly recurrent symptomatic infection
During pregnancy
Renal transplantation
Prior to urologic surgery
Following removal of an indwelling catheter

Prophylaxis Revisited

Primary prophylaxis is designed to prevent the acquisition of infection from small numbers of microbes which originate from a source outside of the urinary tract. The microorganisms might be introduced by instrumentation or acquired from the periurethral flora in females susceptible to recurrent infection. Secondary prophylaxis is designed to prevent emergence of infection from a site within the urinary tract. The focus might be a latent infection in the prostate or kidney or harbored in a urinary calculus. Suppressive therapy is used to decrease the population of microbes already present in the urinary tract.

The potential efficacy of prophylaxis depends upon the characteristics of the host and nature of the invading microbe. A brief exposure to an antimicrobial drug may prevent infection in patients with uncomplicated infections. It may be virtually impossible to eradicate microbes from the urinary tract of patients with complicated infections.

Tactics that might prevent organisms from entering the urinary tract include measures to 1) decrease the population of potential pathogens in the large bowel, 2) prevent colonization of the periurethral zone, 3) eliminate a prostatic focus, 4) prevent attachment and growth of microorganisms once they enter the bladder urine, 5) wash-out of the microorganisms by diuresis, and 6) avoid instrumentation whenever possible.

The indications for prophylaxis are listed in Table 12.7. The most effective measures are those that prevent recurrent infections in susceptible females and in males with a prostatic focus as previously described. The

Table 12.7. Conditions for Which Prophylaxis of Urinary Tract Infections is Often Used

Generally Effective
   Closely spaced, recurrent infections in females
   Peri-coital use in susceptible women
   Infections in men with a persistent prostatic focus
   Renal transplant recipients
   Children with vesico-ureteral reflux
   Single instrumentation of the urethra
   Intermittent catheterization
   After removal of an indwelling catheter
   Before prostatectomy and other urologic procedures
Ineffective
   Long-term indwelling catheters

indications for prophylaxis in children with vesico-ureteral reflux and in patients with a sterile urine before prostatectomy are more controversial.

Urinary Catheters and Instrumentation

Single Instrumentation

Microorganisms may be introduced into the bladder urine by catheterization, cystoscopy and other urologic procedures such as prostatic biopsy. Development of infection depends on the invasive properties of the microorganism and host susceptibility. Turck, Goffe, and Petersdorf (87) found only one instance of infection after single catheterization in 200 otherwise healthy ambulatory men and women, but found 6 cases among 39 elderly bedridden women. Brumfitt et al. (88) reported rates as high as 9.1% after a single catheterization of women with uncomplicated labor and a 22.8% rate in women with complicated or difficult labor. The obvious lesson is to avoid catheterization during labor. A single dose of trimethoprim, nitrofurantoin, or other drugs active against gram negative bacteria may be useful after catheterization of high risk patients such as those with diabetes, urinary calculi, and retention. Flushing the bladder with chlorhexidine has been reported to be useful in preventing postpartum urinary tract infection (89).

Intermittent Catheterization

Conflicting evidence exists as to whether prophylaxis is useful for intermittent catheterization. Some authors report that instilling a neomycin-polymyxin solution after each catheterization is effective, whereas others do not. Some prefer prophylaxis with nitrofurantoin or methenamine mandelate combined with ammonium sulfate to acidify the urine. I see no need to use prophylaxis as long as the patient is asymptomatic.

Long-term Catheterization
Closed drainage systems will delay infection in patients with urinary catheters without the need for antimicrobial prophylaxis. Antimicrobial drugs can delay the onset of colonization, but superinfection with more resistant microorganisms is inevitable. Antimicrobial drugs should not be used in patients with indwelling urinary devices except to treat other infections.

After Removal of Catheters
Treatment is highly effective in women after the catheters are removed (90). A single dose of trimethoprim/sulfamethoxazole given to those who were still bacteriuric at 48 hours after removal of the catheter is as effective as a 10-day course for women younger than 65 years. Longer treatment with a drug to which the microorganism is susceptible should be used in men and older women.

Prostatectomy, Lithotripsy, and Other Urologic Procedures

Preoperative use of antimicrobial drugs before urologic procedures reduces septic complications. Prophylaxis is most useful in patients who are already infected and is of marginal benefit for those with sterile urine. A critical review of the literature by Chodak and Plaut (91) found that most of the earlier studies were flawed by being uncontrolled, not properly randomized, retrospective, or involving a postoperatively-started drug. More recent studies continue to support the efficacy of prophylaxis in transurethral prostatectomy for high-risk patients (92, 93). It is difficult to interpret many of the studies because they often are designed to compare a new agent against an arbitrary "standard" regimen and include too few patients to show a significant difference. It appears that any drug which is broadly active against gram negative enteric bacteria and can achieve adequate concentrations in the urine is potentially effective. Further work is needed to better define the choice of drug, dosage, and duration of prophylaxis. Hopefully this situation will be improved by adherence to more standardized guidelines for clinical trials of antimicrobial drugs (94).

Episodes of severe sepsis have been reported following lithotripsy (95). The microorganisms may be sequestered in stones and released when they are disrupted. There is no advantage to use antimicrobial prophylaxis in patients with sterile urine (96). It is prudent to attempt to eradicate infection before the procedure and anticipate that infection stones often harbor microorganisms. Prophylaxis is used commonly with transrectal prostatic biopsies and appears to be reasonable.

Prevention of Bacterial Endocarditis

Subacute bacterial endocarditis caused by enterococci has become more frequent in recent years among older males. Many patients do not have a clear-cut history of valvular or congenital heart disease. Gram-negative bacteria may also produce endocarditis after urologic procedures. It seems reasonable (but of unproven value) to administer prophylactic antibiotics for enterococcal endocarditis before instrumentation in the older males with a prosthetic heart valve or valvular heart disease. The patient may be given ampicillin (0.5 g) orally and gentamicin (1.5 mg/kg body weight) intravenously about 1 to 2 hours before the procedure to achieve high levels in blood and urine. Vancomycin may be substituted for patients allergic to penicillin. There is no practical means to prevent the rare occurrence of bacterial endocarditis in patients with long-term indwelling catheters.

Children with Vesico-Ureteral Reflux

It has become customary to use long-term prophylaxis with small doses of trimethoprim or nitrofurantoin in young children with vesico-ureteral reflux. Reflux tends to diminish over time and scars usually do not develop in children receiving long-term prophylaxis. Several major trials have demonstrated that medical therapy is as effective as surgical therapy in children with reflux. All of these studies included long-term prophylaxis in both treatment arms. It is therefore difficult to tell whether prophylaxis was really needed. Winberg (97) provides an attractive approach based on a careful review of the data. He reasons that most of the renal damage has already occurred during the initial episode of infection at the time reflux was first discovered. Prevention of recurrent infection is of marginal value. He recommends that it is usually not necessary to use prolonged prophylaxis in boys because they rarely have recurrences after the first year of life and that prophylaxis should be discontinued in girls after the age of 2 years.

Renal Transplant Recipients

The considerable morbidity caused by recurrent urinary tract infections in transplant recipients has led several groups to attempt to prevent these infections by long-term prophylaxis. Excellent results have been obtained with TMP/SMZ. TMP/SMZ is also effective against *Pneumocystis carinii*. Other drugs, including the fluoroquinolones, have also been useful in this regard.

Other Measures

Water Diuresis and Body Habits

Some women have learned that drinking large amounts of fluids combined with frequent voiding can alleviate urinary symptoms. Water diuresis may be effective in some women with uncomplicated infection, but it often delays more effective management with antimicrobial drugs until the patient becomes more ill. The paradoxical effects of water diuresis are discussed elsewhere (see "Effect of Diuresis on the Susceptibility of the Bladder and Kidney to Infection" in Chapter 11). The evidence is too weak to recommend that women change their body habits and menstrual practices or void after intercourse.

In a remarkably designed study, Redjeb et al. (98) reported that they were able to sterilize the urine of patients with symptomatic urinary tract infections using 3 days of treatment with only 10 mg of ampicillin per day combined with intake of 2 liters of fluid each day. Only a few of the controls given water alone were cured of their infection. They attributed their results in part to killing of the organism but raised the possibility that sublethal concentrations of ampicillin were able to prevent adherence or to dislodge the organisms from the bladder wall, thus allowing them to be washed away by the urinary stream.

Cranberry Juice and Ascorbic Acid

Ascorbic acid and cranberry juice are not effective acidifying agents unless taken in very large amounts. The slight antibacterial effect of cranberry juice is caused by excretion of hippuric acid in the urine. Extracts of cranberry and blueberry juices contain lectins that bind type-1 fimbriae, but they may not enter the urine. It is claimed that cranberry juice reduced the frequency of bacteriuria and pyuria in a group of elderly women (99). This study is difficult to interpret because the results are expressed as infection rates for the populations at risk rather than cure rates for individual subjects.

Alteration of the Vaginal Flora and pH

The vagina ordinarily contains low numbers of gram negative enteric bacteria because of competition from the resident microbial flora. Lactobacilli account for the low vaginal pH. Lactobacilli tend to be less abundant in postmenopausal women and after antimicrobial therapy. Vaginal colonization with *E. coli* can be eliminated in monkeys by intravaginal instillation of suspensions of Lactobacilli or vaginal fluid from healthy animals (100). Special strains of Lactobacilli have been developed by Reid and Bruce. They report that intravaginal instillation weekly for 1 year led to a fall in vaginal pH from 5.0 to 4.8 in premenopausal women (101). The rate of recurrences decreased from 6.3 to 1.3 annually. Intravaginal buffer cream (pH 3.0) reduces vaginal pH slightly (4.9 to 4.6), but has no significant effect on colonization of the vaginal introitus by uropathogens (102).

Estrogens in Postmenopausal Women

A group of postmenopausal women with atrophic vaginitis, who experienced frequent urinary tract infections and had failed treatment with antimicrobial therapy and local application of povidone iodine, were treated with monthly cyclic oral estrogen therapy (103). They had fewer recurrent infections during a follow-up ranging from 2 to 8 years. Similar results have been obtained by other investigators (104,105). Intravaginal estriol has also been effective in postmenopausal women with recurrent urinary tract infections (106).

Topical Antimicrobial Ointments

Attempts to prevent recurrent urinary tract infections by applying ointments containing povidone iodine to the periurethral zone are of minimum value and are not recommended. Topical aqueous solutions of povidone iodine applied twice daily to the periurethral zone were less effective than trimethoprim or methenamine hippurate in preventing recurrent urinary infections and did not diminish colonization with enteric gram negative bacteria in the periurethral area (107).

Urinary Analgesics and Antispasmodics

Phenazopyridine (Pyridium™) is sometimes useful to obtain local urinary analgesia. There is no need for routine use. Combinations with antimicrobial drugs tend to be more expensive and are not necessary. Toxic side-effects include phenazopyridine stones, hepatitis, acute renal failure, headache, vertigo, colic, methemoglobinuria and, in high doses, hemolytic anemia. Methylene blue is of no value and should not be used.

A variety of anticholinergic drugs are available as antispasmodics for relief of the acute discomfort of urinary tract infections (dysuria, nocturia, and suprapubic discomfort). I prefer not to use them because eradication of infection is usually accompanied by rapid resolution of symptoms. Cholinergic agents, such as bethanechol and neostigmine, stimulate the smooth muscle of the bladder. They are used often in postoperative and postpartum patients to stimulate voiding and delay or prevent the need for catheterization. These agents should not be used in the presence of obstruction. The efficacy of bethanechol in promoting bladder emptying is controversial (108).

Oral Immunotherapy

Reports on immunostimulating extracts of E. coli claim to reduce the frequency of recurrent infections (109) and decrease the degree of bacteriuria in paraplegic patients (110). These reports are incomprehensible in view of what is known about the immune response to urinary tract infections and the potential for a pyelonephritis vaccine (see "Prospects for a Vaccine" in Chapter 10).

Suppressive Therapy

Suppressive therapy is tried at times in the hope that reducing bacterial counts in urine might be helpful and because nothing else seems to work. Methenamine salts rarely eradicate infection. Attempts at suppression in the face of bacteriologic failure are not only wasteful, but they increase the potential for drug toxicity and superinfection with resistant microorganisms. It is important to recognize failure. The most important measures should be to correct anatomic defects and remove foreign bodies (including catheters) whenever possible.

Treatment of Candida Infections

Patients with urinary and vascular catheters, diabetes, and leukopenia who are intensively treated with antibacterial drugs are at risk of superinfection with Candida and other yeasts. The first step in management of instrumented patients is to remove the device and reevaluate the need for antimicrobial therapy. Candiduria will often clear spontaneously after these simple measures (111). Patients who are leukopenic, immunosuppressed, or have a vascular line should be considered to have systemic candidiasis and must be treated with systemic drugs.

It is not always necessary to treat Candida urinary tract infections. Very little is gained and it may be counterproductive to eradicate Candida from the urine of an asymptomatic patient with a long-term indwelling catheter. The yeasts will inevitably be replaced by new and potentially more virulent microorganisms. Treatment should be reserved for symptomatic patients, for persistent candiduria after the catheter is removed, and for the rare situations in which fungus balls produce obstruction.

Up until recently, amphotericin B was the only satisfactory drug for treatment of Candida urinary tract infections. It can be administered intravenously, but bladder irrigation is preferred because this route is less toxic and highly effective. Fifty mg in a liter of sterile water are instilled daily for 2 to 7 days by continuous irrigation with a three way catheter (112). This amount is usually sufficient and longer treatment is generally not needed. Excellent results have also been obtained by instilling a solution of 20 mg of amphotericin B in 100 ml of sterile water for 2 hours as part of a bladder wash-out procedure (113).

Oral fluconazole is highly effective for candiduria. It has the advantage over bladder irrigation with amphotericin B of not requiring catheterization. The drawback is that not all species are susceptible and resistant strains have emerged. Two randomized clinical trials were completed recently. Oral fluconazole at an initial loading dose of 200 mg followed by 100 mg once daily for 4 more days was compared to a 5-day course of standard bladder irrigation with amphotericin B (114). Two days later, therapy funguria was eradicated from 96% of patients receiving amphotericin B and 73% with fluconazole (P < 0.05), but the proportion of patients without funguria was similar in both groups 1 month after therapy. In another comparative trial, fluconazole 200 mg daily for 7 days was equally effective as 7 days of standard irrigation therapy with amphotericin B (115). Ketoconazole and flucytosine are less effective than fluconazole and are not recommended.

References

1. Stamey TA. Recurrent urinary tract infections in female patients: an overview of management and treatment. Rev Infect Dis 1987;9:S195–S210.
2. Brumfitt W. The Garrod lecture. Progress in understanding urinary infections. Brit Soc Antimicrob Chemother 1991;27:9–22.
3. Harding GKM, Ronald AR. The management of urinary tract infections: what have we learned in the past decade? Int J Antimicrob Agents 1994;4:83–88.
4. Bailey R. Management of uncomplicated urinary tract infections. Int J Antimicrob Agents 1994;4:95–100.
5. Norrby SR. Useful agents in the management of urinary tract infections. Int J Antimicrob Agents 1994;4:129–134.
6. Johnson JR. Treatment and prevention of urinary tract infections. In: Mobley HLT, Warren JW, eds. Urinary tract infections: molecular pathogenesis and clinical management. Washington DC: ASM Press, 1996:95–118.
7. Kunin CM. Resistance to antimicrobial drugs—a worldwide calamity. Ann Intern Med 1993;118:557–561.
8. Wenzel RP, Kunin CM. Should oral antimicrobial drugs be available over-the-counter? J Infect Dis 1994;170:1256–1259.
9. Neu HC. Trimethoprim alone for treatment of urinary tract infection. Rev Infect Dis 1982;4:366–371.
10. Craig WA, Kunin CM. Trimethoprim-sulfamethoxazole: pharmacodynamic effects of urinary pH and impaired renal clearance. Ann Intern Med 1973;78:491–497.
11. Sachs J, Geer T, Noell P, et al. Effect of renal function on urinary recovery of orally administered nitrofurantoin. N Engl J Med 1968;278:1032–1035.
12. Stamey TA, Nemoy NJ, Higgins M. The clinical use of nalidixic acid. A review and some observations. Invest Urol 1969;6:582–592.
13. Crumplin GC, Smith JT. Nalidixic acid: an antibacterial paradox. Antimicrob Agents Chemother 1975;8:251–261.
14. Giamarellou H, Jackson GG. Antibacterial activity of cinoxacin in vitro. Antimicrob Agents Chemother 1975;7:688–692.
15. Hooper DC, Wolfson JS. Treatment of genitourinary tract infections with fluoroquinolones: clinical efficacy in genital infections and adverse effects. Antimicrob Agents Chemother 1989;33:1662–1667.
16. Ryan JL, Berenson CS, Greco TP, et al. Oral ciprofloxacin in resistant urinary tract infections. Am J Med 1987;82(4a)303–306.
17. Fang G, Brennen C, Wagener M, et al. Use of ciprofloxacin versus use of aminoglycosides for therapy of complicated urinary tract infection. Antimicrob Agents Chemother 1991;35:1849–1855.
18. Ena J, Amador C, Martinez C, et al. Risk factors for acquisition of urinary tract infections caused by ciprofloxacin resistant *Escherichia coli*. J Urol 1995;153:117–120.
19. Thomson KS, Sanders WF, Sanders CC. USA resistant patterns among UTI pathogens. J Antimicrob Chemother 1994;33:suppl A 9–15.
20. Iravani A, Tice AD, McCarty J, et al. Short-course ciproflox treatment of acute uncomplicated urinary tract infection in women. Arch Intern Med 1995;155:485–494.
21. Garlando F, Rietiker S, Tauber MG, et al. Single-dose ciprofloxacin at 100 versus 250 mg for treatment of uncomplicated urinary tract infections in women. Antimicrob Agents Chemother 1987;31:354–356.
22. Williams AH, Grüneberg RN. Ciprofloxacin and co-trimoxazole in urinary tract infections. J Antimicrob Chemother 1986;18 suppl D 107–110.
23. Raz R, Genesin J, Gonen E, et al. Single low-dose ofloxacin for the treatment of uncomplicated urinary tract infection in young women. J Antimicrob Chemother 1988;22:945–949.
24. Brumfitt W, Smith GW, Hamilton-Miller JMT, et al. Successful use of reduced dosage of cinoxacin in the treatment of recurrent urinary infection. J Antimicrob Chemother 1985;16:781–788.
25. Daikos GL, Kathpalia SB, Sharifi R, et al. Comparison of ciprofloxacin and beta-lactam antibiotics in the treatment of urinary tract infections and alteration of fecal flora. Am J Med 1987;82(4a):290–294.

26. Tartaglione TA, Johnson CR, Brust P, et al. Pharmacodynamic evaluation of ofloxacin and trimethoprim-sulfamethoxazole in vaginal fluid of women treated for acute cystitis. Antimicrob Agents Chemother 1988;32:1640–1643.

27. Pecquet S, Andremont A, Tancrede C. Effect of oral ofloxacin on fecal bacteria in human volunteers. Antimicrob Agents Chemother 1987;31:124–125.

28. Grüneberg RN. Changes in urinary pathogens and their antibiotic sensitivities, 1971–1992. J Antimicrob Chemother 1994;33:suppl A 1–8.

29. Beunders AJ. Development of antibacterial resistance: the Dutch experience. J Antimicrob Chemother 1994;33:suppl A 17–22.

30. Kunin CM, Finkelberg Z. Oral cephalexin and ampicillin: antimicrobial activity, recovery in urine and persistence in the blood of uremic patients. Ann Intern Med 1970;72:349–356.

31. Norrby SR. Short-term treatment of uncomplicated lower urinary tract infections in women. Rev Infect Dis 1990;12:458–467.

32. Fang LST, Tolkoff-Rubin NE, Rubin RH. Localization and antibiotic management of urinary tract infection. Annu Rev Med 1979;30:225–239.

33. Bailey RR. Single dose therapy of urinary tract infection. Sydney: ADIS Health Science Press, 1983.

34. Osterberg E, Aberg H, Hallander HO, et al. Efficacy of single-dose versus seven-day trimethoprim treatment of cystitis in women: a randomized double-blind study. J Infect Dis 1990;161:942–947.

35. Saginur R, Nicolle LE. Single-dose compared with 3-day norfloxacin treatment of uncomplicated urinary tract infection in women. Arch Intern Med 1992;152:1233–1237.

36. Cardenas J, Quinn EL, Rooker G, et al. Single-dose cephalexin therapy for acute bacterial urinary tract infections and acute urethral syndrome with bladder bacteriuria. Antimicrob Agents Chemother 1986;29:383–385.

37. Fine JS, Jacobson MS. Single-dose versus conventional therapy of urinary tract infections in female adolescents. Pediatrics 1985;75:916–920.

38. Campbell-Brown M, McFadyen IR. Bacteriuria in pregnancy treated with a single dose of cephalexin. Br J Obstet Gynaecol 1983;90:1054–1059.

39. Jakobi P, Neiger R, Merzbach D, et al. Single-dose antimicrobial therapy in the treatment of asymptomatic bacteriuria in pregnancy. Am J Obstet Gynecol 1987;156:1148–1152.

40. Ronald AR, Boutros P, Mourtada H. Bacteriuria localization and response to single-dose therapy in women. JAMA 1976;235:1854–1856.

41. Fihn SD, Johnson C, Roberts PL, et al. Trimethoprim-sulfamethoxazole for acute dysuria in women: a single-dose or 10-day course. Ann Intern Med 1988;108:350–357.

42. Pfau A, Sacks TG. Effective postcoital quinolone prophylaxis of recurrent urinary tract infections in women. J Urol 1994;152:136–138.

43. Iravani A, Richard GA. Single-dose cefuroxime axetil versus multiple-dose cefaclor in the treatment of acute urinary tract infections. Antimicrob Agents Chemother 1989;33:1212–1216.

44. Leibovici L, Wysenbeek AJ. Single-dose treatment of urinary tract infections with and without antibody-coated bacteria: a metaanalysis of controlled trials. J Infect Dis 1991;163:928–929.

45. Kunin CM. A ten-year study of bacteriuria in school girls: final report of bacteriologic, urologic and epidemiologic findings. J Infect Dis 1970;122:382–393.

46. Kraft JK, Stamey TA. The natural history of recurrent bacteriuria in women. Medicine 1977;56:55–60.

47. Wong ES, McKevitt M, Running K, et al. Management of recurrent urinary tract infections with patient-administered single-dose therapy. Ann Intern Med 1985;102:302–307.

48. Vosti KL. Recurrent urinary tract infections: prevention by prophylactic antibiotics after sexual intercourse. JAMA 1975;231:934–980.

49. Stapleton A, Latham RH, Johnson C, et al. Postcoital antimicrobial prophylaxis for recurrent urinary tract infection. JAMA 1990;264:703–706.

50. Kunin CM, Craig WA, Uehling DT. Trimethoprim therapy for urinary tract infection: long-term prophylaxis in a uremic patient. JAMA 1978;239:2588–2591.

51. Nicolle LE, Harding GKM, Thomson M, et al. Efficacy of five years of continuous, low-dose TMP/SMZ prophylaxis for urinary tract infections. J Infect Dis 1988;157:1239–1242.

52. Stamm WE, McKevitt M, Roberts PL, et al. Natural history of recurrent urinary tract infections in women. Rev Infect Dis 1991;13:77–84.

53. Brumfitt W, Hamilton-Miller JMT. Prophylactic antibiotics for recurrent urinary tract infections. J Antimicrob Chemother 1990;25:505–512.
54. Eisenstein BI, Beachey EH, Ofek I. Influence of sublethal concentrations of antibiotics on the expression of the mannose-specific ligand of *Escherichia coli*. Infect Immun 1980; 28:154–159.
55. Dean EA, Kessler RE. Quantitation of effects of subinhibitory concentrations of trimethoprim on P fimbria expression and in vitro adhesiveness of uropathogenic *Escherichia coli*. J Clin Microbiol 1988;26:25–30.
56. Hales BA, Amyes SGB. The effect of a range of antimicrobial drugs on the hemagglutination of two clinical isolates from urinary tract infections. J Antimicrob Chemother 1985;16:671–674.
57. Kovarik JM, Hoepelman IM, Verhoef J. Influence of fluoroquinolones on expression and function of P fimbriae in uropathogenic *Escherichia coli*. Antimicrob Agents Chemother 1989;33:684–688.
58. Kunin CM, Tong HH, Bakaletz LO. Effect of salicylate on expression of flagella by *Escherichia coli* and *Proteus, Providencia* and *Pseudomonas* spp. Infect Immun 1995;63:1796–1799.
59. Stamey TA, Condy M, Mihara G. Prophylactic efficacy of nitrofurantoin macrocrystals and trimethoprim-sulfamethoxazole in urinary infections. Biologic effects on the vaginal and rectal flora. N Engl J Med 1977;296:780–783.
60. Stansfeld JM. Duration of treatment for urinary tract infections in children. Brit Med J 1975;3:65–66.
61. Stamm WE, Counts GW, Wagner KF, et al. Antimicrobial prophylaxis of recurrent urinary tract infections. Ann Intern Med 1980;92:770–775.
62. Nahata MC, Cummins BA, McLeod DC, et al. Effect of urinary acidifiers on formaldehyde concentration and efficacy with methenamine therapy. Eur J Clin Pharmacol 1982;22:281–284.
63. Rosenheim ML. Mandelic acid in the treatment of urinary infections. Lancet 1935;1: 1032–1037.
64. Kass EH, Zangwill DP. Principles in the long-term management of chronic infection of the urinary tract. In: Quinn EL, Kass EH, eds. Biology of pyelonephritis. Boston: Little, Brown and Co., 1960:663–672.
65. Holland NH, West CD. Prevention of recurrent urinary tract infections in girls. Am J Dis Child 1963;105:60–67.
66. Gerstein AR, Okun R, Gonick HC, et al. The prolonged use of methenamine hippurate in the treatment of chronic urinary tract infection. J Urol 1968;100:767.
67. Kasanen A, Kaarsalo E, Hiltunen R, et al. Comparison of long-term, low-dosage nitrofurantoin, methenamine hippurate, trimethoprim and trimethoprim-sulfamethoxazole on the control of recurrent urinary tract infection. Ann Clin Res 1974;6:285–289.
68. Freeman RB, Richardson JA, Thurm RH, et al. Long-term therapy for chronic bacteriuria in men. Ann Intern Med 1975;83:133–147.
69. Kevorkian CG, Merritt J, Ilstrup D. Methenamine mandelate with acidification: an effective urinary antiseptic in patients with neurogenic bladder. Mayo Clin Proc 1984;59: 523–29.
70. Nilsson S. Long-term treatment with methenamine hippurate in recurrent urinary tract infection. Acta Med Scand 1975;198:81–85.
71. Vainrub B, Musher DM. Lack of effect of methenamine in suppression of, or prophylaxis against, chronic urinary infection. Antimicrob Agents Chemother 1977;12:625–629.
72. Lenke RR, VanDorsten JP, Schifrin BS. Pyelonephritis in pregnancy: a prospective randomized trial to prevent recurrent disease evaluating suppressive therapy with nitrofurantoin and close surveillance. Am J Obstet Gynecol 1983;146:953–957.
73. Grüneberg RN, Leigh DA, Brumfitt W. Relationship of bacteriuria in pregnancy to acute pyelonephritis, prematurity and fetal mortality. Lancet 1969;1:1–3.
74. Bint AJ, Hill D. Bacteriuria of pregnancy—an update on significance, diagnosis and management. J Antimicrob Chemother 1994;33:suppl A: 93–97.
75. Angle JL, O'Brian WF, Finan MA, et al. Acute pyelonephritis in pregnancy: a prospective study of oral versus intravenous antibiotic therapy. Obstet Gynecol 1990;76:28–32.
76. Stamm WE, McKevitt M, Counts GW. Acute renal infection in women: treatment with trimethoprim/sulfamethoxazole or ampicillin for two or six weeks. Ann Intern Med 1987;106:341–345.

77. Gleckman R, Crowley M, Natsios GA. Trimethoprim-sulfamethoxazole treatment of men with recurrent urinary tract infections: a double-blind study utilizing the antibody-coated bacteria technique. Rev Infect Dis 1982;4:449.

78. Nicolle LE, Bjornson J, Harding GKM, et al. Bacteriuria in elderly institutionalized men. N Engl J Med 1983;309:1420–1425.

79. Meares EM. Prostatitis: Review of pharmacokinetics and therapy. Rev Infect Dis 1982;4:475–483.

80. Fair WR, Cordonnier JJ. The pH of prostatic fluid: a reappraisal and therapeutic implications. J Urol 1978;120:695–698.

81. Blacklock NJ, Beavis JP. The response of prostatic fluid pH in inflammation. Brit J Urol 1974;46:537–542.

82. Pfau A, Perlberg S, Shapiro A. The pH of prostatic fluid in health and disease: implications of treatment in chronic bacterial prostatitis. J Urol 1978;119:384–387.

83. Weidner W, Schiefer HG, Dalhoff A. Treatment of chronic bacterial prostatitis with ciprofloxacin. Results of a one-year follow-up study. Am J Med 1987;82:280–283.

84. Forland M, Thomas VL. The treatment of urinary tract infections in women with diabetes mellitus. Diabetes Care 1985;8:499–506.

85. Zhanel GG, Harding GKM, Nicolle LE. Asymptomatic bacteriuria in patients with diabetes mellitus. Rev Infect Dis 1991;13:150–154.

86. Ouslander JG, Schapira M, Scnelle JF, et al. Does eradicating bacteriuria affect the severity of chronic urinary incontinence in nursing home residents? Ann Intern Med 1995;122:749–754.

87. Turck M, Goffe B, Petersdorf RG. The urethral catheter and urinary infection. J Urol 1962;88:834–837.

88. Brumfitt W, Davies BI, Rosser E. Urethral catheter as a cause of urinary-tract infection in pregnancy and puerperium. Lancet 1961;2:1059–1062.

89. Gillespie WA, Lennon GG, Linton KB, et al. Prevention of urinary infection in gynaecology. Brit Med J 1964;2:423–425.

90. Harding GKM, Nicolle LE, Ronald AR, et al. How long should catheter-acquired urinary tract infection in women be treated? Ann Intern Med 1991;114 713–719.

91. Chodak GW, Plaut ME. Systemic antibiotics for prophylaxis in urologic surgery: a critical review. J Urol 1979;121:695–699.

92. Cafferkey MC, Falkiner FR, Gillespie WA, et al. Antibiotics in the prevention of septicaemia in urology. J Antimicrob Chemother 1982;9:471–477.

93. Wilson NIL, Lewis HJE. Survey of antibiotic prophylaxis in British urological practice. Brit J Urol 1985;57:478–482.

94. Beam TR Jr, Gilbert DN, Kunin CM. General guidelines for the clinical evaluation of anti-infective drug products. Clin Infect Dis 1992;15(Suppl 1):5–32.

95. Silber N, Kremer I, Gaton DD, et al. Severe sepsis following extracorporeal shock wave lithotripsy. J Urol 1991;145:1045–1046.

96. Rahav G, Strul H, Pode D, et al. Bacteriuria following extracorporeal shock-wave lithotripsy in patients whose urine was sterile before the procedure. Clin Infect Dis 1995;20:1317–1320.

97. Winberg J. Commentary: progressive renal damage from infection with or without reflux. J Urol 1992;148:1733–1734.

98. Redjeb SB, Slim A, Horchani A, et al. Effects of ten milligrams of ampicillin per day on urinary tract infections. Antimicrob Agents Chemother 1982;22:1084–1086.

99. Avorn J, Monane M, Gurwitz JH, et al. Reduction of bacteriuria and pyuria after ingestion of cranberry juice. JAMA 1994;271:751–754.

100. Herthelius M, Gorbach SL, Mollby R, et al. Elimination of vaginal colonization with *E. coli* by administration of indigenous flora. Infect Immun 1989;57:2447–2451.

101. Reid G, Bruce AW. Low vaginal pH and urinary-tract infection. Lancet 1995;346:1704.

102. Moorman CN, Fowler JE Jr. Impact of site release vaginal pH buffer cream on introital colonization by gram-negative bacilli. J Urol 1992;147:1576–1578.

103. Privette M, Cade R, Peterson J, et al. Prevention of recurrent urinary tract infections in postmenopausal women. Nephron 1988;50:24–27.

104. Brandberg Å, Mellström D, Samsioe G. Low dose oral estriol treatment in elderly women with urogenital infections. Acta Obstet Gynecol Scand Suppl 1987;140:33–38.

105. Kirkengen AL, Andersen P, Gjersøe E, et al. Oestriol in the prophylactic treatment of recurrent urinary tract infections in postmenopausal women. Scand J Prim Health Care 1992;10:139–142.
106. Raz R, Stamm WE. A controlled-trial of intravaginal estriol in postmenopausal women with recurrent urinary tract infections. N Engl J Med 1993;329:753–756.
107. Brumfitt W, Hamilton-Miller JMT, Gargan RA, et al. Long-term prophylaxis of urinary infections in women: comparative trial of trimethoprim, methenamine hippurate and topical povidone-iodine. J Urol 1983;130:1110–1114.
108. Finkbeiner AE. Is bethanechol chloride clinically effective in promoting bladder emptying? A literature review. J Urol 1985;134:443–449.
109. Schulman CC, Corbusier A, Michiels H, et al. Oral immunotherapy of recurrent urinary tract infections: a double-blind placebo-controlled multicenter study. J Urol 1993; 150:917–921.
110. Hachen HJ. Oral immunotherapy in paraplegic patients with chronic urinary tract infections: a double-blind, placebo-controlled trial. J Urol 1990;143:759–763.
111. Sobel JD, Vazquez JA. Urinary tract infection due to *Candida* species. In: Mobley HLT, Warren JW, eds. Urinary tract infections: molecular pathogenesis and clinical management. Washington DC: ASM Press, 1996:119–131.
112. Wise GJ. Amphotericin B in urological practice. J Urol 1990;144:215–223.
113. Fong IW, Cheng PC, Hinton NA. Fungicidal effect of amphotericin B in urine: in vitro study to assess feasibility of bladder washout for localization of site of Candiduria. Antimicrob Agents Chemother 1991;35:1856–1859.
114. Jacobs LG, Skidmore EA, Freeman K, et al. Oral fluconazole compared with bladder irrigation with amphotericin B for treatment of fungal urinary tract infections in elderly patients. Clin Infect Dis 1996;22:30–35.
115. Fan-Havard P, O'Donovan C, Smith SM, et al. Oral fluconazole versus amphotericin B bladder irrigation for treatment of candidal funguria. Clin Infect Dis 1995;21:960–965.

Index

DATE DUE

DEC 1 5 1999			
JAN 2 6 2000			
MAY 1 1 2000			
MAY 1 1 2000			
GAYLORD			PRINTED IN U.S.A.